Clinical Gynecologic Endocrinology and Infertility

Second Edition

Clinical Gynecologic Endocrinology and Infertility

Second Edition

Leon Speroff
Robert H. Glass
Nathan G. Kase

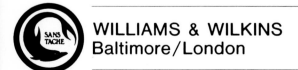

WILLIAMS & WILKINS
Baltimore/London

Copyright 1978
Williams & Wilkins Co.
428 East Preston Street
Baltimore
Maryland 21202
USA

Made in the United States of America

Reprinted July, 1978
Reprinted May, 1979
Reprinted April, 1981
Reprinted June, 1981

Library of Congress Cataloging in Publication Data

Speroff, Leon.
  Clinical gynecologic endocrinology and infertility.

  Bibliography: p.
  Includes index.
  1. Endocrine gynecology. 2. Sterility. I. Glass, Robert
H., joint author. II. Kase, Nathan G., 1930–   joint
author. III. Title. [DNLM: 1. Endocrine diseases. 2.
Gynecologic diseases. 3. Sterility, Male. 4. Sterility,
Female.
WP505 S749c]
RG159.S63 1978   618.1   77-8808
ISBN 0-683-07894-1

Design by Don Moyer

Composed and printed at the Waverly Press, Inc.
Mt. Royal & Guilford Avenues
Baltimore, Maryland 21202 USA

Preface

The second edition of this book follows the guidelines set forth in the first edition: to present the principles and methods which form the basis for the way we manage clinical problems in gynecologic endocrinology and infertility.

This is a field of extremely rapid progress. Concepts emerge quickly from the basic science laboratory into clinical application. An outstanding example is the basic mediator of steroid action, the intracellular receptor. When the first edition of this book was prepared, hormone receptors were mainly topics of conversation among molecular biologists. Today receptor action explains many details of normal ovarian follicular growth and development, as well as illuminating aspects of the previously mysterious polycystic ovary.

Any book of this nature represents a point in time at which accumulation and expansion of knowledge must be interrupted and committed to print. Thus the management of the problem of small pituitary tumors as outlined in this text represents a formulation which was current at the time of writing, but it must be viewed with one eye on the literature for changes dictated by experience. On the other hand, certain clinical problems require little change in approach; for example, the management of dysfunctional uterine bleeding.

We have tried to retain the style and clinical relevance of our first edition. Once again, the book was designed by Don Moyer to achieve an optimum level of readability and utility. Indeed, the success of the book is measured by its usefulness for students, residents, and colleagues.

Leon Speroff, M.D.
Portland, Oregon

Robert H. Glass, M.D.
San Francisco, California

Nathan G. Kase, M.D.
New Haven, Connecticut

Contents

Physiology of Female
Reproduction

Chapter 1:   1
**Hormone Biosynthesis, Metabolism, and
Mechanism of Action**
How hormones are formed and metabolized, and
how hormones work.

Chapter 2:   27
Neuroendocrinology
How reproductive events are perceived, integrated,
and acted upon by the neuroendocrine capability of
the central nervous system.

Chapter 3:   49
Regulation of the Menstrual Cycle
The cyclic changes in ovarian and pituitary
hormones, and what governs the patterns of these
hormonal changes.

Clinical
Endocrinology

Chapter 4:   65
The Ovary from Conception to Senescence
Correlation of morphology with reproductive and
steroidogenic functions. A consideration of the
physiology of the menopause and estrogen
replacement therapy.

✓ **Chapter 5:**   93
Amenorrhea
Differential diagnosis of amenorrhea of all types
Yes utilizing procedures available to all physicians. The
problem of small pituitary tumors.

✓ **Chapter 6:**   123
Anovulation
Yes How loss of ovulation can occur and the clinical
expressions of anovulation. The polycystic ovary.

✓ **Chapter 7:**   135
Hirsutism
The biology of hair growth; the diagnosis and
management of hirsutism.

✓ **Chapter 8:**   151
Dysfunctional Uterine Bleeding
Yes A physiologic basis for medical management
without primary surgical intervention.

Chapter 9:   167
The Breast
The factors involved in physiologic lactation and
the differential diagnosis of galactorrhea. The
endocrinology of breast cancer.

Chapter 10:   185
The Endocrinology of Pregnancy
The steroid and protein hormones of pregnancy,
and the endocrinology of parturition.

✓ **Chapter 11:**   231
ΣH /   **Normal and Abnormal Sexual Development**
Normal and abnormal sexual differentiation, and
the differential diagnosis of ambiguous genitalia.

✓ **Chapter 12:**   253
Abnormal Puberty and Growth Problems
ΣH'   Abnormalities which produce accelerated or
retarded sexual maturation, and growth problems
in normal adolescents.

Chapter 13:   271
Obesity
The physiology of adipose tissue, and the problem
of obesity.

Chapter 14:   283
Steroid Contraception
A survey of potential stresses on physiologic
mechanisms in the patient receiving steroid
contraception. Methods for patient management.

Infertility   ✓ **Chapter 15:**   311
Investigation of the Infertile Couple
Yes   An approach to the problem of infertility. The
proper diagnostic tests and their correct
interpretation.

Chapter 16:   343
Tubal Surgery
NO   Specific techniques and management for tubal
surgery.

Chapter 17:   355
Endometriosis and Infertility
NO   Diagnosis and suitable treatment for the individual
patient.

Chapter 18:   363
Male Infertility
Principles of male infertility, including analysis of
semen, treatment, and artificial insemination.

√ **Chapter 19:**
Induction of Ovulation
A program of clomiphene and HMG
administration.

375

Appendix

Chapter 20:
Clinical Assays
Methods and interpretations of laboratory assays
which are useful in gynecologic endocrine
diagnosis.

393

Read, Sex. Dysfunction
a chapter

1 Hormone Biosynthesis, Metabolism, and Mechanism of Action

To begin a clinical book with a chapter on biochemistry only serves to emphasize that competent clinical judgment is founded upon a groundwork of basic knowledge. On the other hand, clinical practice does not require a technical and sophisticated proficiency in a basic science. *The purpose of this chapter is not therefore to present an intensive course in biochemistry, but rather to present a selective review of the most important principles of how hormones are formed and metabolized, and how hormones work.* This information is essential for the development of the physiologic concepts to follow, and it is intended that certain details which we all have difficulty remembering will be available in this chapter for reference.

The classical definition of a hormone is a substance which travels from a special tissue where it is released into the bloodstream to distant responsive cells where the hormone exerts its characteristic effect. What was once thought of as a simple voyage is now becoming appreciated as an odyssey which becomes more complex as new facets of the journey are unraveled in research laboratories throughout the world. Let us follow an estradiol molecule throughout its career, and in so doing gain an overview of how hormones are formed, how hormones work, and how hormones are metabolized. After this survey, each subject will be considered in detail.

Estradiol begins its lifespan with its synthesis in a specialized cell suited for this task. For this biosynthesis to take place, the proper enzyme capability must be present along with the proper precursors. In the human female the principal sources of estradiol are the theca cells of the developing follicle and the granulosa cells of the corpus luteum. These cells possess the unique ability to respond to a specific stimulus with estradiol production. This stimulus is the gonadotropin, luteinizing hormone (LH). Therefore, an initial step in the process which will give rise to estradiol is the transmission of the message from the stimulating agent, LH, to the steroid-producing mechanism within the cell.

The basic message to stimulate estradiol production must be transmitted through the cell membrane. LH, being a large glycopeptide structure, does not enter the cell, but communicates with the cell by joining with a specific receptor on the cell membrane and in so doing activates a line of communication. A considerable amount of investigation has been devoted to determining the methods by which this communication takes place. E. M. Sutherland received the Nobel Prize in 1971 for proposing the concept of a second messenger.

LH, the first messenger, activates an enzyme in the cell membrane called adenylate cyclase. This enzyme transmits the message by catalyzing the production of a second messenger within the cell, cyclic AMP. The message passes from LH to cyclic AMP, much like a baton in a relay race.

Cyclic AMP, the second messenger, initiates the process of steroidogenesis, leading to the synthesis and secretion of the hormone, estradiol. This process requires protein synthesis, and a least one rate-limiting step is the conversion of cholesterol to pregnenolone within the mitochondria.

Secretion of estradiol into the bloodstream directly follows its synthesis. Once in the bloodstream, estradiol does not necessarily exist in a free-floating state, but a majority of the hormone is bound to a protein carrier, chiefly a beta globulin. The purpose of this binding is not totally clear. The biologic activity of a hormone may be limited by binding in the blood, and potent changes may thus be avoided. In addition, binding may prevent rapid metabolism, allowing the hormone to exist for the length of time necessary to ensure a biologic effect. It is unlikely that specific transportation to a specific site is a function of this binding since distribution of the hormone in the bloodstream is probably homogeneous.

The biologic and metabolic effects of a hormone are determined by a responsive cell's ability to receive and retain a hormone. The estradiol which is not bound to a protein, but floating free in the bloodstream, readily enters cells by rapid diffusion. However, for estradiol to produce its effect, it must be grasped by a receptor within the cell. Thus, only those cells which contain estradiol-specific receptors will respond to estradiol. The job of the receptor is to transport the hormone to the nucleus, resulting in transmission of the hormone's message to the nuclear chromatin. The result is production of messenger RNA leading to protein synthesis and a cellular response characteristic of the hormone.

Once estradiol has accomplished its mission, it is probably released back into the bloodstream. It is possible that estradiol may perform its duty several times before being cleared from the circulation by metabolism. On the other hand, many molecules will be metabolized without ever having the chance of producing an effect. Other hormones, such as testosterone, are metabolized and altered within the cell in which an effect has been produced. In the latter case, a steroid which is then released into the bloodstream is an inactive compound. Clearance of steroids from the blood varies according to the structure of the molecule.

Cells which are capable of clearing estradiol from the circulation accomplish this by biochemical means (conversion to estrone and estriol, moderately effective and very weak estrogens, respectively) and conjugation to products which are water-soluble and excreted in the urine and bile (sulfo- and glucuro-conjugates).

Thus, a steroid hormone has a varied career packed into a short lifetime, and it is now appropriate to review the important segments of this lifespan in greater detail.

Nomenclature	All steroid hormones are of basically similar structure with relatively minor chemical differences leading to striking alterations in biologic activity. The basic structure is the perhydrocyclopentanephenanthrene ring. One ring is benzene, two rings naphthalene, and three rings phenanthrene; add a cyclopentane (5-carbon ring) and you have the perhydrocyclopentanephenanthrene ring or the steroid nucleus.

The sex steroids are divided into three main groups according to the number of carbon atoms. The C-21 series includes the corticoids and the progestins and the basic structure is the pregnane nucleus. The 19-carbon series includes all the androgens and is based on the androstane nucleus, whereas the estrogens are 18-carbon steroids based on the estrane nucleus.

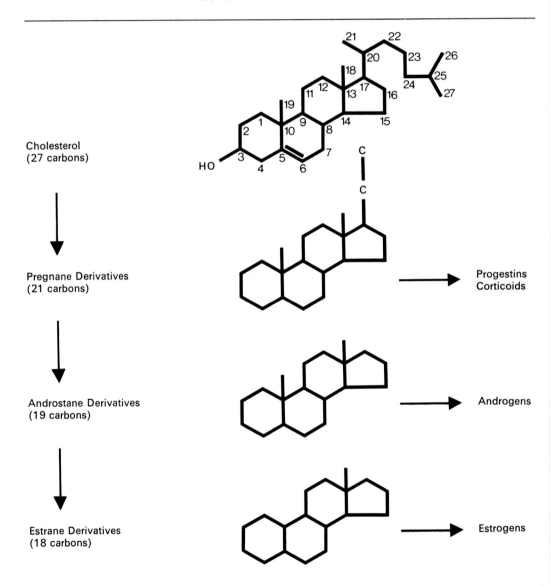

Cholesterol
(27 carbons)

Pregnane Derivatives
(21 carbons)

Progestins
Corticoids

Androstane Derivatives
(19 carbons)

Androgens

Estrane Derivatives
(18 carbons)

Estrogens

There are six centers of asymmetry on the basic ring structure, and there are 64 possible isomers. Almost all naturally occurring and active steroids are nearly flat, and substituents below and above the plane of the ring are designated alpha (dotted line) and beta (solid line), respectively. Changes in the position of only one substituent may lead to inactive isomers. For example, 17-epitestosterone is considerably weaker than testosterone, the only difference being a hydroxyl group in the alpha position at C-17 rather than in the beta position.

Progesterone

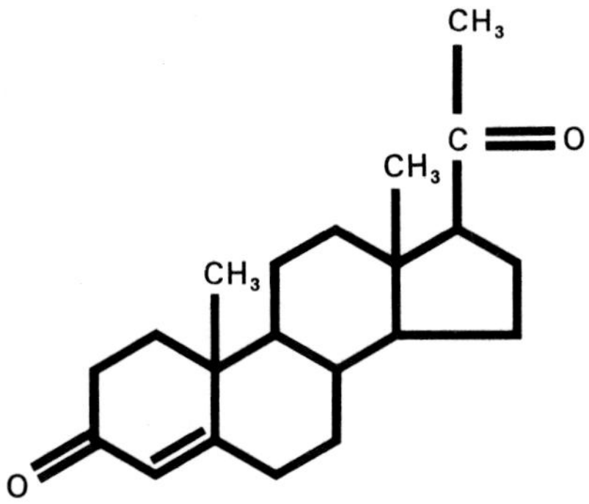

Top View

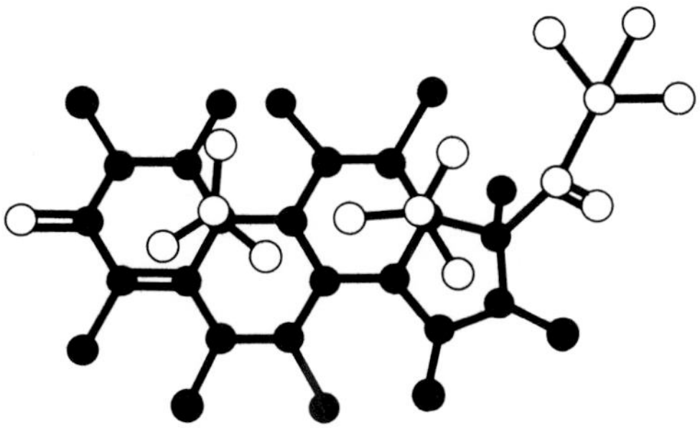

Side View

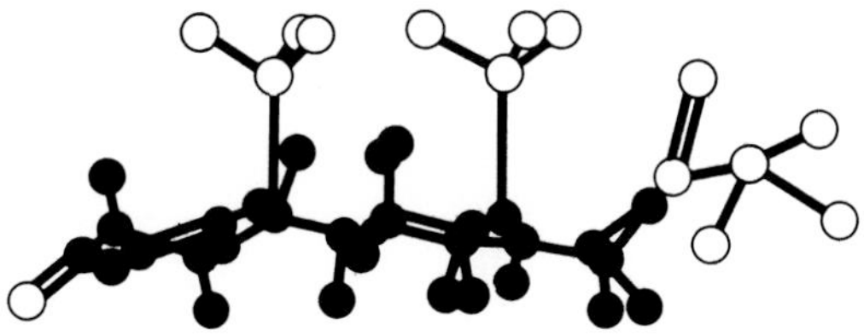

The convention of naming steroids uses the number of carbon atoms to designate the basic name (e.g. pregnane or androstane). The basic name is preceded by numbers which indicate the position of double bonds and the name is altered as follows to indicate 1, 2, or 3 double bonds: -ene, -diene, and -triene. Following the basic name, hydroxyl groups are indicated by the number of the carbon attachment, and 1, 2, or 3 hydroxyl groups are designated -ol, -diol, or -triol. Ketone groups are listed last with numbers of carbon attachments and 1, 2, or 3 groups designated -one, -dione, or -trione. Special designations include: dehydro—elimination of 2 hydrogens; deoxy—elimination of oxygen; nor—elimination of carbon; delta or Δ—location of a double bond.

Estrone
1,3,5(10)-Estratriene-3β-o1-17-one

Testosterone
4-Androstene-17β-o1-3-one

Progesterone
4-Pregnene-3,20-dione

Steroidogenesis

The overall steroid biosynthetic pathway shown in the figure is based primarily on the cumulative work of Ryan and his co-workers (1). These pathways follow the fundamental pattern displayed by all steroid-producing endocrine organs, and it should immediately be emphasized that the normal human ovary produces all three classes of sex steroids: estrogens, progestins, and androgens. The importance of the androgens has only recently been appreciated, not only as obligate precursors to estrogens, but also as clinically important secretory products. The ovary differs from the testis in its functional complement of critical enzymes and, hence, its distribution of secretory products. The ovary is distinguished from the adrenal gland in that it appears to be deficient in 21-hydroxylase and 11 β-hydroxylase enzymes. Glucocorticoids and mineralocorticoids, therefore, are not produced in normal ovarian tissue.

During steroidogenesis, the number of carbon atoms in cholesterol or any other steroid molecule can be reduced but never increased. The following reactions may take place:

1. cleavage of a side chain (desmolase reaction)

2. conversion of hydroxyl groups into ketones or ketones into hydroxyl groups (dehydrogenase reactions)

3. addition of OH group (hydroxylation reaction)

4. creation of double bonds (removal of hydrogen)

Cholesterol is the basic building block in steroidogenesis. All steroid-producing organs except the placenta can synthesize cholesterol from acetate. Progestins, androgens, and estrogens, therefore, may be synthesized *in situ* from a 2-carbon molecule in the various ovarian tissue compartments via cholesterol as the common steroid precursor. An additional resource is blood cholesterol which enters the ovarian cells and can be inserted into the biosynthetic pathway or esterified and thus be available as a stored precursor.

Conversion of cholesterol to pregnenolone involves hydroxylation at the carbon 20 and 22 positions (20-hydroxylase and 22-hydroxylase enzymes), with subsequent cleavage of the side chain (20, 22 desmolase). Conversion of cholesterol to pregnenolone takes place within the mitochondria. It is a rate-limiting step in the steroid pathway and is one of the principal effects of LH stimulation.

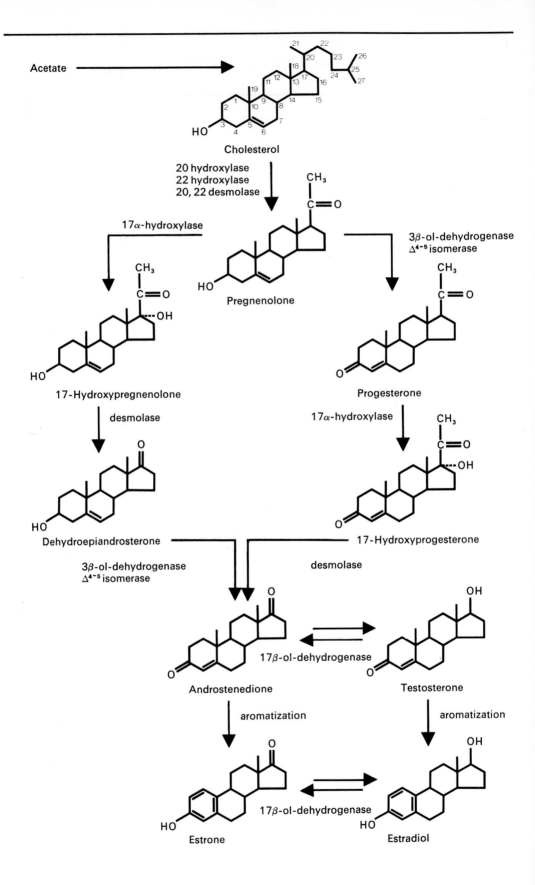

It is important to note that subsequent to pregnenolone, steroid synthesis in the ovary may proceed by one of two pathways: either via Δ^5-3β-hydroxyl steroids or via the Δ^4-3-ketone pathway, the first proceeding by way of pregnenolone and dehydroepiandrosterone (DHA) and the second via progesterone and 17α-hydroxyprogesterone.

The conversion of pregnenolone to progesterone involves two enzyme steps: the 3β-hydroxysteroid dehydrogenase and Δ^{4-5} isomerase reactions which convert the 3β-hydroxyl group to a ketone and transfer the double bond from the 5–6 position to the 4–5 position. Once the Δ^4-3-ketone is formed, progesterone is hydroxylated at the 17α position to form 17α-hydroxyprogesterone. 17α-Hydroxyprogesterone is the immediate precursor of the C-19 (19 carbons) series of androgens in this pathway. By peroxide formation at C-20, followed by epoxidation of the C-17, C-20 carbons, the side chain is split off forming androstenedione. The 17-ketone may be reduced to a 17β-hydroxyl to form testosterone by 17β-hydroxysteroid dehydrogenase. Both C-19 steroids (androstenedione and testosterone) are rapidly converted to corresponding C-18 phenolic steroid estrogens (estrone and estradiol) by microsomal enzymes in a process referred to as aromatization. This process includes hydroxylation of the angular 19-methyl group, followed by oxidation, loss of the 19-carbon as formaldehyde, and ring A aromatization (dehydrogenation).

As an alternative, pregnenolone may be directly converted to the Δ^5-3β-hydroxy C-19 steroid, DHA, by 17α-hydroxylation followed by desmolase cleavage of the side chain. With formation of the Δ^4-3-ketone, DHA is converted into androstenedione. It is thought that conversion of each of the Δ^5 compounds to their corresponding Δ^4 compounds can occur at any step; however, the principal pathways are via progesterone and DHA. Regardless of the precursor source, C-19 Δ^4-3-ketone substrates proceed to estrogens as noted above.

Steroid synthesis in the ovary has been explained in two different ways: the two pathway theory and the two cell hypothesis. According to the two pathway theory, the selection of the Δ^5-3β-hydroxy pathway or the Δ^4-3-ketone pathway is governed by the cell type involved. Whereas the Δ^4-3-ketone pathway seems to be predominant in luteal tissue (granulosal), the Δ^5-3β-hydroxy pathway is characteristic of nonluteinized tissue (theca and stroma). (2, 3) The secretion of estrogen prior to ovulation is then explained on a morphologic basis: limitation of vascularization within the follicular thecal layer ensures that estrogen is the major secretory product. The absence of vascularization in the granulosa layer until after ovulation ensures that progesterone must diffuse toward the theca, where it is utilized for estrogen production. This theory implies that following follicular atresia, the thecal layer loses its ability to aromatize androgens, hence its designation as a new cell type, the stromal tissue.

The two cell hypothesis presents a more modern and logical explanation of the events involved in ovarian follicular steroidogenesis and development. Thecal cells respond to LH and produce androgens. Aromatization of androgens to estrogens is a specific activity within the granulosa layer and is induced by FSH. Androgens produced in the theca layer then must diffuse into the granulosa layer were they are converted to estrogens. The increasing level of estradiol in the peripheral circulation prior to ovulation reflects release of the estrogen back towards the theca layer and into the blood vessels. As the follicle approaches ovulation, LH receptors begin to appear on the granulosa layer and after ovulation the granulosa now responds to LH by secreting both progesterone and estrogen directly into the blood stream. Follicular atresia prior to ovulation is marked by degeneration of granulosa cells, leaving the thecal cells which may persist to secrete androgens.

Savard and his co-workers have shown that the stromal tissue (cells from the theca and surrounding stroma) forms mainly androstenedione, DHA, and testosterone, with androstenedione being the major steroid isolated from *in vitro* incubation studies. This tissue responds to gonadotropins (LH and human chorionic gonadotropin (HCG)) with increased overall steroidogenesis, but especially with secretion of androstenedione and DHA.

There is a midcycle increase in circulating levels of androstenedione and testosterone (4, 5, 6) probably arising from ovarian stromal tissue. Postmenopausally, when only stromal tissue remains, androstenedione is the chief secretory product in the ovarian vein.

Blood Transport of Steroids

While circulating in the blood a majority (about 80%) of the principal sex steroids, estradiol and testosterone, is bound to a protein carrier, a beta globulin known as sex hormone binding globulin (SHBG). Approximately 19% is loosely bound to albumin, leaving about 1% unbound and free. Transcortin, also called corticosterone binding globulin (CBG), is a plasma glycoprotein which binds cortisol, progesterone, deoxycorticosterone, corticosterone and some of the other minor corticoid compounds. Normally about 75% of circulating cortisol is bound to transcortin, 15% is loosely bound to albumin, and 10% is unbound or free. The purpose of this binding is not understood. The biologic activity of a hormone may be limited by binding in the blood, and sudden abrupt hormone effects may thus be avoided or binding may prevent rapid metabolism, allowing the hormone to exist for the length of time necessary to ensure a biologic effect.

The biologic effects of the major sex steroids are determined by the unbound portion, known as the free hormone. In other words, the active hormone is unbound and free while the bound hormone is inactive. Deviations from normal levels of the binding globulins do not seem to affect the biologic efficacy of cortisol, testosterone, or estradiol, indicating that the level of free active hormone is maintained. Routine assays determine the total hormone concentration, bound plus free; and special steps are required to measure the active free level of testosterone, estradiol, and cortisol.

Estrogen Metabolism

Androgens are the common precursors of estrogens. 17β-Hydroxydehydrogenase activity converts androstenedione to testosterone which is not a major secretory product of the normal ovary, but is rapidly demethylated at the C-19 position and aromatized to estradiol, the major estrogen secreted by the human ovary. Estradiol also arises to a major degree from androstenedione via estrone, and estrone itself is secreted in significant daily amounts. Estriol is the peripheral metabolite of estrone and estradiol, and not a secretory product of the ovary. As such, the formation of estriol is typical of general metabolic "detoxification," conversion of biologically active material to less active forms.

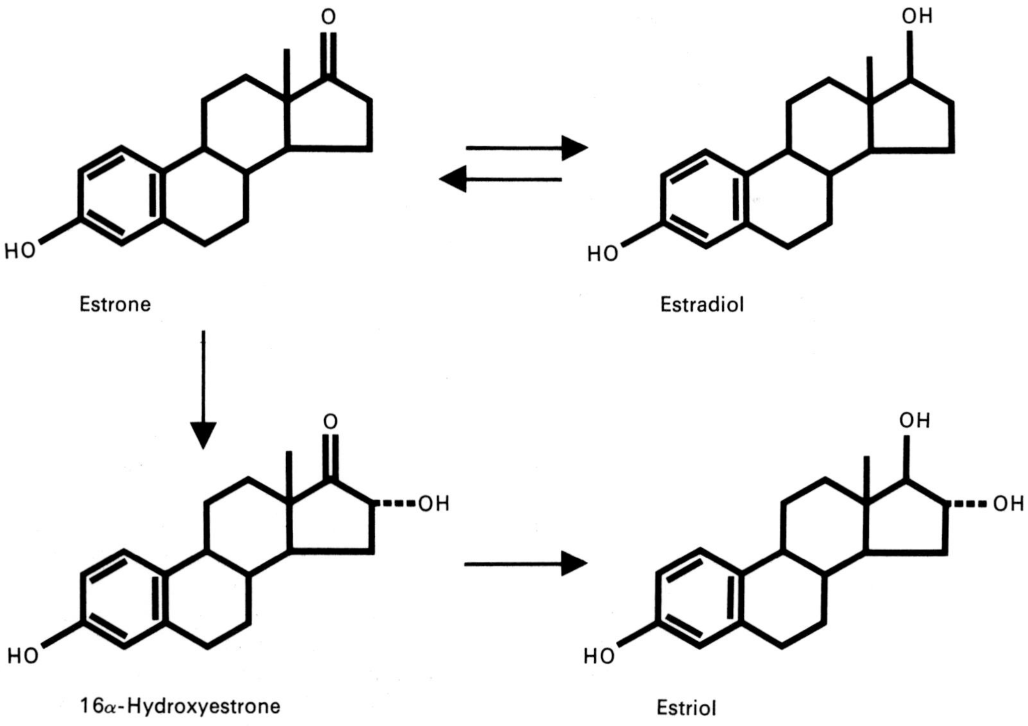

Estrone   Estradiol

16α-Hydroxyestrone   Estriol

The conversion of steriods in peripheral tissues, however, is not always a form of inactivation. Free androgens are peripherally converted to free estrogens; for example in skin and adipose cells. The work of MacDonald and Siiteri (7) has shown that enough estrogen may be derived from circulating androgens to produce bleeding in the postmenopausal woman.

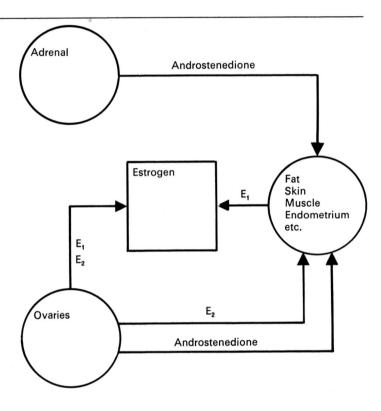

In the male, almost all (if not all), of the circulating estrogens are derived from peripheral conversion of androgens. The adrenal gland remains the major source of circulating androgens, in particular androstenedione.

It can be seen, therefore, that the pattern of circulating steroids in the female is influenced by the activity of various processes outside the ovary. Because of the peripheral contribution to steroid levels, "secretion rate" is reserved for direct organ secretion, whereas "production rate" includes organ secretion plus peripheral contribution via conversion of precursors. The metabolic clearance rate equals the volume of blood which is cleared of the hormone per unit of time. The blood production rate then equals the metabolic clearance rate multiplied by the concentration of the hormone in the blood.

In the normal nonpregnant female, estradiol is produced at the rate of 100–300 μg/day. The production of androstenedione is about 3 mg/day, and the peripheral conversion (about 1% of androstenedione) to estrone accounts for about 20–30% of the estrone produced per day. Since androstenedione is secreted in milligram amounts, even a small percent conversion to estrogens results in a significant contribution to total estrogens, as measured in microgram amounts. Thus the circulating estrogens in the female are principally the sum of direct ovarian secretion of estradiol and estrone, plus peripheral conversion of C-19 precursors.

Premenopausal
Peripheral
Conversion

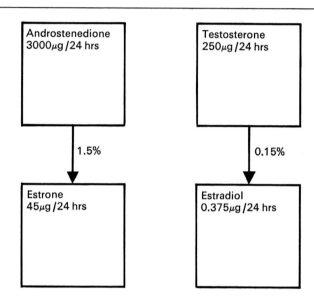

Progesterone Metabolism

Peripheral conversion of steroids to progesterone is not seen in the nonpregnant female, rather the production rate is a combination of secretion from the adrenal and the ovaries. Including the small contribution from the adrenal, the blood production rate of progesterone in the preovulatory phase is about 2–3 mg/day. During the luteal phase, production increases to 20–30 mg/day. The metabolic fate of progesterone, as expressed by its many excretion products, is more complex than estrogen. About 10–20% of progesterone is excreted as pregnanediol.

Pregnanediol glucuronide is present in the urine at concentrations less than 1 mg/day until ovulation. Postovulation pregnanediol excretion reaches a peak of 3–6 mg/day, which is maintained until 2 days prior to menses. The assay of pregnanediol in the urine now has limited use. Newer methods utilizing binding proteins or antibodies to measure plasma levels of progesterone are more rapid, more sensitive, and more precise. From a clinical point of view, however, the basal body temperature continues to be the most practical measure of ovulation and the luteal phase. Plasma progesterone levels might be of some value in the occasional patient with habitual abortion due to inadequate luteal function. In the preovulatory phase in adult females, in all prepubertal females, and in the normal male, the blood levels of progesterone are at the lower limits of assay sensitivity: less than 1 ng/ml. After ovulation, i.e., during the luteal phase, progesterone ranges from 5 to 10 ng/ml. In congenital adrenal hyperplasia, progesterone blood levels may be as high as 50 times above normal.

Pregnanetriol is the chief urinary metabolite of 17α-hydroxyprogesterone, and has clinical significance in the adrenogenital syndrome, where an enzyme defect results in accumulation of 17α-hydroxyprogesterone and increased excretion of pregnanetriol. The plasma or serum assay of 17α-hydroxyprogesterone is a more sensitive and accurate index of an enzyme deficiency. Normally the blood level of 17α-hydroxyprogesterone is less than 1 ng/ml, although after ovulation and during the luteal phase of a normal menstrual cycle, a peak of 2 ng/ml may be reached. In syndromes of adrenal hyperplasia, values may be 50 to 400 times normal.

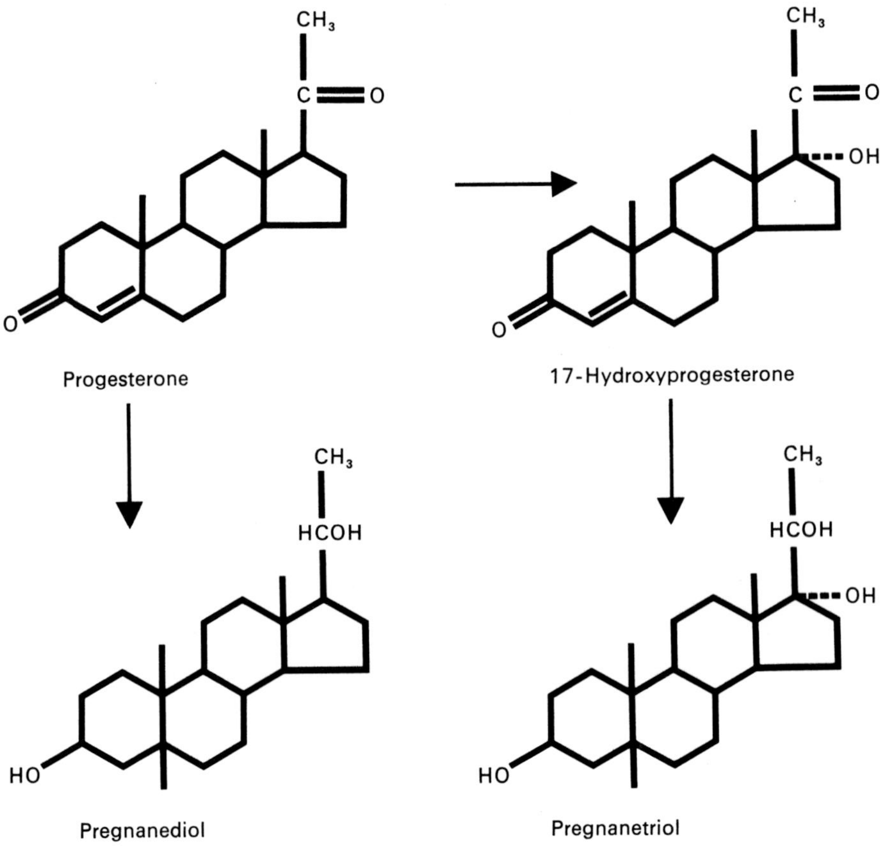

Progesterone

17-Hydroxyprogesterone

Pregnanediol

Pregnanetriol

Androgen Metabolism

The major androgen products of the ovary are dehydro-epiandrosterone (DHA) and androstenedione which are secreted mainly by stromal tissue. With excessive accumulation of stromal tissue or in the presence of an androgen producing tumor, testosterone becomes a significant secretory product. Occasionally a nonfunctioning tumor may induce stromal proliferation and increased androgen production. The normal accumulation of stromal tissue at midcycle results in a rise in circulating levels of androstenedione and testosterone at the time of ovulation. (4, 5, 6)

The adrenal cortex produces three groups of steroid hormones: the glucocorticoids, the mineralocorticoids, and the sex steroids. The sex steroids represent intermediate products in the synthesis of glucocorticoids and mineralocorticoids, and excessive secretion of the sex steroids occurs only with neoplastic cells or in association with enzyme deficiencies. Under normal circumstances adrenal gland production of the sex steroids is less significant than gonadal production of androgens and estrogens.

There is no circadian cycle in the major sex steroids in the female. However, short term variations in the blood levels of testosterone requires multiple sampling for absolutely accurate assessment. Although frequent sampling is necessary for a high degree of accuracy, a random sample is usually sufficient to determine whether a level is within a normal range.

The testosterone binding capacity is decreased by androgens themselves. Hence, the binding capacity in men is lower than that in normal women; the binding globulin level in women with increased androgen production is also depressed. Androgenic effects are dependent upon the unbound fraction which can move freely from the vascular compartment into the target cells. Routine assays determine the total hormone concentration, bound plus free. Thus a total testosterone concentration may be in the normal range in a woman who is hirsute or virilized, but because the binding globulin level is depressed by the androgen effects, the percent free and active testosterone is elevated. The need for a specific assay for the free portion of testosterone can be questioned since the very presence of hirsutism or virilism indicates increased androgen effects. In the face of hirsutism, one can reliably interpret a normal testosterone level as compatible with decreased binding capacity and increased active free testosterone. (8) In only a few women with hirsutism, both total and unbound testosterone are normal. Here, the hirsutism most likely results from an increase in unbound levels of other androgens such as dihydrotestosterone and androstenediol. Therefore, hirsutism which heretofore has been regarded as idiopathic may have a basis in unappreciated and excessive intracellular androgen effects or receptor variability. It should be emphasized that the degree of increased androgen in the circulation does not necessarily parallel the degree of hirsutism.

The production rate of testosterone in the normal female is 0.2–0.3 mg/day, and approximately 50% arises from peripheral conversion of androstenedione to testosterone, while 25% is secreted by the ovary and 25% by the adrenal. Reduction of the Δ^4 unsaturation in testosterone is very significant, producing derivatives very different in their spatial configuration and activity. The 5β derivatives are not androgenic; however, the 5α derivative is extremely potent. Indeed, dihydrotestosterone (DHT), the 5α derivative, is the principal androgenic hormone in a variety of target tissues and is formed within the target tissue itself. (9)

The majority of circulating DHT is derived from testosterone which enters a target cell and is converted by means of a 5α-reductase to DHT. DHT may be reduced by a 3α-keto-reductase to a further metabolite, androstanediol, which is relatively inactive. In tissues sensitive to DHT (which probably includes hair follicles), only DHT enters the nucleus to provide the androgen message. The blood DHT is only about 1/10 the level of circulating testosterone, and it is clear that testosterone is the major circulating androgen.

DHT may perform androgenic actions within cells which do not possess the ability to convert testosterone to DHT. However, not all androgen-sensitive tissues require the prior conversion of testosterone to DHT. In the process of masculine differentiation, the development of the Wolffian duct structures (epididymis, the vas deferens, and the seminal vesicle) appears to be dependent upon testosterone as the intracellular mediator, whereas development of the urogenital sinus and urogenital tubercle into the male external genitalia, urethra, and prostate requires the conversion of testosterone to DHT. (10)

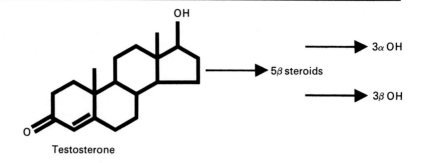

OH

5β steroids

3α OH

3β OH

Testosterone

5α-reductase

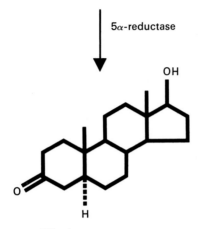

OH

H

Dihydrotestosterone
(DHT)

3α-keto-reductase

3β-keto-reductase

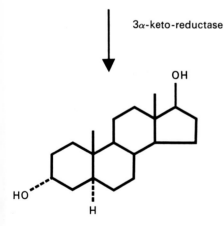

OH

HO

H

3α Androstanediol

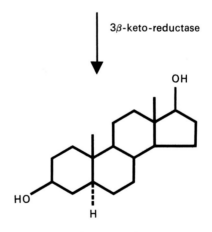

OH

HO

H

3β Androstanediol

17

Excretion of Steroids

Active steroids and metabolites are excreted as sulfo- and glucuro-conjugates. Conjugation of a steroid generally reduces or eliminates the activity of a steroid. This is not completely true, however, since hydrolysis of the ester linkage may occur in target tissues and restore the active form. Furthermore, estrogen conjugates may have biologic activity, and it is known that sulfated conjugates are actively secreted and may serve as precursors. Ordinarily, however, conjugation is a step in deactivation preliminary to and essential for excretion into urine and bile.

Glucosiduronate

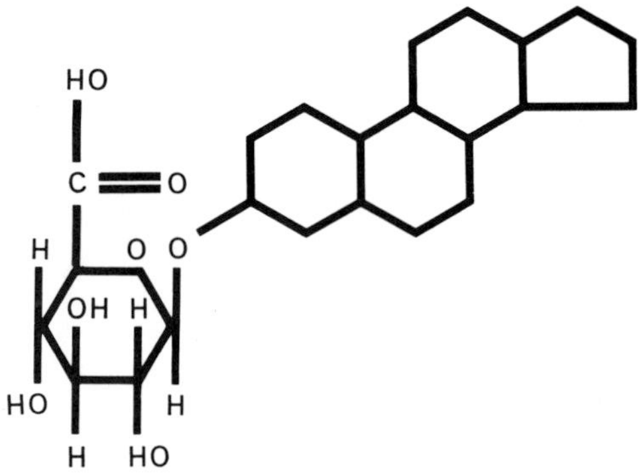

Sulfate

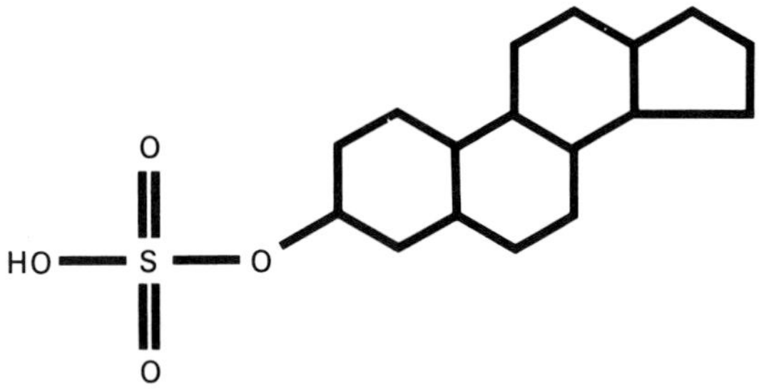

Cellular Mechanism of Action

Hormones circulate in extremely low concentrations and to respond with specific and effective actions, target cells require the presence of special mechanisms. There are two types of hormone action at the cellular level. One mediates the action of tropic hormones (peptide and glycoprotein hormones) at the cell membrane level and involves adenylate cyclase activity. In contrast, the smaller steroid hormones enter cells readily, and the basic mechanism of action involves specific cytoplasm receptor molecules.

Mechanism of Action for Steroid Hormones	The specificity of the reaction of tissues to steroid hormones is due to the presence of intracellular receptor proteins. Different types of tissues, such as liver, kidney, and uterus, respond in a similar manner. The mechanism includes: (1) diffusion across the cell membrane; (2) binding to cytoplasmic receptor protein and transfer of the hormone-receptor complex across the nuclear membrane to the nucleus; (3) binding of a hormone-receptor complex to nuclear DNA; (4) synthesis of messenger RNA (mRNA); (5) transport of the mRNA to the ribosomes; and finally, (6) protein synthesis in the cytoplasm which results in specific cellular activity.

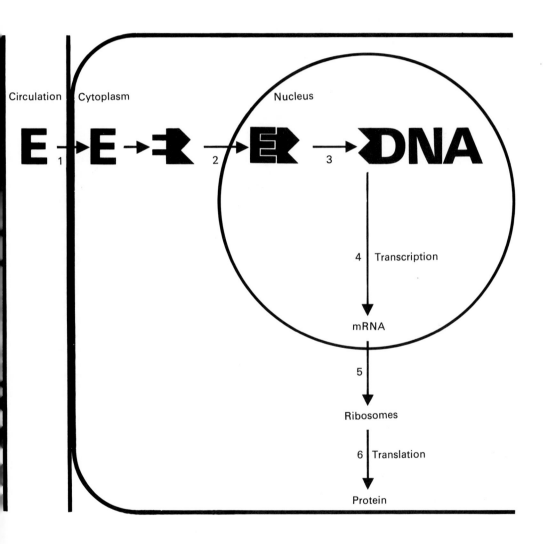

Because the major elucidation of this mechanism has involved estrogens, we will focus on the mechanism of estrogen action. Estrogens are rapidly transported across the cell membrane by simple diffusion. The factors responsible for this transfer are unknown, but the concentration of free (unbound) hormone in the blood stream seems to be an important and influential determinant of cellular function. Once within the cell, assuming the cell is responsive to estrogen (e.g., target tissue such as endometrium), the hormone is quickly bound by a protein receptor. The function of the receptor is to transport the hormone to the nucleus in order to transfer the hormone to the intranuclear environment.

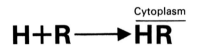

The physiologic response to estrogen requires interaction of the hormone-nuclear receptor with DNA, leading to production of messenger RNA (gene transcription). The nuclear receptor appears to arise from the nuclear relocation of the cytoplasmic receptor. Exactly how the hormone-receptor complex enters the nucleus is unknown; it appears that the shape of the receptor, an elongated ellipsoid, is important in this process. (12) Once in the nucleus, the complex unselectively binds to the chromatin, subsequently moving along the chromosome until the site for gene activation is encountered. At this site, a more specific binding takes place. This specific binding of the hormone-receptor complex with DNA results in RNA polymerase initiation of transcription. Transcription leads to translation, mRNA-mediated protein synthesis in the ribosomes. The principal action of steroid hormones is the regulation of intracellular protein synthesis by means of the receptor mechanism.

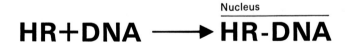

Tissue responsiveness to a hormone is determined not only by the presence of a specific receptor, but also by the intracellular concentration of that receptor. Responsiveness may be modified by affecting receptor concentration. Estrogen, for example, increases target tissue responsiveness to itself and to progesterone by increasing the concentration of its own receptor and that of the intracellular progesterone receptor. Progesterone, on the other hand, limits tissue response to estrogen by inducing a decrease in cytoplasmic estrogen receptors.

Biologic activity is maintained only while the receptor is occupied with the hormone. Therefore, the dissociation rate of the hormone with its receptor is a factor in the biologic response. One reason only small amounts of estrogen need be present in the circulation is the long half-life of the estrogen hormone-receptor complex. Cortisol and progesterone must circulate in larger concentrations because their receptor-complexes have short half-lives.

A hormone effect is also influenced by the half-life of the nuclear chromatin-bound complex. The weaker biologic activity of estriol compared to estradiol is apparently due to its shorter half-life in the nucleus (12).

$$HR_N\text{-}DNA \longrightarrow H+R+DNA$$

Therefore, there are 4 main determinants of biologic response and hormone activity (12):

1. Concentration of the free hormone in the circulation.

2. Concentration of cytoplasmic receptors.

3. The dissociation rate of the hormone-receptor complex.

4. The dissociation rate of the hormone-receptor complex bound to the chromatin.

$$H+R \xrightarrow{\textbf{1}\ \textbf{2}} HR+DNA \rightarrow HR\text{-}DNA \xrightarrow{\textbf{3}\ \textbf{4}} H+R+DNA$$

Pharmacologic agents which interfere with steroid hormone action may do so in the following ways (12):

1. Inhibition of steroidogenesis; e.g., aminoglutethimide (in general — toxic agents).

2. Reduction in the intracellular availability of cytoplasmic receptors; e.g. irreversible covalent binding between the receptor and steroid derivatives (currently experimental).

3. Prevention of translocation of hormone-receptor complex into the nucleus; e.g., spironolactone.

4. Decrease in receptor concentration; e.g., the anti-estrogen effect of progestational agents and clomiphene.

5. Inhibition of transcription; e.g., actinomycin D (nonspecific and toxic).

The mechanism is more complex for androgens. Cellular action of androgens may derive from testosterone itself or it may first require intracellular conversion of testosterone to dihydrotestosterone (DHT). Testosterone may be converted to DHT within the cytoplasm, or possibly a cytoplasmic receptor may carry testosterone to the vicinity of the nuclear membrane, where conversion to DHT occurs. (9) In those cells, which respond only to DHT, only DHT will be found within the nucleus, activating messenger RNA production. Metabolism of DHT to the inactive androstanediol occurs only in the cytoplasm. The syndrome of testicular feminization (androgen insensitivity) represents a congenital abnormality in the androgen intracellular mechanism either as a deficit in receptor production or an abnormality in receptor function. In either event, there is a failure in nuclear binding of androgens. (12)

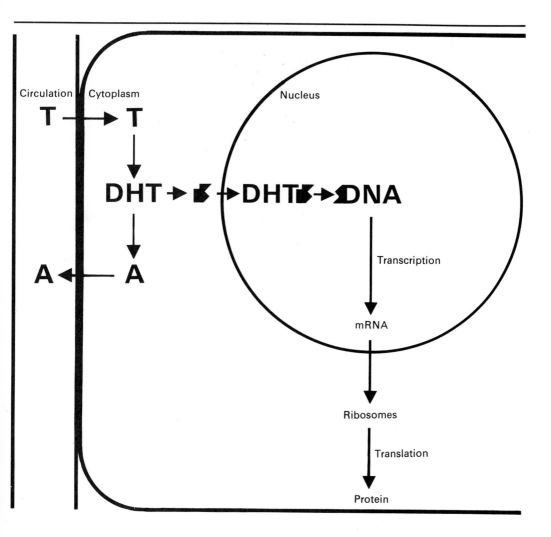

Mechanism of Action for Tropic Hormones

Tropic hormones include a variety of peptides and glycoproteins released by the anterior pituitary gland and the releasing hormones originating in the hypothalamus. The specificity of the tropic hormone depends upon the presence of a receptor in the cell plasma membrane of the target tissue. Tropic hormones do not enter the cell to stimulate physiological events but simply unite with a receptor on the surface of the cell. Union with the receptor activates the adenylate cyclase enzyme within the membrane wall leading to the conversion of ATP within the cell to cyclic AMP (cyclic adenosine 3′5′ monophosphate). The receptor may actually be a functional subunit of a membrane complex which includes adenylate cyclase. Specificity of action and/or intensity of stimulation may be altered by changes in the structure of the receptor at the cell wall binding site. In addition to changes in biological activity due to target cell alterations, changes in the molecular structure of the tropic hormone may interfere with cellular binding and physiologic activity.

The process of tropic hormone activation of cyclic AMP is extremely efficient requiring binding and occupation of only a small quantity of cell wall receptors. The cell's mechanism for sensing the low concentrations of circulating tropic hormone is to have an extremely large number of receptors but to require only a very small percentage (perhaps 1%) to be occupied by the tropic hormone. (13) The cyclic AMP released is specifically bound to a cytoplasm receptor protein, and this cAMP-receptor protein complex activates a protein kinase. The protein kinase is thought to be present in an inactive form composed of a regulatory unit and a catalytic unit. Cyclic AMP frees the catalytic unit by combining with the regulatory unit, and active phosphorylation ensues via the transfer of phosphate from ATP to a variety of substrate proteins by means of the kinase activity. The physiological event follows this cAMP mediated energy-producing event.

Acute responses such as increased steroidogenesis do not operate through gene transcription but rather through phosphorylation. Long-term effects of peptide hormones, such as differentiation and growth, do operate through nuclear activity, and cyclic AMP may also exert an effect on RNA polymerase activity (transcription) as well as on translation. (13) Because LH may stimulate steroidogenesis without apparent changes in cyclic AMP (at low hormone concentrations) it is possible that an independent pathway exists; i.e., a mechanism independent of cyclic AMP.

Prostaglandins have been implicated in this cyclic AMP mechanism. Because prostaglandins stimulate adenylate cyclase activity and cAMP accumulation, a role is implied for prostaglandins in transmitting the message from the exterior cell wall to the interior cell wall and the adenylate cyclase enzyme. Despite this effect on adenylate cyclase, prostaglandins appear to be synthesized after the action of cyclic AMP. (14) This implies that tropic hormone stimulation of cyclic AMP occurs first; cyclic AMP then activates prostaglandin synthesis, and finally intracellular prostaglandin moves to the cell wall to facilitate the response to the tropic hormone.

In addition prostaglandins and cGMP (cyclic guanosine $3'5'$ monophosphate) may participate in an intracellular negative feedback mechanism governing the degree of or direction of cellular activity (e.g., the extent of steroidogenesis or shutting off of steroidogenesis after a peak of activity is reached). In other words, the level of cellular function may be determined by the interaction among prostaglandins, cAMP, and cGMP. (14)

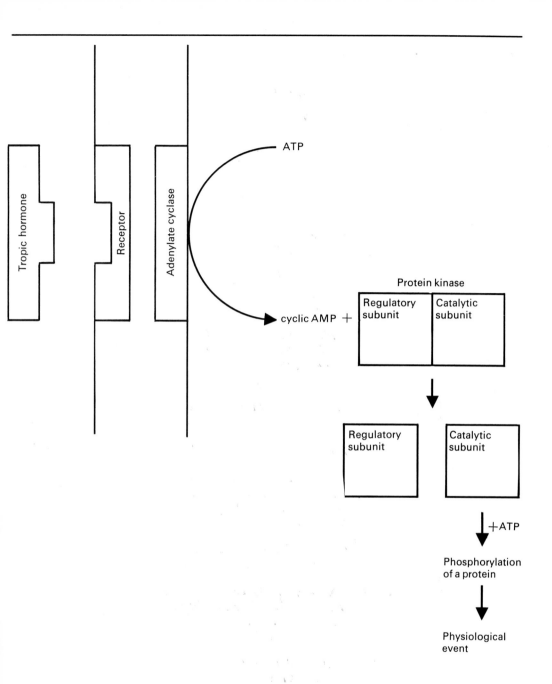

References

1. **Ryan, KJ,** Steroid Hormones and Prostaglandins, in Reid, DE, Ryan, KJ, and Benirschke, K, *Principles and Management of Human Reproduction,* W. B. Saunders Co, Philadelphia, 1972.

2. **Kase, N,** Steroid Synthesis in Abnormal Ovaries, III. Polycystic Ovaries, Am J Obstet Gynecol 90:1268, 1964.

3. **Ryan, KJ, Petro, Z, and Kaiser, J,** Steroid Formation by Isolated and Recombined Ovarian Granulosa and Thecal Cells, J Clin Endocrinol Metab 28:355, 1968.

4. **Judd, HL, and Yen, SSC,** Serum Androstenedione and Testosterone Levels During the Menstrual Cycle. J Clin Endocrinol Metab 36:475, 1973.

5. **Abraham, GE,** Ovarian and Adrenal Contribution to Peripheral Androgens During the Menstrual Cycle, J Clin Endocrinol Metab 39:340, 1974.

6. **Vermeulen, A, and Verdonck, L,** Plasma Androgen Levels During the Menstrual Cycle, Am J Obstet Gynecol 125:491, 1976.

7. **Siiteri, PK, and MacDonald, PC,** Role of Extraglandular Estrogen in Human Endocrinology, in Geiger, SR, Astwood, EB, and Greep, RO, eds, *Handbook of Physiology,* Section 7, Endocrinology, American Physiology Society, Washington, DC, 1973, pp. 615–629.

8. **Rosenfield, RL,** Plasma Testosterone Binding Globulin and Indexes of the Concentrations of Unbound Plasma Androgens in Normal and Hirsute Subjects, J Clin Endocrinol Metab 32:171, 1971.

9. **Wilson, JD,** Recent Studies on the Mechanism of Action of Testosterone, New Eng J Med 287:1284, 1972.

10. **Walsh, PC, Madden, JD, Harrod, MJ, Goldstein, JL, MacDonald, PC, and Wilson, JD,** Familial Incomplete Male Pseudohermaphrodism, Type 2, New Eng J Med 291:944, 1974.

11. **Jensen, EV, and DeSombre, ER,** Estrogen-Receptor Interaction, Science 182:126, 1973.

12. **Chan, L, and O'Malley, BW,** Mechanism of Action of the Sex Steroid Hormones, New Eng J Med 294:1322, 1372, 1430, 1976.

13. **Catt, KJ, and Dufau, ML,** Basic Concepts of the Mechanism of Action of Peptide Hormones, Biol Reprod 14:1, 1976.

14. **Kuehl, FA, Jr.,** Prostaglandins, Cyclic Nucleotides and Cell Function, Prostaglandins 5:325, 1975.

2 Neuroendocrinology

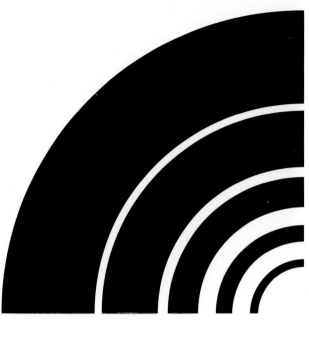

That neuroendocrine mechanisms are basic factors in the reproductive cycle is no longer a matter for debate. Rather, the larger and more difficult task of unraveling the complex interactions by which the brain controls anterior pituitary function is the current challenge of research in reproductive biology. This fascinating topic has attracted intense interest on the part of numerous able investigators. As a result, an enormous and rapidly expanding volume of data has appeared in a relatively short period of time. A transducer concept has evolved in which specialized neural cells of the hypothalamus function as the final common pathway by which the entire spectrum of internal and external environmental signals are recognized, integrated, and reduced to neuro-humoral directions which guide anterior pituitary hormonal responses appropriate to the body's physiologic needs.

A full understanding of this pivotal feature of reproductive biology will benefit the clinician who daily faces problems in gynecologic endocrinology. With this understanding he or she can comprehend the hitherto mysterious but significant effects of stress, diet, activity, and diverse diseases on the pituitary-gonadal axis. Furthermore, he or she will be prepared to make advantageous use of the impending availability of numerous neuropharmacologic agents that are the anticipated dividends of neuroendocrine research. *To these ends, this chapter offers a review of the current status of reproductive neuroendocrinology.*

Hypothalamic-Hypophyseal Portal Circulation

In order to influence the anterior pituitary gland, the brain requires a means of transmission or connection between the two organ systems. A direct nervous connection does not exist. The blood supply of the anterior pituitary, however, originates in the capillaries which richly lace the median eminence area of the hypothalamus. The direction of the blood flow in this hypopyseal portal circulation is from the brain to the pituitary. Section of the neural stalk combined with interruption of this portal circulation leads to inactivity and atrophy of the gonads, along with decreased adrenal and thyroid activity to basal levels. With regeneration of the portal vessels, anterior pituitary function is restored. Regeneration of the neural connection to the posterior pituitary is not required. Anatomic evidence suggests that specific aggregates of hypothalamic cells are linked with specific areas of the anterior pituitary by the portal vessels. An individual portal vessel may convey blood containing specific neurohumors to its specific site, allowing precise anatomic control over pituitary secretion.

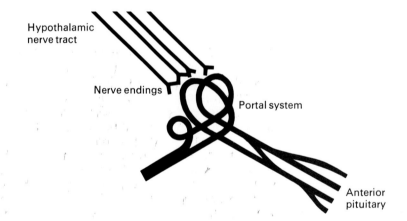

Neurochemo-transmitter Concept

A considerable body of diverse biologic evidence has accumulated indicating that control of the pituitary by the hypothalamus is achieved by materials secreted in the cells of the hypothalamus and transported to the pituitary by the portal vessel system. In addition to the stalk section experiments cited above, transplantation of the pituitary to ectopic sites (e.g. under the kidney capsule) results in failure of gonadal function. With retransplantation to an anatomic site under the median eminence, followed by regeneration of the portal system, normal pituitary function is regained. This retrieval of gonadotropic function is not accomplished if the pituitary is transplanted to other sites in the brain. Hence there is something very special about the blood draining the basal hypothalamus. An exception to this overall pattern of positive influence is the control of prolactin secretion. Stalk section and transplantation cause release of prolactin from the anterior pituitary, implying a negative hypothalamic control. Furthermore, anterior pituitary tissue culture release of prolactin occurs in the absence of hypothalamic tissue or extracts.

Other classical experiments which emphasize the importance of hypothalamic control include the following: electrical stimulation of the median eminence in animals leads to ovulation, while destruction of this area of the hypothalamus results in gonadal atrophy; crude extracts of median eminence cause gonadotropin release after injection into intact animals, and from tissue culture preparations of anterior pituitary.

Using tissue culture reactions as an assay, crude hypothalamic extracts have been chromatographed and materials with relatively specific effects have been isolated. The individual portions of the extract have positive stimulatory impact on growth hormone, thyroid-stimulating hormone (TSH), ACTH, as well as gonadotropins, and represent the individual neurotransmitters of the hypothalamus. The neurotransmitter which controls gonadotropins is called gonadotropin-releasing hormone, GnRH. The neurotransmitter which controls prolactin is called prolactin inhibiting factor. Behavioral effects within the brain have been demonstrated for several of the releasing factors. Thyrotropin releasing hormone antagonizes the sedative action of a number of drugs and also has a direct antidepressant effect in humans. GnRH evokes mating behavior in male and female animals.

Antagonists for these factors would be useful for investigational work as well as for certain clinical situations, such as contraception. Antagonists have been developed by changing or removing amino acids. These analogues will require considerable testing before clinical usefulness can be established.

Gonadotropin Releasing Hormone—
a decapeptide

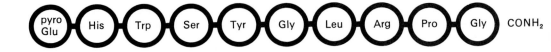

There has been controversy over whether there are separate releasing hormones for LH and FSH, or a single neurotransmitter for both gonadotropins. Initially it was believed that two hormones existed, but this has been questioned by the finding that purified and synthesized GnRH stimulated both LH and FSH secretion. The argument in favor of one releasing hormone is further supported by the finding that histologic stains and immunostaining cannot differentiate between FSH and LH producing cells in the pituitary. (1) In the presence of a single GnRH, the divergent patterns of FSH and LH secretion are thought to represent modulating influences of the endocrine environment in the hypothalamus and the pituitary gland.

The Hypothalamus

The hypothalamus is the part of the diencephalon, at the base of the brain, which forms the floor of the third ventricle and part of its lateral walls. The hypothalamus can be considered as the final pathway for endocrine and nervous system coordination. Within the hypothalamus are peptidergic neural cells which secrete the releasing and inhibiting hormones. These cells share the characteristics of both neurons and endocrine gland cells. They respond to signals in the blood stream, as well as to neurotransmitters within the brain, in a process known as neurosecretion. In neurosecretion, a neurohormone or neurotransmitter is synthesized on the ribosomes in the cytoplasm of the neuron, packaged into a granule in the Golgi apparatus, and then transported by active axonal flow to the neuronal terminal for secretion into a blood vessel or across a synapse.

There are several pathways within the hypothalamus by which brain centers may influence the pituitary gland. These pathways include the following anatomic and physiologic systems for neurosecretion:

1. The tonic and cyclic centers for secretion of gonadotropin releasing hormone.

2. Tanycytes, neuronal cells which connect the portal system with the cerebrospinal fluid.

3. The posterior pituitary pathway.

The Tonic and Cyclic Centers. It is useful to consider gonadotropin function to be under the control of two distinct centers in the hypothalamus, a tonic center responsible for the day-to-day basal level of gonadotropins and responsive to the negative feedback effects of steroids, and a cyclic center responsible in the female brain for the midcycle surge of gonadotropin and responsive to a positive feedback of estrogen. Studies in the rat have indicated that the tonic center with relatively short axons is located in the medial basal hypothalamus.

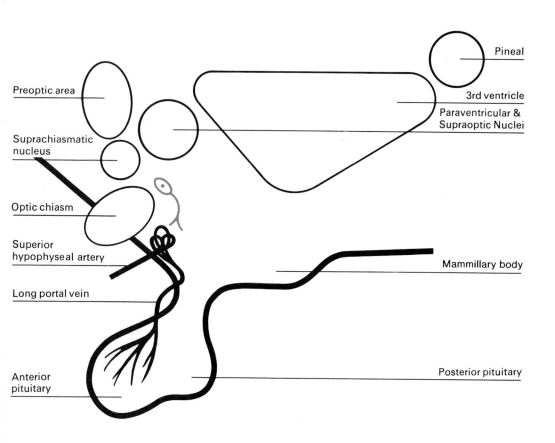

Preoptic area

Suprachiasmatic nucleus

Optic chiasm

Superior hypophyseal artery

Long portal vein

Anterior pituitary

Pineal

3rd ventricle

Paraventricular & Supraoptic Nuclei

Mammillary body

Posterior pituitary

The cyclic center with long axons is thought to be located in the anterior portion of the hypothalamus, in the preoptic area. Neurons sensitive to the positive feedback of estrogen may directly transmit GnRH to the portal system, or influence the tonic neurons to liberate GnRH.

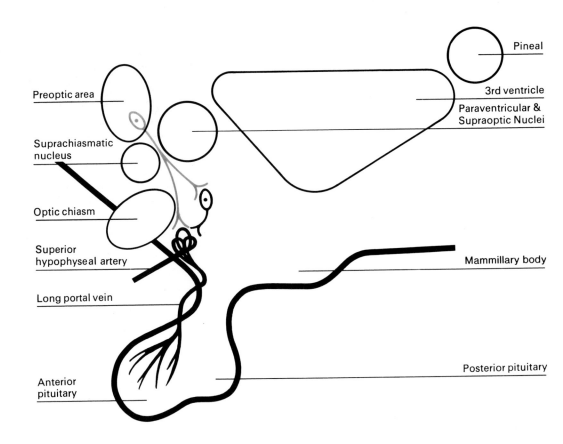

Preoptic area

Suprachiasmatic nucleus

Optic chiasm

Superior hypophyseal artery

Long portal vein

Anterior pituitary

Pineal

3rd ventricle

Paraventricular & Supraoptic Nuclei

Mammillary body

Posterior pituitary

Studies in the monkey have suggested that there are differences in the primate brain, particularly in the location and function of the cyclic center. Utilizing surgical techniques to isolate the medial basal hypothalamus, the cyclic and tonic centers could not be separated, suggesting that both centers reside within the medial basal hypothalamus. (2) However other investigators claim that the monkey brain is similar to the rat brain, containing distinct and separate tonic and cyclic centers. (3) Functionally it is useful to maintain the concept of separate centers when considering aberrations of the menstrual cycle.

Classic studies in rodents have indicated that the cyclic center in the male is permanently abolished by the exposure to testosterone during a critical time period of hypothalamic differentiation. This effect is in accord with the principle of sexual differentiation, i.e. the appearance of testosterone imposes masculine differentiation while the absence of testosterone allows feminine development.

If the hypothalamus of primates is influenced by androgens, in the same manner as in rats, then estrogen should not be able to elicit a gonadotropin surge in an adult male monkey. In other words, during male development the cyclic center should have been permanently abolished by testosterone. However castrated male monkeys, given estrogen chronically to maintain levels of gonadotropins characteristic of intact adults, respond to large doses of estradiol with surges of LH indistinguishable from those observed during normal cycles. (4) Thus, when these adult male monkeys were deprived of circulating levels of testosterone by castration, the cyclic center became operative. It appears that the continuous presence of androgens is necessary in primates to inhibit the function of the cyclic center in the hypothalamus.

Tanycytes. A significant pathway for hypothalamic influence may be via the cerebrospinal fluid. Tanycyctes are specialized ependymal cells whose ciliated cell bodies line the third ventricle over the median eminence. The cells terminate on portal vessels and they can transport materials from ventricular CSF to the portal system, e.g. substances from the pineal gland. Tanycytes change morphologically in response to steroids, and exhibit morphological changes with the ovarian cycle.

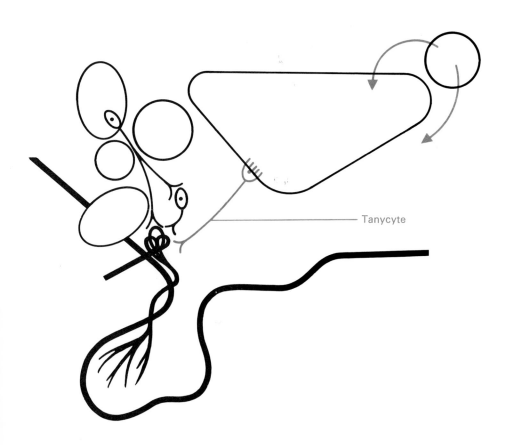

Tanycyte

The Posterior Pituitary Pathway. The posterior pituitary is a direct prolongation of the hypothalamus via the pituitary stalk. Cells in both the supraoptic and paraventricular nuclei make vasopressin, oxytocin, and a newly appreciated peptide, neurophysin. Neurophysin as well as vasopressin and oxytocin are transported along the length of the pituitary stalk to the posterior pituitary where they are stored in the axonal terminals which in aggregate make up the posterior pituitary.

Besides secretion into the posterior pituitary, vasopressin, oxytocin, and neurophysin are also secreted into the cerebrospinal fluid and into the portal system for the anterior pituitary. Their function in the CSF is unknown, but in the anterior pituitary, vasopressin may assist in ACTH and growth hormone secretion, while oxytocin may be involved in gonadotropin secretion.

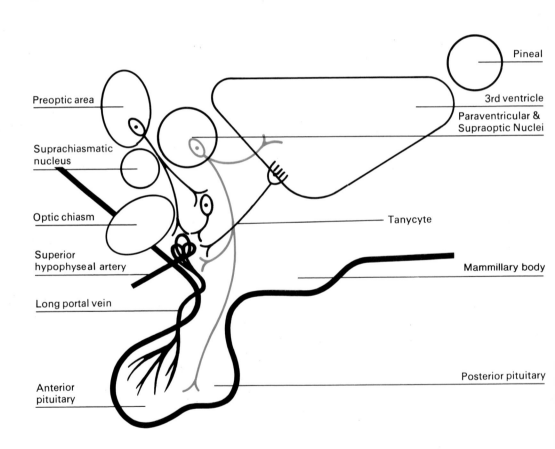

Preoptic area

Suprachiasmatic nucleus

Optic chiasm

Superior hypophyseal artery

Long portal vein

Anterior pituitary

Pineal

3rd ventricle

Paraventricular & Supraoptic Nuclei

Tanycyte

Mammillary body

Posterior pituitary

There appear to be two distinct neurophysins. (5) One is called nicotine neurophysin because hemorrhage or the administration of nicotine increases the circulating levels of this neurophysin. The other is called estrogen neurophysin because estrogen administration will increase the levels in the peripheral blood, and a peak is found at midcycle at the time of the LH surge. The rise in estrogen neurophysin begins 10 hours after the rise in estrogen and precedes that of the LH surge. The elevated levels of neurophysin also last longer than the LH surge. Large amounts of neurophysin along with GnRH, have been detected in the portal blood of the monkey. It is thought that nicotine neurophysin is specifically related to vasopressin, while estrogen neurophysin accompanies oxytocin. (5) Because GnRH and oxytocin are competing substrates for hypothalamic degradation enzymes, it has been hypothesized that oxytocin in the portal blood at the midcycle may inhibit the metabolism of the GnRH, thus increasing the amount of GnRH available for stimulation of gonadotropins. (5)

Control of GnRH Secretion

The half-life of GnRH is only a few minutes. Therefore control of the reproductive cycle depends on variable but constant release of GnRH. This function in turn depends upon the complex and coordinated interrelationship among this releasing hormone, other neurohormones, the pituitary gonadotropins, and the gonadal steroids. The interplay among these substances is governed by feedback effects, both positive stimulatory and negative inhibitory. The long feedback loop refers to the feedback effects of circulating levels of target gland hormones, and this occurs both in the hypothalamus and in the pituitary. The short feedback loop indicates a negative feedback of gonadotropins on pituitary secretion, via inhibitory effects on GnRH in the hypothalamus. Ultrashort feedback refers to inhibition by the releasing hormone of its own synthesis. These various feedback loops provide information from the internal body environment for the GnRH mechanism. Signals from the external environment as well as from higher centers in the central nervous system may modify GnRH activity through an array of neurotransmitters, primarily dopamine and norepinephrine, but also serotonin and melatonin.

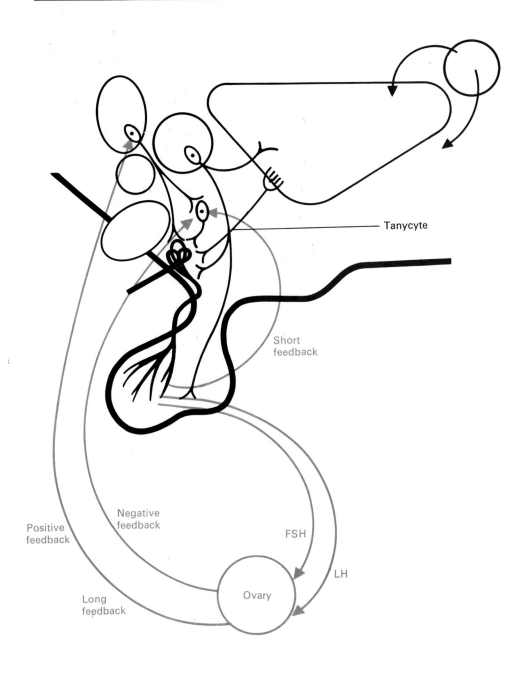

Tanycyte

Short
feedback

Positive
feedback

Negative
feedback

FSH

LH

Long
feedback

Ovary

Role of Catecholamines. The mechanism for the transmission of feedback effects at the hypothalamic level seems to involve a dopamine-norepinephrine system. Dopamine is synthesized in the nerve terminal by decarboxylation of dihydroxyphenylalanine (DOPA), which in turn is synthesized by hydroxylation of tyrosine. Dopamine is the immediate precursor of norepinephrine, but dopamine itself may be the key neurotransmitter in the hypothalamic regulation of gonadotropins.

In the presence of median eminence tissue *in vitro,* dopamine increases the release of LH and FSH from the anterior pituitary, while norepinephrine and serotonin have no effect. Portal perfusion of the rat anterior pituitary *in vivo* with monoamines has no effect. Injection of dopamine into the third ventricle of the rat, however, produces an increase in plasma LH and FSH within 3 minutes. Following third ventricle injection of dopamine, GnRH is markedly increased in hypophyseal stalk plasma, and this effect can be blocked by estradiol.

These data suggest that the tonic center for GnRH secretion is dopamine-dependent and it is at this site that inhibitory negative feedback of estradiol is exerted. The response to the third ventricle injection is thought to be due to the rapid transport of the material to the median eminence at the base of the ventricle. The administration of dopamine by intravenous infusion to men and women is associated with a suppression of circulatory prolactin and LH levels. (6) Here the effect may be at the pituitary as well as in the hypothalamus.

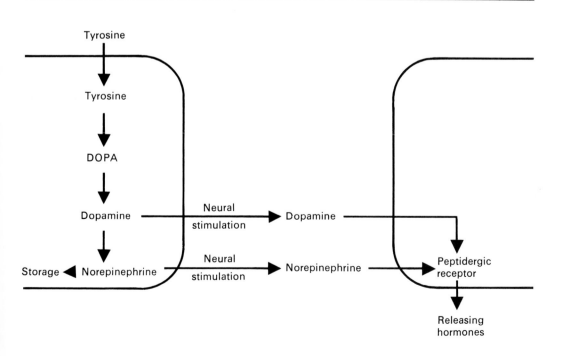

McCann proposes that norepinephrine may still be the GnRH inducer. (7) The effects of dopamine may be due to conversion to norepinephrine and norepinephrine release. Ineffectiveness of injected norepinephrine may reflect rapid catabolism.

Whereas the sequence catecholamine → hypothalamic peptide → pituitary tropic hormone applies to gonadotropins, in the control of prolactin secretion, dopamine itself may be the prolactin inhibiting factor. Dopamine directly inhibits the in vitro secretion of prolactin by the pituitary. (8) Ergot derivatives, used clinically to treat high prolactin levels, activate dopaminergic receptors and directly inhibit the secretion of newly synthesized prolactin.

Pituitary Response to GnRH

Responses of LH and FSH to GnRH suggest the presence of two pools of pituitary gonadotropins; one of which is released immediately and one which requires continued stimulation. (9) "Secretion" may be used to refer to the first pool and "reserve" to the second. Secretion and reserve change during the cycle. At the beginning of the cycle when estrogen levels are low, both secretion and reserve are low, but with increasing levels of estradiol, a greater increase occurs in reserve when compared to secretion. This suggests that the rate of synthesis exceeds the rate of release, setting the stage for the midcycle surge. During the late follicular phase until the midcycle surge there is a more rapid increase in pituitary secretion in response to GnRH. During this phase, subsequent responses to GnRH are greater than initial responses, suggesting that each response not only induces release of the first pool of gonadotropins, but also *activates* the reserve pool for the next response. At midcycle, there is maximal sensitivity to GnRH resulting in the well-known surge-like release of gonadotropins.

Estradiol has both a positive action on pituitary synthesis and storage (reserve) and an inhibitory action on secretion. (10). As the midcycle is approached, premature release of gonadotropins is prevented by the inhibitory action of estrogen on pituitary secretion. The midcycle surge of gonadotropins, therefore, is due to an outpouring of GnRH in response to the positive feedback action of estradiol on the cyclic center of the hypothalamus. This large amount of GnRH overpowers the inhibitory action of estradiol on the pituitary.

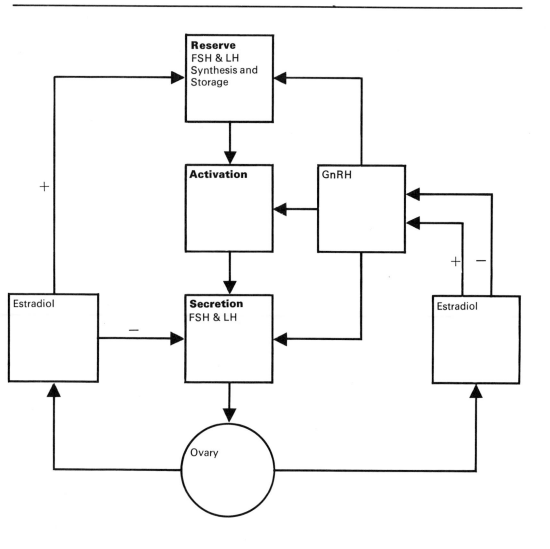

After the midcycle, both secretion and reserve decline. Progesterone at high levels does not seem to impair pituitary secretion or reserve, thus its effect must be principally on the hypothalamus. Indeed, high levels of progesterone exert a profound negative feedback on the hypothalamus and can block the midcycle LH surge responsible for ovulation. This negative feedback effect of progesterone requires the presence of estrogen, however, since progesterone given alone to an ovariectomized monkey will not lower gonadotropin secretion. (11) This effect of the combination of progesterone and estrogen is utilized in the birth control pill to inhibit ovulation.

Progesterone at low levels increases pituitary secretion and reserve in the presence of estrogen (12), thus enhancing the response to GnRH. The degree of enhancement is dependent upon previous estrogen priming. This effect of progesterone is consistent with a facilitory role during the midcycle surge of gonadotropins, acting primarily on the pituitary. (13)

The steroid actions on pituitary response to GnRH are reminiscent of steroid influences on tropic hormone receptors in the ovarian follicle. The mechanism for steroid modulation of GnRH effects may involve the pituitary cell wall receptor sites.

Heterogeneity of the Peptide Hormones

Many of the glycoprotein and polypeptide hormones exist in several forms within their secreting glands and also as they circulate in the blood. Differences in the amino acid content may exist. There may also be differences in the carbohydrate content of the glycoprotein hormones especially the sialic acid content of LH, FSH, and HCG. Such heterogeneity may be an expression of pathophysiology, but in at least one instance, it reflects a normal state: the α and β subunits of the glycoprotein hormones.

FSH, LH, TSH, and HCG consist of two nonidentical subunits. These two subunits are designated as α and β and are bound non-covalently. The α subunits of all of the glycoprotein hormones are similar in chemical structure and are interchangeable with one another. The specificity of glycoprotein hormones, both biologically and in radioimmunoassays, is given by the β subunit. The α and β subunits have little biological activity when compared to the intact hormone. Biologic activity can be recovered by combining the two units.

The common α subunit of the glycoprotein hormones circulates in the blood independently of the intact hormones. (14) It is present in developing follicles, but does not affect viability or steroidogenesis. As α and β subunits are added to granulosa cells, they recombine and stimulate steroid production. (14) The placenta secretes and produces larger amounts of the α subunit than the β subunit, and it appears that the limiting factor in HCG production by the placenta is a low level of β subunit synthesis. (15)

There is an excess of free α subunits in the pituitary gland, in the blood, and in the urine. It has been hypothesized that LH is synthesized as a prohormone with a connecting piece similar to the α subunit. (16) The terminal α unit and the β unit bind by noncovalent forces, then the intermediate connecting piece may be cleaved yielding the native hormone and an excess of α-like material. The advantage of such a procedure would be to provide ordered synthesis, avoiding the synthesis of hybrid units, e.g. α units combining with β TSH units when the physiologic demand is for LH.

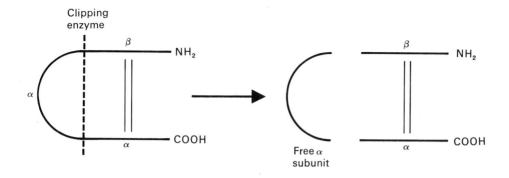

Free α
subunit

Pineal Gland

The reproductive functions of the hypothalamus may also be under inhibitory control of the brain via the pineal gland. The pineal arises as an outgrowth of the roof of the third ventricle, but soon after birth it loses all afferent and efferent neural connections with the brain. Instead the parenchymal cells receive a new and unusual sympathetic innervation.

The neural pathway begins in the retina and passes through the inferior accessory optic tracts and the medial forebrain bundle to the upper cord. Preganglionic fibers terminate at the superior cervical ganglion, and postganglionic sympathetic nerves terminate directly on pineal cells. Interruption of this pathway gives the same effect as darkness, which is an increase in pineal biosynthetic activity.

Hydroxyindole-*o*-methyl transferase (HIOMT) is found mainly in pineal parenchymal cells, and its products, therefore, are essentially unique to the pineal. Norepinephrine stimulates tryptophan entry into the pineal cell and also adenylate cyclase activity in the membrane. The resulting increase in cyclic AMP leads to *N*-acetyl transferase activity, the rate-limiting step in melatonin synthesis. Thus, melatonin synthesis is controlled by norepinephrine stimulation of adenylate cyclase, and the norepinephrine is liberated by sympathetic stimulation due to the absence of light.

The association of pineal tumors with decreased gonadal function, and destructive tumors with precocious puberty, suggested that the pineal is a source of gonadal inhibiting substances. However, pineal mechanisms cannot be absolutely essential for gonadal function. Several weeks after pinealectomy, normal reproductive function returns to the pinealectomized rat.

41

A rat in constant light develops a small pineal with decreased HIOMT and melatonin, while the ovarian weight increases. A rat in constant dark has the opposite result, increased pineal size, HIOMT, and melatonin, with decreased ovarian weight and pituitary function. A rhythm is established in pineal HIOMT activity by the presence or absence of light. Short days and long nights result in gonadal atrophy, and this may be a mechanism governing seasonal breeding. Possible roles in humans may be to give circadian rhythmicity to other functions such as temperature and sleep.

The pituitary implantation of pineal products gives no significant effects. Implants in the median eminence, on the other hand, have a characteristic pattern: serotonin and 5-methoxyindoleacetic acid decrease FSH pituitary stores, while melatonin and 5-hydroxytryptophol decrease LH stores. Melatonin and 5-methoxyindoleacetic acid may be the important agents since methoxy indoles are produced only by pineal HIOMT.

The pineal, therefore, may play a role in inhibiting reproductive function with melatonin participating in regulation of LH and 5-methoxyindoleacetic acid of FSH. These substances may reach the hypothalamus by way of the cerebrospinal fluid and tanycyte transport. Persistent curiosity over the role of the pineal in neuroendocrine mechanisms is shown in recent research.

Pineal glands have been found to contain large amounts of TRH and GnRH. Perhaps the pineal serves as a reservoir for these releasing hormones, important for the tonic maintenance levels of pituitary secretion. (17) The pineal does have intracellular steroid receptors and may be responsive to changes in the ovarian cycle. The pineal also contains one or more polypeptides which have antigonadotropic activity. (18) Melatonin may serve within the pineal itself to regulate production of an antigonadotropin peptide.

Despite a variety of suggestive leads, there is little evidence for a role of the pineal in humans. However a melatonin-like substance has been detected in the plasma of men during the darkness hours and not during the daytime. (19) Another possible influence of the pineal gland may be the synchronization of menstrual cycles noted among women who spend time together. A significant increase in synchronization of cycles among roommates and among closest friends occurred in the first 4 months of residency in a dormitory of a women's college. (20)

**Gonadotropin
Secretion Through
Fetal Life,
Childhood and
Puberty**

Gonadotropin production has now been documented throughout fetal life, during childhood, and into the adult years. Remarkable levels of FSH and LH, similar to postmenopausal levels, can be measured in the fetus. The peak concentrations of FSH and LH occur at about 20 weeks of intrauterine life. (21, 22)

The production of gonadotropins until midgestation reflects the growing ability of the hypothalamic-pituitary axis to perform at full capacity. Beginning at midgestation there is an increasing sensitivity to inhibition by steroids, i.e. a maturation of the negative feedback system. Full sensitivity to steroids is not reached until late in infancy. The rise in gonadotropins after birth reflects loss of the high levels of placental steroids.

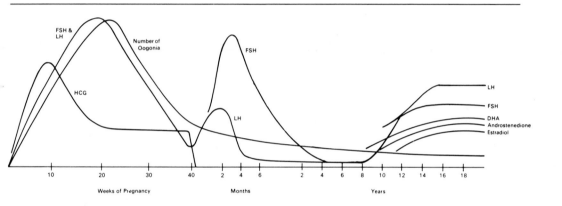

43

Testicular function in the fetus can be correlated with the fetal hormonal patterns. (21, 22, 23) Initial testosterone production and sexual differentiation is in response to the high fetal levels of HCG, while further testosterone production and differentiation appear to be maintained by the fetal pituitary gonadotropins. Decreased testosterone levels in late gestation despite continued significant gonadotropin levels may be due to heterogeneity of the gonadotropins (and thus decreased biologic activity), the decrease in gonadotropins due to placental steroids, interference with steroidogenesis by prolactin, or interference with Leydig cell function by the placental steroids, particularly estrogen. In the female, the peak of oogenesis and the onset of atresia appear to coincide with peak production of pituitary gonadotropins in the fetus. (23)

There is a sex difference in gonadotropin levels. In fetal life there are higher FSH and LH levels in female fetuses. The lower male levels may be due to elevated testosterone levels. In infancy the postnatal FSH rise is more marked and more sustained in females, while LH values are not as high. (22)

The precise signal which initiates the events of puberty is unknown. In girls, the very first steroid to rise in the blood is dehydroepiandrosterone (DHA), beginning at 6 to 8 years of age. (24) This is followed by a rise in androstenedione at 8 to 10 years of age. The estrogens do not begin to rise until 10 to 12 years of age. A positive correlation can be demonstrated between bone age and the rise in the adrenal steroids. (24) If the onset of puberty is triggered by the first hormone to increase in the circulation, then a role for adrenal steroids must be considered. Perhaps DHA in some unknown manner evokes a change in the hypothalamic-pituitary-gonadal feedback system

Puberty is associated with the development of episodic LH secretion associated with sleep. (25) At the time of the appearance of secondary sex characteristics, the mean LH levels are 2 to 4 times higher during sleep than during wakefulness, and the number of LH spurts corresponds to the number of sleep cycles of rapid and non-rapid eye movements (REM and NREM). This pattern is not present before or after puberty, and is an early sign of changes taking place in the hypothalamus. FSH levels plateau by mid-puberty while LH and estradiol levels continue to rise until late puberty.

The trend toward lowering of the menarcheal age and the period for acceleration of growth appears to have halted. In a 10 year prospective study of middle-class contemporary American girls, the mean age of menarche was 12.83 with a range of 9.14 to 17.70. (26) The age of onset of puberty is variable and influenced by genetic factors, socioeconomic conditions, and general health. The earlier menarche in this decade when compared to past decades is probably due to improved nutrition and better health. It has been suggested that initiation of growth and menarche occur at a particular body weight. (27) Although the hypothesis of a critical weight is a helpful concept, the extreme variability in onset of menarche indicates that there is no particular age or size at which an individual girl should be expected to experience menarche. In fact weight appears as a correlate of menarche, not as a determinent. (26).

In the female the typical sequence of events is growth initiation, thelarche, pubarche, and finally menarche. (28) This generally begins sometime between 8 and 14 years of age. The length of time involved in this evolution is usually 2–4 years. During this time-span puberty is said to occur. Individual variation in the order of appearance of this sequence, however, is great. For example, growth of pubic hair and breast development are not always correlated.

If the systems are potentially responsive, what holds function in check until puberty? The hypothalamic-pituitary-gonadal feedback system is operative prior to puberty, but extremely sensitive to steroids and therefore suppressed. (29, 30) The changes at puberty are due to gradually increasing gonadotropin secretion which takes place because of a decrease in the sensitivity of the hypothalamic centers to the negative inhibitory feedback of gonadal steroids. This can be pictured as a slowly rising set point of decreased sensitivity resulting in increasing gonadotropin production leading to increasing ovarian stimulation, and finally increasing estrogen levels. The development of the positive feedback response to estrogens occurs later, thus the well known finding of anovulation in the first months of menstruation. The overall result of this decrease in hypothalamic sensitivity is the development of secondary sex characteristics, attainment of adult set point levels, and the ability to reproduce. Neoplastic and vascular disorders which alter hypothalamic sensitivity probably reverse the prepubertal threshold restraint and lead to precocious puberty.

References

1. **Herbert, DC,** Immunocytochemical Evidence that Luteinizing Hormone (LH) and Follicle Stimulating Hormone (FSH) are Present in the Same Cell in the Rhesus Monkey Pituitary Gland, Endocrinology 98:1554, 1976.

2. **Krey, LC, Butler, WR, and Knobil, E,** Surgical Disconnection of the Medial Basal Hypothalamus and Pituitary Function in the Rhesus Monkey, I. Gonadotropin Secretion, Endocrinology 96:1073, 1975.

3. **Norman, RL, Resko, JA, and Spies, HG,** The Anterior Hypothalamus: How It Affects Gonadotropin Secretion in the Rhesus Monkey, Endocrinology 99:59, 1976.

4. **Karsch, FJ, Dierschke, DJ, and Knobil, E,** Sexual Differentiation of Pituitary Function: Apparent Difference Between Primates and Rodents, Science 179:484, 1973.

5. **Robinson, AG, Ferin, M, and Zimmerman, EA,** Plasma Neurophysin Levels in Monkeys: Emphasis on the Hypothalamic Response to Estrogen and Ovarian Events, Endocrinology 98:468, 1976.

6. **LeBlanc, H, Lachelin, GCL, Abu-Fadil, S, and Yen, SSC,** Effects of Dopamine Infusion on Pituitary Hormone Secretion in Humans, J Clin Endocrinol Metab 43:668, 1976.

7. **Donoso, AO, Bishop, W, Fawcett, CP, Krulich, L, and McCann, SM,** Effects of Drugs that Modify Brain Monoamine Concentrations on Plasma Gonadotropin and Prolactin Levels in the Rat, Endocrinology 89:774, 1971.

8. **Macleod, RM, and Lehmeyer, JE,** Studies on the Mechanism of the Dopamine Mediated Inhibition of Prolactin Secretion, Endocrinology 94:1077, 1974.

9. **Wang, CF, Lasley, BL, Lein, A, and Yen, SSC,** The Functional Changes of the Pituitary Gonadotropins During the Menstrual Cycle, J Clin Endocrinol Metab 42:718, 1976.

10. **Yen, SSC, Vandenberg, G, and Siler, TM,** Modulation of Pituitary Responsiveness to LRF by Estrogen, J Clin Endocrinol Metab 39:170, 1974.

11. **Yamaji, T, Dierschke, DJ, Bhattacharya, AN, and Knobil, E,** The Negative Feedback Control by Estradiol and Progesterone of LH Secretion in the Ovariectomized Rhesus Monkey, Endocrinology 90:771, 1972.

12. **Lasley, BL, Wang, CF, and Yen, SSC,** The Effects of Estrogen and Progesterone on the Functional Capacity of the Gonadotropins, J Clin Endocrinol Metab 41:820, 1975.

13. **Shaw, RW, Butt, WR, and London, DR,** The Effect of Progesterone on FSH and LH Response to LH-RH in Normal Women, Clin Endocrinol 4:543, 1975.

14. **Hagen, C, McNatty, KP, and McNeilly, AS,** Immunoreactive α and β Subunits of Luteinizing Hormone in Human Peripheral Blood and Follicular Fluid Throughout the Menstrual Cycle, and Their Effect on the Secretion Rate of Progesterone by Human Granulosa Cells in Tissue Culture, J Endocrinol 69:33, 1976.

15. **Franchimont, P, Gaspard, U, Reuter, A, and Heynen, G,** Polymorphism of Protein and Polypeptide Hormones, Clin Endocrinol 1:315, 1972.

16. **Prentice, LG, and Ryan, RJ,** LH and Its Subunits in Human Pituitary, Serum, and Urine, J Clin Endocrinol Metab 40:303, 1975.

17. **White, WF, Hedlund, MT, Weber, GF, Rippel, RH, Johnson, ES, and Wilbur, JF,** The Pineal Gland: A Supplemental Source of Hypothalamic-Releasing Hormones, Endocrinology 94:1422, 1974.

18. **Matthews, MJ, and Benson, B,** Inactivation of Pineal Antigonadotropin by Proteolytic Enzymes, J Endocrinol 56:339, 1973.

19. **Pelham, RW, Vaughan, GM, Sandock, KL, and Vaughan, MK,** Twenty-four-hour Cycle of a Melatonin-like Substance in the Plasma of Human Males, J Clin Endocrinol Metab 37:341, 1973.

20. **McClintock, MK,** Menstrual Synchrony and Suppression, Nature 229:244, 1971.

21. **Kaplan, SL, and Grumbach, MM,** The Ontogenesis of Human Fetal Hormones. II. Luterinizing Hormone and Follicle Stimulating Hormone, Acta Endocrinologica 81:808, 1976.

22. **Winter, JSD, Hughes, IA, Reyes, FI, and Faiman, C,** Pituitary-gonadal Relations in Infancy: 2. Patterns of Serum Gonadal Steroid Concentrations in Man From Birth to Two Years of Age, J Clin Endocrinol Metab 42:679, 1976.

23. **Reyes, FI, Boroditsky, RS, Winter, JSD, and Faiman, C,** Studies on Human Sexual Development. II. Fetal and Maternal Serum Gonadotropin and Sex Steroid Concentrations, J Clin Endocrinol Metab 38:612, 1974.

24. **Ducharme, JR, Forest, MG, DePeretti, E, Sempe, M, Collu, R, and Bertrand, J,** Plasma Adrenal and Gonadal Sex Steroids in Human Pubertal Development, J Clin Endocrinol Metab 42:468, 1976.

25. **Boyar, R, Rosenfield, RS, Finkelstein, JW, Kapen, S, Roffwarg, HP, Weitzman, EO, and Hellman, L,** Ontogeny of Luteinizing Hormone and Testosterone Secretion, J Steroid Biochem 6:803, 1975.

26. **Zacharias, L, Rand, WM, and Wurtman, RJ,** A Prospective Study of Sexual Development and Growth in American Girls: The Statistics of Menarche, Obstet Gynec Survey 31:325, 1976.

27. **Frish, RE, and Revelle, R,** Height and Weight at Menarche and a Hypothesis of Critical Body Weights and Adolescent Events, Science 169:397, 1970.

28. **Marshall, WA, and Tanner, JM,** Variations in Pattern of Pubertal Changes in Girls, Arch Dis Child 44:291, 1969.

29. **Kulin, HE, Grumbach, MM, and Kaplan, SL,** Changing Sensitivity of the Pubertal Gonadal Hypothalamic Feedback Mechanism in Man, Science 166:1012, 1969.

30. **Sizonenko, PC, Burr, IM, Kaplan, SL, and Grumbach, MM,** Hormonal Changes in Puberty. II. Correlation of Serum Luteinizing Hormone and Follicle Stimulating Hormone with Stages of Puberty and Bone Age in Normal Girls, Pediatr Res 4:36, 1970.

3 Regulation of the Menstrual Cycle

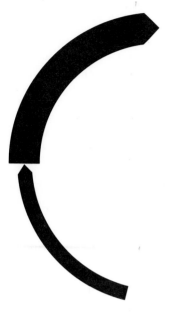
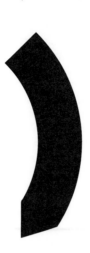

Diagnosis and management of abnormal menstrual function must be based upon an understanding of the physiologic mechanisms involved in the regulation of the normal cycle. Dynamic relationships exist between the pituitary and gonadal hormones which allow for the cyclic nature of normal reproductive processes. These hormonal changes are correlated with morphologic changes in the ovary, making the coordination of this system one of the most remarkable events in biology.

The menstrual cycle can be best described by dividing the cycle into three phases: the follicular phase, ovulation, and the luteal phase. We will examine each of these phases, *concentrating on the changes in ovarian and pituitary hormones, what governs the pattern of hormonal changes, and the effects of these hormones on the ovary, pituitary, and hypothalamus in regulating the menstrual cycle.*

Follicular Phase

During the follicular phase an orderly sequence of events takes place which ensures that the proper number of follicles is ready for ovulation. In the human ovary the end result of this follicular development is (usually) one surviving mature follicle. This process, which occurs over the space of 10–14 days, features a series of sequential actions of hormones on the follicle, leading the follicle destined to ovulate through a period of initial growth, a mid-follicular stage and finally the preovulatory phase.

Initial Follicular Growth (Days −2 to 6)

Follicular growth is a process, best described by Peters (1) as a continuum. Until their numbers are exhausted, follicles begin to grow under practically all physiologic circumstances. Growth is not interrupted by pregnancy, ovulation, or periods of anovulation. Growth continues at all ages, including infancy and around the menopause.

The number of follicles which start growing each cycle is probably dependent upon the size of the residual pool of inactive follicles. (1) Reducing the size of the pool (e.g. unilateral oophorectomy) causes the remaining follicles to redistribute their availability over time. The mechanism for determining which follicles or how many will develop during any one cycle is unknown. It is possible that the follicle which is singled out to play the leading role in a particular cycle is the beneficiary of a timely match of follicle "readiness" and appropriate tropic hormone stimulation. The first follicle able to respond to stimulation may achieve an early lead which it never relinquishes.

The initiation of follicular growth appears to be independent of gonadotropin stimulation. In the vast majority of instances this growth is limited and rapidly followed by atresia. This general pattern is interrupted at the beginning of the menstrual cycle when a group of follicles responds to a hormonal change and is propelled to further growth. The most important hormonal event at this time is a rise in follicle-stimulating hormone (FSH). Indeed follicular growth may have begun in the waning days of the previous luteal phase, when the regressing corpus luteum secretes diminishing amounts of steroids. The decline in luteal phase steroidogenesis allows a rise in the gonadotropins, FSH and luteinizing hormone, (LH).

At the beginning of the cycle FSH, but not LH, is found in the follicular fluid of small follicles. (2) It is useful to consider FSH as the gonadotropin responsible for growth while LH serves to stimulate steroidogenesis. However, such a classification may be an over-simplification. The interrelationships among estradiol, FSH, and LH are such that growth and steroidogenesis depend upon a cooperative effort from all of these hormones.

FSH receptors are probably confined to the granulosa cells. FSH may contribute to steroidogenesis by specifically stimulating the aromatizing system within granulosa cells (3, 4). However, such a direct effect on the steroidogenic capability of the follicle is probably not the major role for FSH. In terms of steroidogenesis, the principal contribution of FSH is to increase the activity or the number of LH receptors.

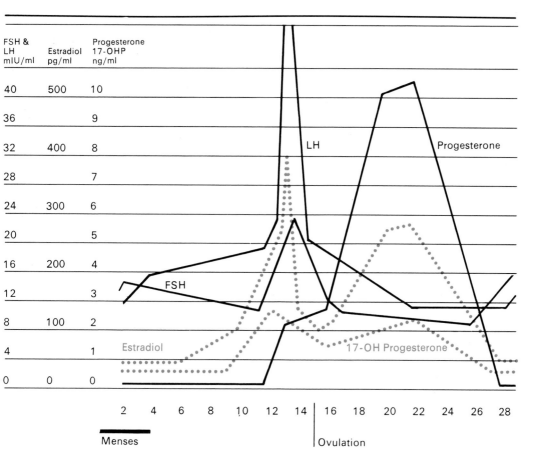

FSH & LH mIU/ml	Estradiol pg/ml	Progesterone 17-OHP ng/ml
40	500	10
36		9
32	400	8
28		7
24	300	6
20		5
16	200	4
12		3
8	100	2
4		1
0	0	0

LH   Progesterone

FSH

Estradiol   17-OH Progesterone

2   4   6   8   10   12   14   16   18   20   22   24   26   28

Menses   Ovulation

During this early period of FSH-stimulated follicular growth there is little, if any, detectable change in the plasma levels of gonadal hormones. A rise in LH also occurs during menses, but no specific function can be assigned to LH at the beginning of the cycle, other than to maintain low levels of steroidogenesis. The period of initial follicular growth ends when a significant increase in plasma estrogen is detectable 7 or 8 days before the preovulatory LH surge.

The Mid-follicular Stage (Days 7 to 10)

Continued follicular growth is dependent upon gonadotropins and is correlated with increasing production of estradiol. As the follicle matures the number of gonadotropin receptors increases. This continued growth is not an expression of an increased affinity for the gonadotropins, but an increased ability to respond because of an increase in receptors. (5) The stimulus for the increased number of receptors for FSH appears to be FSH, itself, in an action enhanced by estradiol.

The early production of estradiol is necessary to ensure a continued response to FSH. Estradiol itself may stimulate granulosa cell proliferation, probably by increasing the ovarian uptake of FSH. It is likely that this interaction of estradiol and FSH is tightly and mutually interdependent. Estradiol increases the number of FSH receptors, and FSH may allow a greater estradiol response by indirectly increasing steroidogenesis through the induction of LH receptors. (7, 8) This action of FSH is enhanced by estradiol, but estradiol alone does not increase LH receptors. (9) Thus estradiol and FSH act synergistically to prepare follicles to respond to LH, both in terms of ovulation and luteinization.

The sequence of events is as follows:

1. Initial follicular growth.

2. FSH stimulation into the mid-follicular stage.

3. Estradiol production, increasing the sensitivity to FSH by enhancing FSH action.

4. FSH induction of LH receptors (enhanced by estradiol).

5. Theca cell differentiation with even greater estradiol production.

The Feedback Systems. The interaction between estrogen and FSH and between estrogen and LH is complex, and is best understood by attention to the following theoretical model. As one increases estradiol in a hypergonadotropic state (postmenopause), the effect of graded increments of estradiol is first seen as suppression of LH, followed at higher levels of estradiol by a suppression of FSH. At still higher doses of estradiol, FSH remains low, but LH secretion is now stimulated. The changes in hormonal levels are regulated, therefore, by feedback mechanisms. In the case of FSH, there is a negative inhibitory feedback relationship with estradiol (the most potent and effective estrogen in the human), while in the case of LH there is a negative inhibitory feedback at low levels of estradiol and a positive stimulatory feedback at high levels of estradiol. Thus, in the early part of the cycle as estrogens rise, one would expect a decrease in FSH due to a negative feedback effect. A concomitant decrease in LH does not occur since the positive hypothalamic center is responding to the rising levels of estrogen and overriding the negative feedback center. The negative feedback of estrogens upon LH secretion therefore operates at a very low level and is probably maximal throughout the cycle. Accordingly, fluctuations in LH reflect the positive feedback of estradiol during the follicular and ovulatory phases, and during the luteal phase LH secretion is suppressed by the negative feedback of progesterone. In contrast FSH levels are regulated throughout the cycle by the negative feedback of estrogen.

The positive feedback system is activated by an increase in circulating estradiol. There are two critical features in this mechanism: (1) the concentration of estradiol and (2) the length of time during which the estradiol elevation is sustained. In women the estradiol concentration necessary to achieve a positive feedback is over 200 pg/ml, and this concentration must be sustained for approximately 50 hours. (10) In contrast a change in circulating estradiol (in the Rhesus monkey) of only 20 pg/ml will activate the negative feedback system within minutes. (11)

The negative feedback system may consist of two components: (1) a major system within the hypothalamus involving the tonic center, and (2) a modulating system governing the response of the pituitary to GnRH. A rapid increase in circulating estradiol results in a direct inhibitory effect of the pituitary response to GnRH. (12) In the monkey, physiologic doses of estradiol which depressed circulating levels of LH did not decrease levels of GnRH in blood collected from the pituitary stalk. (13) The increasing concentration of estradiol at midcycle augments the pituitary response to GnRH in women (14), while, as noted, acute increases in estradiol inhibit the response to GnRH. Thus the nature of the steroid present in the circulation (estradiol, progesterone, androgens), the steroid concentration, and the time course all influence behavior of the hypothalamic-pituitary system.

The short feedback system refers to a negative (inhibiting) effect of the gonadotropins on GnRH. This mechanism may involve activation (by FSH and LH) of hypothalamic enzymes which degrade GnRH. (15)

The Preovulatory Phase (Days 10 to 14)

During the late follicular phase, estrogens rise slowly at first, then rapidly, reaching a peak just before ovulation. Concomitant with the rise in estrogens there is a decline in FSH. In contrast, LH increases steadily, and then rapidly in a surge-like burst at midcycle. The rapid growth of the follicle late in the follicular phase when FSH levels are actually decreasing indicates that as the follicle matures it becomes increasingly sensitive to FSH. The follicle destined to ovulate protects itself from premature atresia by its own hormone production. High local estradiol concentration increases follicular sensitivity to FSH by promoting follicular binding of FSH. The concentration of FSH remains high in those follicles in which the concentration of estradiol exceeds 1 μg/ml. (2) The decrease in the circulating level of FSH (brought about by the negative feedback effect of the rising estradiol) would then be significant in terms of a loss of growth stimulation to the smaller less differentiated follicles which are producing less estrogen. A wave of atresia is therefore seen to parallel the rise in estrogen.

LH is not detectable in follicular fluid until luteinization of the granulosa cells begins about 24–36 hours before the LH peak. (2) This occurs in response to an increase in LH receptors (induced by FSH and enhanced by estradiol) and the rising levels of LH (stimulated by the positive feedback effects of the rising estradiol). As a result there is a high concentration of progesterone in the preovulatory follicles.

Atresia and Androgens. During follicular growth, the surrounding stromal cells are organized into a theca layer. LH binds to theca cells and promotes steroidogenesis. These cells become the principle source for estradiol until ovulation.

Most of the estradiol at midcycle is produced by the follicle destined to ovulate. When the remaining follicles fail to achieve full maturity, atresia occurs, marked by a loss of receptors for estradiol, FSH, and LH. During and after the process of atresia, the thecal cells return to their origin as a component of stromal tissue, retaining, however, an ability to respond to LH with steroid production.

It should be emphasized that stromal tissue is not truly atretic in that steroid production continues to be significant. Rather than estrogen, however, the principal stromal products are androgens, especially androstenedione and testosterone. The increase in stromal tissue in the late follicular phase is associated with a rise in androgen levels in the peripheral plasma at midcycle, a 15% increase in androstenedione and a 20% increase in testosterone. (16, 17)

Androgen production at this stage in the cycle may serve two purposes: (1) a local role within the ovary to enhance the process of atresia, and (2) a systemic effect to stimulate libido.

Intraovarian androgens accelerate granulosa cell death and follicular atresia. (18, 19) The mechanism for this action may be suppression of granulosa cell receptors for estradiol. Therefore androgens may play a regulatory role in ensuring that the proper number of follicles reaches the point of ovulation.

It is well known that libido can be stimulated by androgens. If the midcycle rise in androgens affects libido, then an increase in sexual activity should coincide with this rise. Previous studies failed to demonstrate a consistent pattern in coital frequency in women because of the effect of male partner initiation. If only sexual behavior initiated by women is studied, a peak in female-initiated sexual activity is seen during the ovulatory phase of the cycle, and no such peak is noted in users of birth control pills. (20) A hormone effect is indicated by the loss of the midcycle peak in pill users. Therefore the midcycle raise in androgens may serve to increase sexual activity at the time most likely to achieve pregnancy.

Occasionally nonendocrine tumors of the ovary (such as Brenner, Krukenberg, cystadenoma), derived from germinal epithelial cells, will be associated with stromal hyperplasia. Extraglandular conversion of the androgen secreted by the hyperplastic stroma may result in estrogenic manifestations such as endometrial hyperplasia; androgenic signs and symptoms may prevail if androstenedione and testosterone production are very high. (21)

Ovulation

The available information strongly supports the theory that the rise in estradiol during the late follicular phase is the trigger that sets off the gonadotropin surge. Administration of estrogen to humans and monkeys has demonstrated stimulation of gondadotropin release. This positive feedback stimulatory effect of estrogen requires a "female" hypothalamus, centers in the hypothalamus which respond to rapidly increasing levels of estradiol with an outpouring of GnRH. The presence of abnormal levels of androgens may prevent this response by suppressing function of the cyclic center.

As noted, there are two critical requirements for stimulation of the midcycle gonadotropin surge: a minimal concentration of estradiol (over 200 pg/ml) and exposure of the cyclic center to estradiol for a critical time period (approximately 50 hours). Careful analysis of the time relationships between estradiol and LH in the monkey indicates that the LH surge is initiated prior to withdrawal of estrogen. Thus the gonadotropin surge is not a response to removal from negative feedback inhibition.

The simultaneous modest rise in FSH at midcycle probably represents a response to the common releasing factor, GnRH. The functional importance of the midcycle increase in FSH has only been recently appreciated. The ability of LH to bring about the process of ovulation and luteinization is dependent upon the presence of LH receptors. Because FSH induces the appearance of LH receptors (8), the midcycle rise in FSH may be necessary to produce a normal corpus luteum. Indeed, a short luteal phase in women has been associated with lower midcycle levels of FSH. (22)

A full gonadotropin surge involves not only an adequate response in the hypothalamus, but also the proper pituitary response to GnRH. At midcycle there is a maximal sensitivity to GnRH, involving both FSH and LH release. (12) This response is largely influenced by the high levels of estradiol, but the slightly elevated concentrations of progesterone also play a role.

Progesterone under certain conditions will stimulate gonadotropin release, e.g. in estrogen-suppressed postmenopausal women or in anovulatory women. But a careful analysis of the sequence of events during the human menstrual cycle indicates that the levels of progesterone do not rise prior to the gonadotropin surge (as do the levels of estradiol). However there is a small increase in progesterone levels during the ovulatory period, probably a consequence of LH and luteinization. It is likely that the small rise in progesterone during this period has a central facilitative feedback to enhance gonadotropin secretion. This effect may center on the pituitary response to GnRH. (23) However with increasing levels of progesterone, the effect on LH secretion becomes inhibitory. This inhibitory effect requires the presence of estrogen, and while there may be an action at both hypothalamic and pituitary levels, the major inhibition is probably in the hypothalamus.

The ovulatory period is also associated with a rise in plasma levels of 17α-hydroxyprogesterone. This steroid does not appear to have a role in cyclic regulation, and its appearance in the blood may simply represent the secretion of an intermediate product.

The high levels of gonadotropins persist for approximately 24 hours, then decrease during the luteal phase to nadir values. The secretion of gonadotropins is not smooth, but oscillatory with a regular episodic release by the pituitary, which is most pronounced with LH. Collection of pituitary stalk blood in monkeys reveals that GnRH release into the portal system is pulsatile in nature (13) indicating that the episodic pituitary secretion is in response to a similar pattern in GnRH secretion. The purpose of this pulse-like function is not clear. The rapid changes may play a role in transmission of stimulatory and inhibitory feedback messages.

The mechanism that shuts off the LH surge is unknown. Within hours after the rise in LH, there is a precipitous drop in the plasma estrogens. The drop in LH may be due to a loss of the positive stimulating action of estradiol. This decrease in estrogen is probably secondary to luteinization of the follicle. This morphologic change is associated with a shift from estrogen-secreting thecal dominance to progesterone-secreting granulosa cell dominance. The abrupt fall in LH levels may also reflect a depletion in pituitary LH content. Finally, LH may further be controlled by "short" negative feedback of LH upon the hypothalamus. Direct LH suppression of hypothalamic releasing hormone production has been demonstrated.

An adequate gonadotropin surge does not ensure ovulation. The follicle must be at the appropriate stage of maturity in order for it to respond to the ovulating stimulus. In the normal cycle gonadotropin release and final maturation of the follicle coincide because the timing of the gonadotropin surge is controlled by the level of estradiol, which in turn is a function of follicular growth and maturation. Therefore gonadotropin release and morphologic maturity are usually coordinated and coupled in time.

Rupture of the follicle occurs within the 24 hour period after the LH peak. (24) In the majority of human cycles, the requisite feedback relationships in this system allow only one follicle to reach the point of ovulation. Multiple births may in part reflect the random statistical chance of more than one follicle fulfilling all the requirements for ovulation.

The mechanism which results in the rapid dissolution of the ovum's physical confinement remains unknown. An increase in intrafollicular pressure is not responsible for the release of the ovum. Rather the escape of the ovum is associated with degenerative changes of the collagen in the follicular wall so that just prior to ovulation the follicular wall becomes thin due to passive stretching. (25) The augmented blood flow which accompanies vascularization of the granulosa layer in response to LH leads to an increase in clearance of blood constituents through the capillary walls with passage into the antrum. Ovulation occurs with no change in pressure because elasticity reaches a minimal value. With the increase in antral volume, the follicular wall ruptures. These events are in some way related to the surge-like rise in the secretion of LH.

The actual physical expulsion of the oocyte is related to an LH-induced acute rise in the prostaglandin content within the follicle. (26) Inhibition of this rise in prostaglandins in a variety of animals results in corpus luteum formation with an entrapped oocyte.

Luteal Phase

After rupture of the follicle and release of the ovum, the granulosa cells increase in size, soon assuming a characteristic vacuolated appearance associated with the accumulation of a yellow pigment, lutein, which lends its name to the process of luteinization and the new anatomical subunit, the corpus luteum. During the first 3 days after ovulation, the granulosa cells enlarge. Capillaries penetrate into the granulosa layer, reaching the central cavity and often filling it with blood. By day 8 or 9 after ovulation, a peak of vascularization is reached, associated with peak levels of progesterone and estradiol in the blood. The primate corpus luteum is unique in that it synthesizes all 3 classes of sex steroids: androgens, estrogens, and progestins. A plasma level of progesterone over 3 ng/ml is reliable evidence of ovulation. (27)

57

Beginning about 10–12 days after ovulation, the corpus luteum enters into a stage of regression first noted by a gradual decrease of blood in the capillaries, followed by decreasing progesterone secretion. During this period of time, large follicles are seen once again within the ovary. (2) These follicles probably appear in response to a growth stimulus due to the midcycle surge in FSH. Continued growth is impossible however due to the diminished levels of FSH during this phase. Indeed the large follicles present in the luteal phase do not appear to be functional as estrogen levels and mitotic activity are low. (2)

In the normal cycle the time period from the LH midcycle surge to menses is consistently close to 14 days. It is well-known that the variability in cycle length among women is due to the varying number of days required for follicular growth and maturation in the follicular phase.

It had been thought that the lifespan of the corpus luteum in the human was independent of the secretion of gonadotropins, and that once formed, the corpus luteum functioned autonomously. LH and FSH fall to their lowest levels when progesterone and estradiol secretion are maximal in the luteal phase, probably due to the negative feedback effects of these steroids. Studies in hypophysectomized women, however, have clearly demonstrated that normal corpus luteum function requires the continuous presence of small amounts of LH. (28) This reaffirms the principle that ovarian steroidogenesis is impossible without LH. There is no evidence that other luteotropic hormones, such as prolactin, play a role in the human menstrual cycle.

The corpus luteum rapidly declines 9–11 days after ovulation, and the mechanism of this degeneration remains unknown. In certain nonprimate mammalian species, a luteolytic factor originating in the uterus (probably prostaglandin $F_{2\alpha}$) regulates the lifespan of the corpus luteum. No definite luteolytic factor has been identified in the primate menstrual cycle; however the morphologic regression of luteal cells may be induced by the estradiol produced by the corpus luteum. The concentration of estradiol within the monkey corpus luteum increases late in the luteal phase when progesterone is decreasing. (29) During this time period the corpus luteum becomes increasingly sensitive to the luteolytic effect of administered estrogen. The mechanism of this estrogen effect may involve prostaglandins. (30)

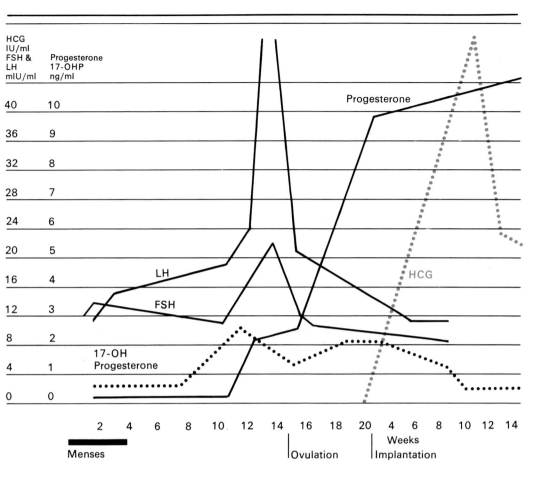

HCG IU/ml FSH & LH mlU/ml	Progesterone 17-OHP ng/ml		
40	10		
36	9		
32	8		
28	7		
24	6		
20	5		
16	4		
12	3		
8	2		
4	1		
0	0		

Progesterone

LH

FSH

HCG

17-OH Progesterone

2   4   6   8   10   12   14   16   18   20   4   6   8   10   12   14

Menses

Ovulation

Weeks
Implantation

Degeneration of the corpus luteum is inevitable unless pregnancy intervenes. With pregnancy, survival of the corpus luteum is prolonged by the emergence of a new stimulus of rapidly increasing intensity, human chorionic gonadotropin (HCG). This new stimulus first appears at the peak of corpus luteum development (9 to 13 days after ovulation), just in time to prevent luteal regression. (31) HCG serves to maintain the vital steroidogenesis of the corpus luteum until approximately the 9th or 10th week of gestation, by which time placental steroidogenesis is well-established. In some pregnancies placental steroidogenesis will be sufficiently established as early as the 6th or 7th week of gestation.

The short or inadequate luteal phase has received considerable attention as a possible cause of infertility. The short luteal phase is characterized by a low secretion of progesterone, early regression and demise of the corpus luteum, with menses occurring 6 to 9 days after the LH peak. Subnormal levels of estradiol during the follicular phase and a lower midcycle surge of FSH indicate that the etiology of this condition is inadequate stimulation and response prior to ovulation. (22) An inadequate luteal phase may also be due to elevated prolactin levels, a specific situation associated with infertility which may be effectively treated with ergot derivatives (see Chapter 9).

The luteal phase is associated with increased circulating levels of aldosterone, a direct effect of the sex steroids. Progesterone interferes with aldosterone action at the renal tubule, leading to a secondary rise in aldosterone secretion. Estradiol stimulates an increase in liver synthesis of angiotensinogen, leading to an elevation in the renin-angiotensin-aldosterone system. Even higher levels of aldosterone during the luteal phase have been noted in women with cyclic edema. (32)

Key Events in Human Menstrual Cycle

The human menstrual cycle is a recycling system dependent upon essential changes in estradiol levels at key moments in time. Estradiol plays a principal role in the following events:

1. The beginning of the cycle is initiated by a rise in FSH which occurs in response to the decline in estradiol in the preceding luteal phase.

2. Estradiol maintains follicular sensitivity to FSH by inducing FSH receptors.

3. Estradiol enhances follicular response to LH by working synergistically with FSH to induce LH receptors.

4. Ovulation is triggered by the rapid rise in estradiol at midcycle.

5. Regression of the corpus luteum may depend upon its own estradiol production and a local luteolytic effect.

The coordination of this complex system can be understood therefore, by an appreciation for the essential role of estrogen. The interplay between the follicle and the hypothalamus depends upon estradiol functioning as a classic hormone, i.e. to transmit the messages of negative and positive feedback, and also upon the local effect of estradiol within the follicle to insure gonadotropin sensitivity. Events which prevent estrogen production or obtund the necessary fluctuations in circulating levels will interfere with the normal reproductive cycle.

References

1. **Peters, H, Byskov, AG, Himelstein-Graw, R, and Faber, M,** Follicular Growth: The Basic Event in the Mouse and Human Ovary, J Reprod Fertil 45:559, 1975.

2. **McNatty, KP, Hunter, WM, McNeilly, AS, and Sawers, RS,** Changes in the Concentration of Pituitary and Steroid Hormones in the Follicular Fluid of Human Graafian Follicles Throughout the Menstrual Cycle, J Endocrinol 64:555, 1975.

3. **Moon, YS, Dorrington, JH, and Armstrong, DT,** Stimulatory Action of Follicle-stimulating Hormone on Estradiol-17β Secretion by Hypophysectomized Rat Ovaries in Organ Culture, Endocrinology 97:244, 1975.

4. **Erickson, GF, and Ryan, KJ,** The Effect of LH/FSH, Dibutyryl Cyclic AMP, and Prostaglandins on the Production of Estrogens by Rabbit Granulosa Cells in Vitro, Endocrinology 97:108, 1975.

5. **Kammerman, S, and Ross, J,** Increase in Numbers of Gonadotropin Receptors on Granulosa Cells During Follicle Maturation, J Clin Endocrinol Metab 41:546, 1975.

6. **Goldenberg, RL, Vaitukaitis, JL, and Ross, GT,** Estrogen and Follicle-stimulating Hormone Interactions on Follicle Growth in Rats, Endocrinology 90:1492, 1972.

7. **Goldenberg, RL, Reiter, EO, Vaitukaitis, JL, and Ross, GT,** Hormone Factors Influencing Ovarian Uptake of Human Chorionic Gonadotropin, Endocrinology 92:1565, 1973.

8. **Zeleznik, AJ, Midgley, AR, Jr., and Reichert, LE, Jr.,** Granulosa Cell Maturation in the Rat: Increased Binding of Human Chorionic Gonadotropin Following Treatment with Follicle-stimulating Hormone in vivo, Endocrinology 95:818, 1974.

9. **Richards, JS, and Midgley, AR, Jr.,** Protein Hormone Action: A Key to Understanding Ovarian Follicular and Luteal Cell Development, Biol Reprod 14:82, 1976.

10. **Young, JR, and Jaffe, RB,** Strength-duration Characteristics of Estrogen Effect On Gonadotropin Response to Gonadotropin-releasing Hormone in Women. II. Effects of Varying Concentrations of Estradiol, J Clin Endocrinol Metab 42:432, 1976.

11. **Karsch, FJ, Weick, RF, Butler, WR, Dierschke, DJ, Krey, LC, Weiss, G, Hotchkiss, J, Yamaji, T, and Knobil, E,** Induced LH Surges in the Rhesus Monkey: Strength-duration Characteristics of the Estrogen Stimulus, Endocrinology 92:1740, 1973.

12. **Yen, SSC, Vandenberg, G, and Siler, TM,** Modulation of Pituitary Responsiveness to LRF by Estrogen, J Clin Endocrinol Metab 39:170, 1974.

13. **Carmel, PN, Araki, S, and Ferin, M,** Pituitary Stalk Portal Blood Collection in Rhesus Monkeys: Evidence for Pulsatile Release of Gonadotropin-releasing Hormone (GnRH), Endocrinology 99:243, 1976.

14. **Jaffe, RB, and Keye, WR, Jr.,** Estradiol Augmentation of Pituitary Responsiveness to Gonadotropin-releasing Hormone in Women, J Clin Endocrinol Metab 39:850, 1974.

15. **Kuhl, H, and Taubert, HD,** Short-loop Feedback Mechanism of Luteinizing Hormone: LH Stimulates Hypothalamic L-cystine Arylamidase to Inactivate LH-RH in the Rat Hypothalamus, Acta Endocrinologica 78:649, 1975.

16. **Judd, HL, and Yen, SSC,** Serum Androstenedione and Testosterone Levels during the Menstrual Cycle, J Clin Endocrinol Metab 38:475, 1973.

17. **Abraham, GE,** Ovarian and Adrenal Contribution to Peripheral Androgens During the Menstrual Cycle, J Clin Endocrinol Metab 39:340, 1974.

18. **Schreiber, JR, and Ross, GT,** Further Characterization of a Rat Ovarian Testosterone Receptor with Evidence for Nuclear Translocation, Endocrinology 99:590, 1976.

19. **Febres, F, Gondos, B, and Siiteri, P,** Androgen-induced Ovarian Follicular Atresia in the Rat, Gynec Invest 7:52, 1976.

20. **Adams, DB, Gold, AR, and Burt, AB,** Rise in Female Initiated Sexual Activity at Ovulation and its Suppression by Oral Contraceptives, Personal Communication.

21. **MacDonald, PC, Grodin, JM, Edman, CD, Vellios, F, and Siiteri, PK,** Origin of Estrogen in a Postmenopausal Woman with a Nonendocrine Tumor of the Ovary and Endometrial Hyperplasia, Obstet and Gynec, 47:644, 1976.

22. **Sherman, BM, and Korenman, SG,** Measurement of Plasma LH, FSH, Estradiol and Progesterone in Disorders of the Human Menstrual Cycle: The Short Luteal Phase, J Clin Endocrinol Metab 38:89, 1974.

23. **Shaw, RW, Butt, WR, and London, DR,** The Effect of Progesterone on FSH and LH Response to LH-RH in Normal Women, Clin Endocrinol 4:543, 1975.

24. **Pauerstein, CJ, Eddy, CA, Croxatto, HD, Hess, R, and Croxatto, HB,** Temporal Relationships of Estrogen, Progesterone, and Luteinizing Hormone Levels to Ovulation in Women and Infrahuman Primates, Am J Obstet Gynec, in press.

25. **Lipner, H,** Mechanism of Mammalian Ovulation, in Greep, RO and Astwood, EB, eds., *Handbook of Physiology, Section 7, Endocrinology Vol II. Female Reproductive System, Part 1*, American Physiological Society, Washington DC, 1973 pp 409–438.

26. **Lemaire, WJ, Yang, NST, Behrman, HR, and Marsh, JM,** Preovulatory Changes in the Concentration of PGS in Rabbit Graafian Follicles, Prostaglandins 3:367, 1973.

27. **Israel, R, Mishell, DR, Jr., Stone, SC, Thorneycroft, IH, and Meyer, DL,** Single Luteal Phase Serum Progesterone Assay as an Indicator of Ovulation, Am J Obstet Gynec 112:1043, 1972.

28. **Vande Wiele, RL, Bogumil, J, Dyrenfurth, I, Ferin, M, Jewelewicz, R, Warren, M, Rizkallah, R, and Mikhail, G,** Mechanisms Regulating the Menstrual Cycle in Women, Rec Prog Hor Res 26:63, 1970.

29. **Karsch, FJ, and Sutton, GP,** An Intra-ovarian Site for the Luteolytic Action of Estrogen in the Rhesus Monkey, Endocrinology 98:553, 1976.

30. **Auletta, FJ, Caldwell, BV, and Speroff, L,** Estrogen-induced Luteolysis in the Rhesus Monkey: Reversal with Indomethacin, Prostaglandins 11:745, 1976.

31. **Catt, KJ, Dufau, ML, and Vaitukaitis, JL,** Appearance of HCG in Pregnancy Plasma Following the Initiation of Implantation of the Blastocyst, J Clin Endocrinol Metab 40:537, 1975.

32. **Schwartz, UD, and Abraham, GE,** Corticosterone and Aldosterone Levels During the Menstrual Cycle, Obstet Gynec 45:339, 1975.

4

The Ovary from Conception to Senescence

The physiologic responsibilities of the ovary are the periodic release of gametes (eggs) (oocytes) and the production of the steroid hormones, estradiol and progesterone. Both activities are integrated in the continuous repetitive process of follicle maturation, ovulation, and corpus luteum formation and regression. The ovary, therefore, cannot be viewed as a relatively static endocrine organ whose size and function expand and contract depending on the vigor of stimulating tropic hormones. Rather, the female gonad is an envelope containing subunits (follicle, corpus luteum, stroma) with different and variable biologic properties, a heterogeneous everchanging tissue whose cyclicity is measured in weeks, rather than hours. As a result the activity of the human ovary at any given time is defined by a single subunit during the brief period of its dominance.

In this chapter, the development and differentiation of the ovary will be described with emphasis on that most critical functioning subunit of the gonad, the follicle. Events within the ovary will be traced from early embryonic formation to final senescent atrophy. Correlations of morphology with reproductive and steroidogenic functions will be emphasized. Finally, the menopause and the rationale for therapy of this physiologic state will be re-examined in the light of information on endogenous estrogen production and the impact of estrogen on nonreproductive functions of the female.

Embryology and Differentiation of the Ovary

During fetal life, the development of the human ovary can be traced through four stages. These include: (1) the indifferent gonadal stage; (2) the differentiation and cortical supremacy state; (3) the period of oogonal multiplication; and finally (4) the stage of follicle formation.

Indifferent Gonadal State

At approximately 5 weeks of intrauterine life, the paired gonads are structurally consolidated prominences overlying the mesonephros, forming the gonadal ridge. At this point, although sexual characterization of this tissue is possible by nuclear sex chromatin studies, the gonad is morphologically indistinguishable as a primordial testis or ovary. The gonad is composed of primitive germ cells intermingled with coelomic surface epithelial cells and an inner core of medullary mesenchymal tissue. Just below this ridge lies the mesonephric duct. The germ cells originate in the primitive endoderm of the yolk sac and hindgut, and are recognizable at this site before the mesonephros is formed. They migrate to the gonadal ridge, the one and only site where they survive, in a journey which is completed by the 5th week. The germ cells are the direct precursors of sperm and ova, and by the 6th week, on completion of the indifferent stage, these germ cells have multiplied by mitosis to a total of 100,000.

Differentiation and Cortical Supremacy Stage

If the indifferent gonad is destined to become a testis, differentiation along this line will take place at 4–6 weeks. The absence of testicular evolution (formation of medullary primary sex cords, primitive tubules, and incorporation of germ cells) gives implicit evidence of the existence of a primitive, albeit momentarily quiescent, ovary. Despite inactivity, the cortical dominance over the medulla has been asserted. These events are related to the genetic constitution of the germ cells and the territorial receptivity of the mesenchyme. If either factor is deficient or defective, improper development occurs. As has been noted, primitive germ cells appear unable to survive in locations other than the gonadal ridge. If partial or imperfect gonadal tissue is formed, the resulting abnormal nonsteroidal and steroidal events have wide ranging morphologic, reproductive, and behavioral effects. In this indifferent stage, therefore, the Müllerian duct system is preserved and the Wolffian potential is unrealized.

Stage of Oogonal Multiplication and Maturation

At 6–8 weeks, the first signs of ovarian differentiation are expressed by the onset of rapid mitotic multiplication of oogonal endowment reaching 6–7 million germ cells by 20 weeks. This represents the maximum oogonal content of the gonad. From this point in time germ cell content will irretrievably decrease until, some 50 years later, the store of germ cells will be finally exhausted. The egg depletion process by atresia begins at about 15 weeks gestation when evidence of nuclear maturation is first seen. The oogonia are transformed to oocytes as they enter the first meiotic division and arrest in prophase.

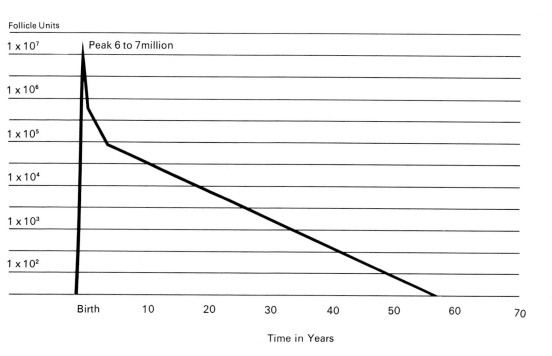

Follicle Units

1 x 10⁷   Peak 6 to 7 million

1 x 10⁶

1 x 10⁵

1 x 10⁴

1 x 10³

1 x 10²

Birth   10   20   30   40   50   60   70

Time in Years

Stage of
Follicle
Formation

When nuclear maturation within germ cells becomes noticeable, the gonad is composed of an expanded dense sheet of oogonia and oocytes in huge numbers. At 20 weeks, this highly cellular cortex is gradually perforated by vascular channels originating in the deeper medullary areas. As the finger-like vascular projections enter the cortex, the cortex takes on the appearance of secondary sex cords. As the blood vessels invade and penetrate, they divide the previously solid cortical cell mass into smaller and smaller segments. Drawn in with the blood vessels are perivascular cells which are both mesenchymal and epithelial in origin. These cells surround the oocyte in layers. The resulting unit is the primordial follicle – an oocyte arrested in prophase of meiosis enveloped by a single layer of pregranulosa (primitive epithelial) and an outer less organized matrix of mesenchymal cells, (the pretheca cells). Eventually all oocytes are covered in this fashion. Residual mesenchyme not utilized in primordial follicle formation is noted in the interstices between follicles, forming the primitive ovarian stroma.

As soon as the oocyte is surrounded by the rosette of pregranulosa cells it may resume meiosis and the entire follicle undergoes variable degrees of maturation before arresting and becoming atretic. These events include in sequence: oocyte cytoplasmic enlargement, eccentric migration of the nucleus, and proliferation of several layers of granulosa cells by mitosis. As a result a primary follicle is formed. Less frequently, but by no means rarely, further differentiation is expressed as more complete granulosa proliferation, Call-Exner body formation, coalescence to form the antrum, and occasionally a minor thecal layer system may be seen.

Even in fetal life, the cycle of follicle formation, variable ripening, and atresia occurs. Although these steps are precisely those typical of adult reproductive life, full maturity, as expressed in ovulation, does not occur. However, the ovary at birth may contain several cystic follicles of varying size.

The initiation of follicle maturation and atresia has a profound effect on germ cell endowment. As a result of prenatal follicle differentiation, the total cortical content of germ cells has fallen to 1–2 million by birth. This huge depletion of germ call mass (close to 4–5 million) has occurred over as short a time as 20 weeks. No similar rate of depletion will be seen again. Studies with the scanning electron microscope have indicated that the major mechanism for the loss of eggs during intra-uterine life is elimination through the surface of the ovary into the peritoneal cavity. (1) Clusters of oogonias and oocytes make their way through the ovarian stroma and can be seen emerging from the ovarian surface. Due to the fixed initial endowment of germ cells the newborn female enters life, still far from reproductive potential, having lost 80 percent of her oocytes.

Neonatal Ovary

At birth, the ovary is approximately 1 cm in diameter, although sizable cystic follicles may exist and enlarge the total dimensions. Compartmentalization of the gonad into cortex and a small residual medulla has been achieved. In the cortex almost all the oocytes are involved in primordial follicle units. Varying degrees of maturation in some units can be seen as in the prenatal state.

Adult Ovary

At the onset of puberty, the germ cell mass has been reduced to 300,000 units. During the next 35–40 years of reproductive life, these units will be depleted further to a point at menopause where only a few thousand units remain. In this period of time the typical cycle of follicle maturation, including ovulation and corpus luteum formation will be realized. This results from the complex but well-defined sequence of hypothalamic-pituitary-gonadal interactions in which follicle and corpus luteum steroid and pituitary gonadotropin production are integrated to yield ovulation. These important events are described in detail in Chapter 3. For the moment, our attention will be exclusively directed to a description of the events as the gonad is driven inexorably to final and complete exhaustion of its germ cell supply. The major feature of this reproductive period of the adult ovary's existence is the full maturational expression of some follicle units in ovulation and corpus luteum formation, and the accompaniment of varying steroidal output of estradiol and progesterone. For every follicle which ovulates, close to 1000 will pursue abortive growth periods of variable length.

Follicle
Growth

In the adult ovary, the two stages of follicle development noted even in the prenatal period are repeated, but to a more complete degree. Initially the oocyte enlarges and the granulosa cells markedly proliferate. A solid sphere of cells encasing the oocyte is formed. At this point the theca interna is noted in initial stages of formation. The zona pellucida begins to form. In this stage of development gonadotropins must be available, but these events are not the result of an input of gonadotropin (follicle-stimulating hormone (FSH)) activity. Meiosis I, which has been suspended since formation of the follicle, is resumed. If gonadotropin increments are available, as may be seen early in the cycle, a second, gonadotropin-dependent stage of follicle maturation is seen. The numbers of follicles maturing in any one cycle and the degree of morphologic and biochemical maturity achieved by these follicles (as expressed in estrogen secretion) are dependent on the amount of FSH and luteinizing hormone (LH) available to the gonad and the sensitivity of the follicles to gonadotropins.

The sequence of maturation in this second phase of follicle growth proceeds in the following order. The antrum appears as a coalescence of numerous intragranulosa cavities (Call-Exner bodies). Whether this represents liquefaction or granulosa cell secretion is uncertain. At first the cavity is filled with a coagulum of cellular debris. Soon a liquor accumulates, which is essentially a transudation of blood filtered through the avascular granulosa from the thecal vessels. With antral formation, the theca interna develops more fully, expressed by increased cell mass, increased vascularity, and the formation of lipid rich cytoplasmic vacuoles within the theca cells. As the follicle expands, the surrounding stroma is compressed and is called the theca externa.

At any point in this development individual follicles become arrested and eventually regress in the process known as atresia. At first the granulosa component begins to disrupt. The antral cavity constituents are resorbed, and the cavity collapses and obliterates. The oocyte degenerates *in situ*. Finally, a ribbon-like scarred streak surrounded by theca is seen. Eventually this theca mass loses its lipid and becomes indistinguishable from the growing mass of stroma. Prior to regression, the cystic follicle may be retained in the cortex for variable periods of time.

The ovary has the capability of making steroids via two major pathways: the Δ^5-3β-hydroxy pathway through DHA and the Δ^4-3-ketone pathway through progesterone. Clearly one pathway (Δ^5-3β-hydroxy) avoids preliminary synthesis of progesterone as a precursor to estradiol, while in the other (Δ^4-3-ketone) progesterone is a required essential precursor. From *in vitro* experiments it seems likely that the theca interna makes estrogen via the pregnenolone, DHA, estradiol pathway, whereas the granulosa makes estrogen via the formation of progesterone. In yet another example of integration of anatomy and biochemistry, it is apparent that the tissue (theca) which is vascularized and making lipid precursor is the main steroid producer of the follicle, making estrogen but not progesterone. On the other hand, the corpus luteum, in which the granulosa now has the vascularization and lipid to express its steroidogenic potential, makes estrogen via the progesterone pathway.

Ovulation

Of the several follicle units thrust to varying degrees of maturity, one unit will advance to ovulation if gonadotropin stimulation is adequate. Morphologically these events include distension of the antrum by increments of antral fluid, and compression of the granulosa against the limiting membrane separating the avascular granulosa and the luteinized and vascularized theca interna. In addition, the antral fluid increment gradually pinches off the tongue of granulosa enveloping the oocyte as the cumulus oophorus. The events associated with the thinning of the theca over the surface of the now protruding distended follicle, the creation of an avascular area weakening the ovarian capsule, and the final acute distension of the antrum with rupture and extrusion of the oocyte in its cumulus are unknown at this time. Repeated evaluation of intrafollicular pressures has failed to indict an explosive factor in this crucial event.

In a variety of animal experiments the physical expulsion of the oocyte appears to be dependent upon a preovulatory surge in prostaglandin synthesis within the follicle. (2) Inhibition of this prostaglandin synthesis produces a corpus luteum with an entrapped oocyte.

As uncertain as the factors which "choose" the follicles for maturity in any particular cycle, so is the mechanism by which, in most cases, only a single unit is selected for the final burst of maturity expressed as ovulation. Recent evidence has implicated local concentrations of estrogen within a follicle unit as an important organizational factor. As FSH quantities diminish prior to ovulation, it appears that the most mature follicle, and hence the most efficient estrogen producer, selectively binds available FSH better than its less successful sisters. As a result the limited FSH supplies are directed to a single maturing follicle. As ovulation occurs, in still another event of exquisitely delicate synchrony, the first polar body is extruded.

Corpus Luteum

Shortly after ovulation profound alterations in cellular organization occur in the ruptured follicle that go well beyond simple repair. After tissue integrity and continuity are retrieved, the granulosa cells hypertrophy markedly, gradually filling in the cystic, sometimes hemorrhagic, cavity of the early corpus luteum. In addition, for the first time the granulosa becomes markedly luteinized by incorporation of lipid rich vacuoles within its cytoplasm. Also for the first time vascularization occurs in the granulosa. Both these properties had been the exclusive features of the theca prior to ovulation. For its part, the theca of the corpus luteum becomes less prominent, vestiges being noted eventually only in the interstices of the typical scalloping of the mature corpus luteum. As a result a new yellow body is formed now dominated by the enlarged, lipid rich, fully vascularized granulosa. In the 14 days of its life, dependent on the low but important quantities of LH available in the luteal phase, this unit produces estrogen and progesterone. Failing a new enlarging source of LH-like human chorionic gonadotropin (HCG) from a successful implantation, the corpus luteum rapidly ages. Morphologically its vascularity and lipid content wanes, and the sequence of scarification (albicantia) ensues.

Correlation of Follicle Maturation, Follicle Availability and Estrogen Production

If one considers the effects of increments of endogenous estrogen production on the body, certain categorical effects can be seen as varying estrogen thresholds are reached. As biologic levels of estrogen increase, the sequence of formation and maintenance of secondary sexual characteristics, cervical mucus and vaginal cornification, endometrial proliferation and menses, and finally ovulation, is achieved. Each event requiring quantum increments in estrogen production is bound to the evolving, increased maturation of the follicle units.

As we trace estrogen effects over a lifespan, with increased follicle maturation, female phenotype is asserted early, growth spurt is stimulated, and appearance of secondary sex characteristics is also seen. As individual follicles undergo greater and greater maturity, menarche and the first ovulation are achieved in short order. For the next 30 years estrogen production and follicle maturation work hand in hand to sustain adult reproductive efficiency via repeated monthly ovulations. At this level of steroid production all other estrogen-dependent systems are more than sufficiently sustained.

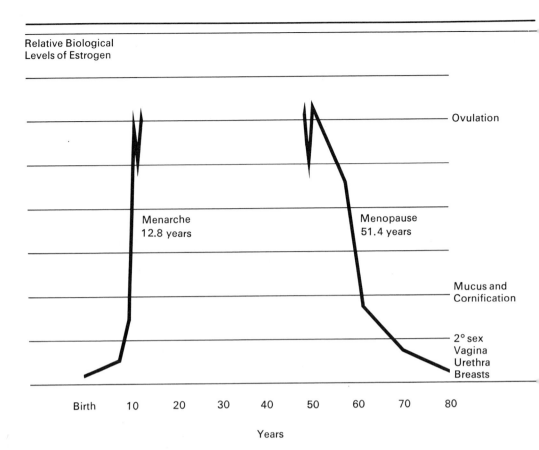

Relative Biological
Levels of Estrogen

Ovulation

Menarche
12.8 years

Menopause
51.4 years

Mucus and
Cornification

2° sex
Vagina
Urethra
Breasts

Birth   10   20   30   40   50   60   70   80

Years

At approximately age 38–42, ovulation is clinically known to reduce in frequency. It has been suggested that the residual follicle units, now only a few thousand in number are the least sensitive to gonadotropin stimulation, and hence are less likely to achieve successful and complete maturation. As numbers of follicle units decrease and resistant factors increase, less and less estrogen is produced from the surviving stimulated units. Eventually the recession in estrogenicity no longer proliferates endometrium to yield menstruation, and menopause ensues. Further retreat in estrogen production threatens even the most basic tissues which are estrogen dependent.

At one point enough follicle maturation has yielded sufficient estrogen to cause the first period (menarche). Menarche therefore is one point on a curve of ascending estrogen production. Similarly, the climacteric defines a more prolonged period of estrogen withdrawal, starting with the first decreases in frequency of ovulation, and ending in atrophy of secondary sex characteristics. A single point in that curve, when insufficient follicle maturity results in inadequate estrogen and no menses, is the menopause.

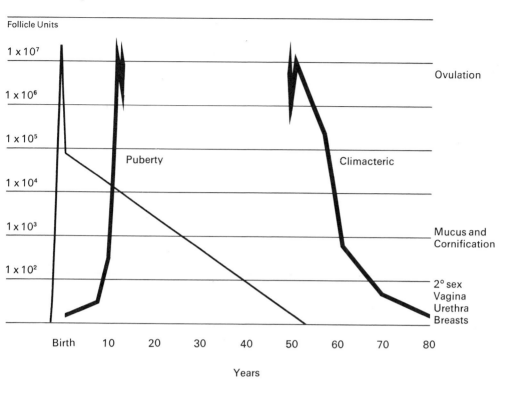

Relative Biological
Levels of Estrogen

Follicle Units

1 x 10⁷

1 x 10⁶   Ovulation

1 x 10⁵

Puberty   Climacteric

1 x 10⁴

1 x 10³   Mucus and
                                                          Cornification

1 x 10²

                                                          2° sex
                                                          Vagina
                                                          Urethra
                                                          Breasts

Birth   10   20   30   40   50   60   70   80

Years

Hormone Production after Follicle Exhaustion

Some residual follicles exist within the gonads even after the menopause is reached. Their performance in terms of both steroidogenesis and morphological change is a matter of degree. Even prior to the menopause, the remaining follicles begin to perform less well. During the perimenopausal period, women who are having regular periods may have lower estradiol levels and higher levels of FSH, and the cycle begins to change, mainly because of a shortening of the follicular phase. (3) This is a time period during which postmenopausal levels of FSH (greater than 40 mIU/ml) may be seen despite continued menstrual bleeding, while LH levels usually remain in the normal range. It is likely that the elevated FSH levels are an indicator of a significant reduction in the number of follicles remaining, and those remaining have diminished ability to produce estrogen. However, FSH may also be regulated in part by the negative feedback action of a nonsteroid substance produced by granulosa cells, a situation which would be similar to the action in the male of inhibin, a peptide produced in the testicular Sertoli cells. Occasionally corpus luteum formation and function occurs. As cycles become irregular, vaginal bleeding occurs at the end of an inadequate luteal phase or after a peak of estradiol without subsequent ovulation or corpus luteum formation. Eventually there is a 10–20 fold increase in FSH and approximately a 3 fold increase in LH, reaching a maximum level 1–3 years after menopause, after which there is a gradual and slight decline. Elevated levels of both FSH and LH appear to be conclusive evidence of ovarian failure.

After menopause, the circulating level of androstenedione is about one half that seen prior to menopause. (4, 5) Most of this postmenopausal androstenedione is derived from the adrenal gland, with only a small amount secreted from the ovary. Testosterone levels do not fall appreciably, and in fact the postmenopausal ovary secretes more testosterone than the premenopausal ovary. (4, 5) With the disappearance of follicles and estrogen, the elevated gonadotropins probably drive the remaining stromal tissue in the ovary to a level of increased testosterone secretion.

The circulating estradiol level after menopause is approximately 10–20 pg/ml, most of which is probably derived from peripheral conversion of testosterone and estrone. The circulating level of estrone in the postmenopausal women is higher than that of estradiol, the mean level being approximately 30 pg/ml. (5) The average production rate of estrogen is approximately 45 μg/24 hours; almost all, if not all, being estrone derived from the peripheral conversion of adrostenedione. (6) The percent conversion of estrone from androstenedione correlates with age. (7) While the amount of precursor, androstenedione, decreases by about one half, the percent conversion approximately doubles in the postmenopausal woman as she grows older. These changes compensate for each other maintaining estrogen production at a relative stable level of 45 μg/24 hours.

The percent conversion of androstenedione to estrogen also correlates with body weight. (5, 6) Increased production of estrogen from androstenedione with increasing body weight is probably due to the ability of fat to aromatize androgens. (8) This fact may be the basis for the well-known association between obesity and the development of endometrial cancer.

Estrogen production by the ovaries does not continue beyond the menopause. However, estrogen levels in postmenopausal women continue to be significant, principally due to the extraglandular conversion of androstenedione to estrone. The clinical impact of this estrogen will vary from one postmenopausal individual to another, depending upon the degree of extraglandular production, probably modified by a variety of factors.

Postmenopausal
Peripheral
Conversion

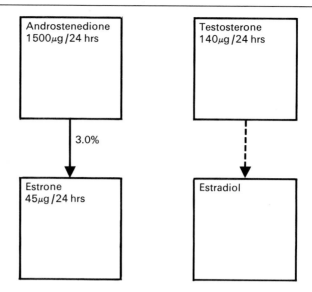

Androstenedione
1500μg/24 hrs

Testosterone
140μg/24 hrs

3.0%

Estrone
45μg/24 hrs

Estradiol

The two major influences are:

1. An increase in substrate (e.g. stress induced increases in adrenal production of androstenedione).

2. An increase in the percent conversion of androstenedione to estrone (e.g. with an accumulation of adipose tissue).

Estrogen derived from these sources may be sufficient to sustain breasts and estrogen-stimulated surfaces such as urethra and vagina.

Eventually the ovarian stroma is exhausted and despite huge reactive homeostatic increments in FSH and LH no further steroidogenesis of importance results from gonadal activity. With increasing age the adrenal contribution of precursors for estrogen production proves inadequate. In this final state of estrogen availability, levels are insufficient to sustain secondary sex tissues.

Problems Associated with Reproductive Years

It is commonly recognized that behavioral changes may be associated with the menstrual cycle. Suicides and suicidal attempts are more frequent in the immediate premenstrual and menstrual phases. Half of the inmates in a woman's prison committed their crimes during menstruation or in the immediate premenstrual phase. (9)

Occasionally the gynecologist is consulted by a psychiatrist for advice regarding a patient with cyclic emotional disturbances. Presumably these behavioral problems are due to cyclic changes in hormone levels, and an empiric approach to eliminating hormonal changes is worth considering. While depression and mood liability may be associated with oral contraceptive use, an opposite stabilizing effect may also be achieved. In extreme circumstances, complete elimination of sex steroid variability may be achieved with the daily use of an oral contraceptive, as in the treatment of endometroisis, or with administration of Depo Provera, 150 mg intramuscularly every three months. On occasion, we have experienced beneficial and gratifying results in patients with incapacitating emotional swings.

The irritability and depression that many women experience just prior to the menstrual period have been attributed to fluid retention and to changes in the levels of estrogen and progesterone. This premenstrual tension is frequently accompanied by a slight increase in weight and varying degrees of edema. Diuretic therapy, however, is not uniformly effective. Indeed therapy of premenstrual tension is not precise due to lack of knowledge concerning the basic causes of the problem. The judicious use of a mild tranquilizer may be helpful; however, inhibition of ovulation with an oral contraceptive may be still more beneficial.

It now appears very likely that primary dysmenorrhea is due to myometrial contractions induced by prostaglandins originating in the endometrium. (10) Endometrial production of prostaglandins is higher in the luteal phase of the cycle, and with the onset of menstruation, prostaglandin levels rise even higher. Thus the correlation of dysmenorrhea with ovulation is probably due to the higher prostaglandin production in secretory endometrium. The beneficial effect of oral contraceptives can be explained, therefore, by the presence of decidualized, atrophic endometrium with lower prostaglandin levels. Relief of dysmenorrhea has been achieved with the administration of potent inhibitors of prostaglandin biosynthesis. However, because these inhibitors affect prostaglandin synthesis throughout the body, their use requires extensive evaluation for safety and toxicity.

Climacteric (Menopause and Postmenopause): Clinical Implications And Rationale For Estrogen Replacement Therapy

After 3 decades of ovulatory menstrual function, accompanied by full biologic estrogen maintenance of dependent tissues, at approximately 40 years of age, the frequency of ovulation decreases. This initiates a period of waning ovarian function called climacteric, which will last as long as 20 years, and will carry the woman through decreased fertility, menopause, and manifestations of progressive tissue atrophy and aging. It is likely that the major factor in this evolving picture is the diminution of estrogen production associated with this period of life. Menopause occurs in the United States between ages 48–55 with the median age being 51.4.

In this section, the clinical implications of estrogen withdrawal will be reviewed. A policy supporting replacement therapy, consistent with cautious medical practice and based on supporting data, will be offered.

Although estrogen does not wane in a straight line function as depicted in several diagrams in this chapter, its progressive diminution over time leads to a sequential loss of estrogenic dependent functions: ovulation, menstrual function, vaginal and vulvar tissue strength, and finally generalized atrophy of all estrogen-dependent tissues.

This estrogen loss is due to the continued attrition in the numbers of residual follicle units in the 5th decade of life. Since fewer follicles are available, less and less estrogen production is possible. It must be remembered that these oldest follicle units have perhaps remained in the ovary unstimulated by gonadotropin not entirely by chance, but possibly due to their inherent refractoriness to otherwise appropriate gonadotropin stimulation. When these are finally activated, the degree of differentiation each is likely to experience is limited. Thus each follicle growth period will be increasingly blunted, with less estrogen produced. Eventually even the older and sluggish follicles are exhausted, and estrogen production is now at a lower level of efficiency resulting almost entirely from indirect resources, the peripheral conversion of ovarian stromal and adrenal precursors to active estrogen in nonendocrine tissue sites.

Finally the gonadal resource becomes defunct: the ovary shrivels to an atrophic mass of fibrous tissue. Estrogenicity, now at marginally sustaining levels, is the product of inadvertent dietary intake, and adrenal activity. As peripheral tissues age (now in the 7th, 8th and 9th decade) even these low levels wane still further.

The symptoms frequently seen and related to estrogen loss in this protracted climacteric are:

1. Disturbances in menstrual pattern, including anovulation and reduced fertility, decreased flow, hypermenorrhea, and irregular frequency of menses.

2. Vasomotor instability, (hot flashes and sweats). Hot flashes are not well-understood, but apparently are the result of instability between the hypothalamus and the autonomic nervous system, brought about by a decline in estrogen. Hot flashes are wave-like sensations of heat that move up the chest to the head, frequently followed by profuse perspiration. The flashes may last a few seconds or as long as 30 minutes or 1 hour. They are especially disturbing at night, perhaps because the hypothalamus is relatively unoccupied.

3. Psychological symptoms, including anxiety, increased tension, mood depression, and irritability.

4. Atrophic conditions: atrophy of vaginal epithelium, urethral caruncles, dyspareunia and pruritus due to vulvar, introital, and vaginal atrophy, general skin atrophy, urinary difficulties such as urgency and cystitis.

5. A variety of complaints such as headaches, insomnia, myalgia, changes in libido, and palpitations. Lower back pain may be due to osteoporosis.

A precise understanding of the symptom complex the individual patient may display is often difficult to achieve. Some patients will show severe multiple reactions that may be disabling. Others will show no reactions, or minimal reactions which go unnoticed until careful medical evaluation. The majority of patients (50–60%) require medical assistance and support for intermittent difficulties of moderate severity.

It appears that three factors are at work in all climacteric women. The symptomatic reaction is the sum of impact of these three components:

1. The amount of estrogen depletion and the rate at which estrogen is withdrawn.

2. The collective inherited and acquired propensities to succumb or withstand the impositions of the overall aging process.

3. The psychologic impact of aging and the individual's reaction to the emotional implications of "a change of life."

Although menopause, the last menstrual period, is only a single point in the protracted unfolding of the climacteric, only the most stoical, objective, and rationally composed human can dismiss it as a minor physiologic event. For most women, it signals an end to the known, the accustomed and expected, and the beginning of an era of insidiously diminishing competence, leading irretrievably to aging and death. Add to this gloomy prospect the almost obsessive cultish pursuit of youthful sexual femininity that our society espouses, and one can only wonder why more postmenopausal women do not complicate their physiologic deficits with great emotional burdens.

Clearly good medical practice obligates the concerned physician to support patients in all aspects of the prolonged and possibly difficult climacteric period. We have found it helpful to classify these needs according to events of the "early" and "late" climacteric.

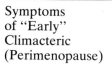

The degree of symptomatology experienced by women as they proceed through early estrogen withdrawal appears to depend on the speed of that withdrawal. If occasioned by surgical or radiation castration, the resulting abrupt estrogen loss is very symptomatic. Often the worst expressions of vasomotor flushes and sweats, globus hystericus, palpitations, etc., are displayed in these circumstances. Accompanying emotional reactions, depressions, anxiety, irritability, also appear to be the most virulent under these conditions. Our practice is to administer 25 mg conjugated estrogens intramuscularly in the recovery room, immediately following surgical castration.

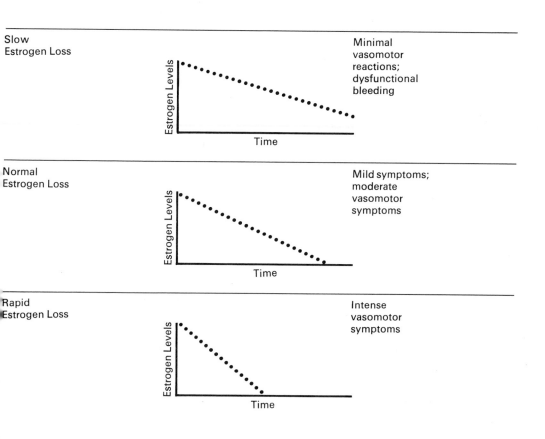

If estrogen loss is very slow, vasomotor reactions are minimal, but abnormal and often prolonged uterine bleeding becomes the worrisome factor. Appropriately, both the patient and her physician are concerned about an underlying malignant process resulting in this abnormal expression. Reassurance on this score may require operative investigation.

A large middle group of women undergo depletion of estrogen at an intermediate rate, so that menopause is accompanied by mild periodic flushes. Obviously the factors which influence the slope of estrogen withdrawal are unknown. Gonadotropin sensitivity, numbers of follicles, the degree of peripheral estrogen production, the amount of retained ovarian stromal activity, and the organic and emotional health of the patient are certainly involved.

Symptoms of "Late" Climacteric

The effects of the late climeracteric (extremely low estrogen production) depend on many factors, including the general resistance to aging of target tissues, the overall health, quality of diet and level of activity. Also important is the amount of estrogen produced by the peripheral nonendocrine routes.

With extremely low estrogen production, not enough estrogen is available to sustain, even marginally, any estrogen dependent tissue. Pruritus, vaginitis, dyspareunia, urinary difficulties (dysuria, urge incontinence, urethritis), and osteoporosis are the likely results of this situation. Somewhat higher function may marginally sustain tissues. It is not infrequent to find estrogenized cervical mucus and vaginal epithelium in a woman 10–15 years postmenopause. Finally, periodic stress may yield spikes of estrogen production competent to produce sufficient endometrial activity to produce bleeding.

Postmenopausal Estrogen Replacement Therapy

In view of the above considerations, our opinion is as follows: There is little question that women who suffer from hot flushes or atrophy of reproductive tract tissues can and should be relieved of their problems by use of estrogens. It also is likely that the long term disabilities of osteoporosis can be ameliorated by therapy with estrogen. The protective effects afforded by estrogen must be weighed against the apparent increased incidence of endometrial cancer that may be associated with hormone use. Until further information is available we suggest treatment with estrogen for all women showing any stigmata of hormone deprivation. The lowest dose of estrogen that reverses the deficiency should be used and monthly addition of a short course of progestin is advised. In practice, we exclude from therapy those patients in whom estrogen is specifically contraindicated (estrogen dependent tumors, impaired liver metabolism, and, in a matter of clinical judgement, patients with thromboembolic problems or conditions predisposing to thromboembolism). The decision to use or not to use estrogen belongs to the patient and it should be based on the information available in this chapter.

1. **Control of Vasomotor Reations.** Although there is only a little evidence to implicate autonomic nervous system dysfunction in the production of the vasomotor reactions, the immediate and sustained response of these symptoms to estrogen replacement is clinically very impressive and persuasive.

2. **Reduction of Emotional Reactions to Climacteric.** Whether directly due to estrogen withdrawal or indirectly due to the implications of the menopause, anxiety, depression, and mood swings will often respond to estrogen. Recent double blind studies have indicated that depression and psychological performance can be significantly improved with estrogen therapy. (11, 12) Significant reductions have been noted in insomnia, irritability, headaches, anxiety, urinary frequency, and improvements have been recorded in memory and mood, when an estrogen treated group was compared to a placebo group. (13) Of course estrogen therapy does not always eliminate these problems, and additional sedation, counseling or psychotropic drugs may be required.

3. **Preventive Medicine.** As a result of these immediate responses in early climacteric symptoms, the patient enters the climacteric more confident of herself emotionally, sexually, and physically. In our view, this establishes or cements good patient-physician interchange and relations. The follow-up of the patient on effective estrogen replacement is more secure and certain. The practitioner offering estrogen replacement has a better and more reliable opportunity to act as primary physician for these aging women. All monitoring of health systems will be improved as a result of this single involvement. Bowel, breast, cardiac, and various metabolic functions are scrutinized periodically as consistent with good health practice.

4. **Osteoporosis.** Osteoporosis is a reduction in the quantity of bony material resulting in structural fragility. The statistics relating the problems of osteoporosis to the postmenopausal woman are very impressive (14):

   Approximately 25% of white women over 60 have spinal compression fractures due to osteoporosis. There are racial differences; black women have a greater quantity of bone and rarely develop osteoporosis.

   Symptomatic spinal osteoporosis is 5 times as common in women as in men.

   80% of all hip fractures are associated with osteoporosis.

   17% of all hip fracture patients die within 3 months.

   An increase in distal forearm fractures in women begins at about age 45, and by 60, the female to male ratio is 10 to 1.

There is now sufficient evidence to make the judgment that estrogen replacement therapy has significant prophylactic value in retarding osteoporosis. The mechanism of action is thought to be an interference with parathyroid hormone action on the bone (15).

There are two significant studies in the literature. Long-term followup (4 to 10 years) of postmenopausal and castrated women revealed a significantly lower rate of bone mineral loss in those women on estrogen therapy (0.625 and 1.25 mg conjugated estrogens). (16) Interestingly, only 20% of castrated women and only 30% of women with a natural menopause did not lose bone, indicating that a minority of women would not benefit from estrogen for osteoporosis prophylaxis.

A double blind prospective study in England, using densitometric and photon absorption measurements, has reached the 5 year mark. (17) Mestranol (in a dose of 20 μg) was associated not only with a reduction in the rate of bone loss, but there was actually a positive gain in mineral content in the treated group. In women who are treated with estrogen, the incidence of fractures is reduced (18).

Therefore the prevention of osteoporosis is a substantial advantage for the use of estrogen replacement therapy in both postmenopausal women and women with premature menopause.

5. **Coronary Heart Disease.** The apparent sex difference between men and women in respect to coronary heart disease is a phenomenon characteristic only of affluent populations with a high incidence of other risk factors such as hyperlipidemia, diabetes, cigarette smoking, and hypertension. In fact, closer inspection of this apparent difference reveals that there is no change in the incidence of coronary mortality in women at the time of menopause. (19) The decreasing ratio of male to female mortality rates is due principally to a slower acceleration with increasing age in the male population. Nevertheless, this apparent difference prompted a series of studies in which estrogen was given for secondary prophylaxis of myocardial infarction. High doses of estrogen (clearly pharmacological) were associated with an increase in mortality from cardiovascular disease while low doses did not differ when compared to a placebo group. (19) Therefore, there is no evidence that estrogen plays a prophylactic role when given to men, and a retrospective study has failed to detect a preventive effect for replacement estrogen in postmenopausal women. (20) On the other hand, retrospective studies have also failed to find an increase risk for coronary heart disease or stroke in postmenopausal women using estrogen (20, 21)

However, in women who are castrated prior to the menopause, studies indicate that premature loss of estrogen is associated with a higher incidence of coronary heart disease. (22, 23, 24, 25) There is one study in conflict; however, the incidence of heart disease was very high in the control group. (26) When women who were castrated when young and treated with estrogen were compared with a similar group not treated, there was an increased incidence of cardiovascular disease in the non-treated group. (18) Therefore in women subjected to premature menopause (before age 40) estrogen replacement therapy probably reduces the risk of coronary heart disease.

6. **Reversal of Atrophy.** After loss of estrogen, the epidermis becomes thinner and the number of mitoses becomes low. Estrogen therapy causes the epidermis to thicken with an increase in the number of mitoses. (27) Such thickening may reduce the susceptibility to skin changes and irritations.

Genitourinary atrophy leads to a variety of symptoms which affect the ease and quality of living. Urinary frequency and urgency may be secondary to urethral atrophy which leads to narrowing and inflammation of the distal urethra, and eventually stricture formation. (28) Vaginal atrophy with dyspareunia, pruritus, and discomfort during pelvic exams responds well to estrogen therapy. Relief from these problems often results in significant improvements in general well-being.

Disadvantages of Estrogen Replacement, Therapy

1. **Cancer.** Estrogen replacement therapy may increase the risk of breast cancer in postmenopausal women. In a long-term followup study of postmenopausal women treated with conjugated estrogens (mostly 0.625 and 0.3 mg) there was a 30% increase in the observed number of breast cancers when compared with the expected number. (29) However, this observation was only of borderline statistical significance, and the excess number of cases was seen only after 10–12 years of estrogen therapy. Although the number of cases was small, a statistically significant increase in risk was associated with higher dose levels, and with treatment regimens which were other than daily administration. (29) The relative risk was 1.3 which increased to 2.0 after 15 years of treatment. It is by no means established that the use of exogenous estrogens causes breast cancer. In view of many negative retrospective studies, and one negative study with a longterm followup (30), the above positive study must be viewed as a suggestion that a possible risk exists, and further evaluation is necessary.

The association of estrogen with cancer of the endometrium is more impressive. Estrogen promotes growth of the endometrium. Progression of growth associated with estrogen can be divided into the following histologic stages: cystic hyperplasia, adenomatous polyps, adenomatous hyperplasia, atypical hyperplasia, carcinoma-in-situ, and adenocarcinoma. It is said that 10% of atypical hyperplasia goes on to carcinoma (31). The practicing gynecologist is obviously impressed with this potential change, as seen in the frequent performance of hysterectomy because of the presence of endometrial hyperplasia.

Attention has only recently focused on the relationship of these histologic changes to the use of exogenous estrogen. Retrospective studies have estimated that the risk of endometrial cancer in women on replacement estrogen therapy is increased by a factor ranging from 4 to 8 (32, 33, 34). The risk estimate appears to increase with the duration of exposure, (32) and the dose of estrogen (34). When adjusted for the recognized risks of obesity, hypertension, and diabetes, the increased risk with estrogen matched the risk for those reasons. (33) In other words, the increased risk with estrogen was not additive to the other risks. In one of these studies, (34) the data suggest a latent period of 4 to 8 years. If these figures are accurate, the actual incidence of endometrial cancer in America would increase from 1 per 1000 postmenopausal women per year to 4 to 8 per 1,000 per year.

Additional reports have supported the contention that exogenous estrogen increases the risk of endometrial cancer. A retrospective study of women with breast cancer indicated that the group of women receiving estrogen treatment had a 3-fold increased risk of developing endometrial cancer. (35). Young women on sequential oral contraception and patients with genetic ovarian failure on estrogen replacement therapy have been reported with endometrial cancer. It should be noted that in these last two categories, large doses of estrogen were utilized.

The amount of estrogen replacement therapy in the United States more than doubled from 1965 to 1974. (36) If exogenous estrogen is associated with an increased risk of endometrial cancer then one would expect the national incidence to reflect the increased use of estrogen. Early reports failed to do so (37), perhaps reflecting a failure to correct for those who had hysterectomies, and also not covering the recent years when the increased incidence would be noticeable. A later study has indicated an increase in the rate of endometrial cancer in various parts of the United States. (38) Not resolved, however, is the contention that such an increased incidence may reflect better diagnostic ability. Furthermore, the increased incidence of endometrial cancer was also noted in premenopausal women not on estrogen therapy. (38)

The data on this issue do not need to be conclusive. The indications are that estrogen is associated with an increased risk, even though the degree of risk and the impact in terms of mortality and morbidity remain to be determined. Therefore the clinician must make a judgment as to whether the benefits of estrogen therapy outweigh the risks. It is our contention that there are selective clinical indications for the use of estrogen, and that the risk can be minimized by the addition of a progestational agent to the treatment regimen.

While estrogen promotes growth of the endometrium, progesterone inhibits growth. In addition to the morphologic changes associated with conversion to a secretory endometrium, progestins interfere with the estrogen stimulus to growth by reducing the quantity of cytoplasmic estrogen receptors available. (39, 40) Therefore the number of estrogen receptor complexes that are translocated and retained in the endometrial nuclei is decreased. Hence, periodic exposure of the endometrium to a progestational agent will interfere with mitotic changes, and produce an interruption to growth. In addition, progestational agents increase the activity of an enzyme in endometrium which converts estradiol to estrone. (41) The estrone rapidly leaves the tissue; thus the intracellular level of estradiol is decreased. For these reasons we advocate the addition of a progestational agent as outlined in our method of treatment.

2. **Side Effects of Estrogen.** Despite careful support of the patient the appearance of side effects (usually due to injudicious dosage) reopens the fears and concerns of the patient. Side effects include breast tenderness, intermittent uterine breakthrough bleeding, an increase in vaginal discharge, edema, and weight gain. Each requires careful responses in terms of concern, investigation, revision of dosage, and where necessary specific ancillary therapy.

3. **Metabolic Effects.** Estrogens, again particularly when used in injudicious dosage regimens, may have a serious impact on total health. Major concerns include diabetes, hypertension and atherosclerosis. The details of the manner by which high doses of synthetic estrogens affect the metabolic process are dealt with in Chapter 14. It is our opinion that the usual dose formulations used in the climacteric are probably below provocative concentrations. Nevertheless, careful medical history, family history, and followup surveillance are necessary in all patients on estrogen replacement. Our practice involves an annual visit including general history, physical examination, and PAP smear, with emphasis on breast, pelvic, and rectal examination, blood pressure, urinalysis, and complete blood count.

Which Drug Should Be Used? There currently is no evidence that one form of estrogen is superior to another. It has been argued that estrone may be a specific oncogenic agent. (42) It appears more appropriate to view a relationship between estrone and cancer as derived from the fact that estrone is the major circulating estrogen in the postmenopausal years. The specific estrogen does not appear to be as important as the duration, dose, and continuity of exposure in the absence of progesterone. Which estrogen is administered may not be as significant as the method with which it is used. For example, the administration of estradiol does not insure that estradiol (rather then estrone) reaches estrogen sensitive tissues as there is conversion of the estradiol to estrone within the body and the blood level of estrone rises faster and higher than that of estradiol. (43) It is also difficult to know the equivalent potency within the human body of the various estrogen preparations. A daily dose of 10 μg of ethinyl estradiol is necessary to produce a consistent suppression of LH and FSH. (44) A similar dose of conjugated estrogens is probably 1.25 mg. However any estrogen properly monitored and administered is acceptable.

When Should Treatment Begin? Our policy, which advocates early initiation of therapy, is to begin estrogen approximately 1 year postmenopausal in the patient who does not produce withdrawal bleeding when challenged with progestin administration. A complete dialogue assessing risks and benefits is a necessary initial step.

How Do We Treat? If a uterus is present, estrogens are administered on a cyclic basis, either 3 weeks on, 1 week off, or as a convenient method from the 1st through the 24th of each month. For the last 7 days of estrogen administration, a daily dose of 10 mg of medroxyprogesterone acetate (Provera) is added. Some practitioners do not see the need to use cyclic administration or a progestational agent in the absence of a uterus. However, in view of a possible impact on the breast, it seems appropriate to adhere to a cyclic schedule including the terminal use of a progestin for the reasons we have already noted.

The dose of estrogen utilized is that which will provide sufficient estrogen to sustain physiologic functions, yet short of provoking a return of menstrual flow. An important principle of treatment is that relief of symptoms can usually be achieved by sub-bleeding doses of estrogen. For early climacteric where there is still considerable endogenous estrogen present, the usual effective dose is 0.625 mg conjugated estrogens per day. In late climacteric where endogenous estrogen may be very low at best, a higher dose, 1.25 mg, may be necessary depending on symptoms.

Spotting and bleeding require evaluation to rule out uterine malignancy. The liberal use of endometrial aspiration biopsy with a paracervical block is encouraged. If endometrial hyperplasia is encountered, it is worthwhile to consider a reduction or discontinuation of the estrogen medication, with endometrial biopsy followup.

When estrogen is contraindicated, Depo Provera (starting dose of 150 mg every 3 months) is effective in relieving vasomotor symptoms. The mechanism of action is unknown, but it is not due to metabolism of the progestational agent into estrogens. The effect of this progestational agent on the other problems associated with menopause (e.g. osteoporosis) is also unknown.

Occasionally a patient will remain symptomatic, particularly showing decreased libido. We have found that the addition of androgen (methyltestosterone, up to 5 mg daily) in addition to the estrogen, may provide an increased sense of well-being, along with an increase in libido. The patient should be cautioned that hirsutism may develop.

We find no need to monitor dosage by any means other than symptoms and bleeding; assessing vaginal cytology is not useful.

Conclusion: No one can hope to stay young forever, and hormones certainly will not prevent aging. There should be no misconceptions here. Some of the difficulties of aging, however, can be softened with estrogen therapy, and several potentially disabling problems can be avoided. However, unanswered questions remain. Practical clinical means are needed to identify which patients require estrogen. Controlled clinical studies are necessary in order to determine which form of estrogen is best, what schedule of estrogen should be used, how much progestational agent is necessary, and how long a progestational agent should be given. Until these questions are answered, close clinical surveillance of our patients is necessary.

References

1. **Bonilla-Musoles, F, Renau, J, Hernandez-Yago, J, and Torres, YJ,** How Do Oocytes Disappear? Arch Gynak 218:233, 1975.

2. **LeMaire, WJ, Yang, NST, Behrman, HR, and Marsh, JM,** Preovulatory Changes in the Concentration of Prostaglandins in Rabbit Graafian Follicles, Prostaglandins 3:367, 1973.

3. **Sherman, BM, West, JH, and Korenman, SG,** The Menopausal Transition: Analysis of LH, FSH, Estradiol, and Progesterone Concentrations During Menstrual Cycles of Older Women, J Clin Endocrinol Metab 42:629, 1976.

4. **Vermeulen, A,** The Hormonal Activity of the Postmenopausal Ovary, J Clin Edocrinol Metab 42:247, 1976.

5. **Judd, HL,** Hormonal Dynamics Associated with the Menopause, Clin Obstet Gynec 19:775, 1976.

6. **Siiteri, PK, MacDonald, PC,** Role of Extraglandular Estrogen, in Human Endocrinology, in Geiger, SR, Astwood, EB, and Greep, RO, eds *Handbook of Physiology, Section 7, Endocrinology*, American Physiology Society, Washington DC, 1973.

7. **Hemsell, DL, Grodin, JM, Brenner, PF, Siiteri, PK, and MacDonald, PC,** Plasma Precursors of Estrogen, II. Correlation of the Extent of Conversion of Plasma Androstenedione to Estrogen With Age, J Clin Endocrinol Metab 38:476, 1976.

8. **Schindler, AEE, Ebert, A, and Friedrich, E,** Conversion of Androstenedione to Estrogen by Human Fat Tissue, J Clin Endocrinol Metab 35:627, 1972.

9. **Dalton, K,** Menstruation and Crime, Br Med J 2:1752, 1961.

10. **Halbert, DR, Demers, LN, and Jones, DED,** Dysmenorrhea and Prostaglandins, Obstet Gynec Survey 31:77, 1976.

11. **Aylward, M,** Estrogens, Plasma Tryptophan Levels in Perimenopausal Patients, in Campbell, S, Editor, *The Management of the Menopause and Postmenopausal Years*, University Park Press, Baltimore, 1976, pp 135–147.

12. **Kantor, HI, Michael, CM, and Shore, H,** Estrogen for Older Women, Am J Obstet Gynec 116:115, 1973.

13. **Campbell, S,** Double Blind Psychometric Studies on the Effects of Natural Estrogens on Postmenopausal Women, in Campbell, S, Editor, *The Management of the Menopause and Postmenopausal Years*, University Park Press, Baltimore, 1976, pp 149–158.

14. **Heaney, RP,** Estrogens and Postmenopausal Osteoporosis, Clin Obstet Gynec 19:791, 1976.

15. **Riggs, BL, Jowsey, J, Goldsmith, RS, Kelly, PJ, Hoffman, DL, and Arnaud, CD,** Short-and-Long-Term Effects of Estrogen and Synthetic Anabolic Hormone in Postmenopausal Osteoporosis, J Clin Invest 51:1659, 1972.

16. **Meema, S, Bunker, ML, and Meema, HE,** Preventive Effect of Estrogen on Postmenopausal Bone Loss, Arch Intern Med 135:1436, 1975.

17. **Lindsay, R, Aitken, JM, Anderson, JB, Hart, DM, MacDonald, EB, and Clarke, AC,** Long-Term Prevention of Postmenopausal Osteoporosis by Estrogen, Lancet 1:1038, 1976.

18. **Johansson, BW, Kaij, L, Kullander, S, Lenner, HC, Svanberg, L, and Astedt, B,** On Some Late Effects of Bilateral Oophorectomy in the Age Range 15–30 Years, Acta Obstet Gynec Scand 54:449, 1975.

19. **Furman, RH,** Coronary Heart Disease and the Menopause, in Ryan, KJ, and Gibson, DC, eds, *Menopause and Aging,* DHEW Publication No. (NIH) 73-319, US Government Printing Office, Washington, D.C., 1971, pp. 39–55.

20. **Rosenberg, L, Armstrong, B, and Jick, H,** Myocardial Infarction and Estrogen Therapy in Postmenopausal Women, New Eng J Med 294:1256, 1976.

21. **Pfeffer, RI, and VanDenNoort, S,** Estrogen Use and Stroke Risk in Postmenopausal Women, Am J Epidemiology 103:445, 1976.

22. **Wuest, J, Dry, TJ, and Edwards, JE,** The Degree of Coronary Sclerosis in Bilaterally Oophorectomized Women, Circulation 7:801, 1953.

23. **Parrish, HM, Carr, CA, Hall, DG, and King, TM,** Time Interval From Castration in Perimenopausal Women to Development of Excessive Coronary Atherosclerosis, Am J Obstet Gynec 99:155, 1967.

24. **Oliver, MF,** The Menopause and Coronary Heart Disease, in Campbell, S, Editor, *The Management of the Menopause and Postmenopausal Years,* University Park Press, Baltimore, 1976, pp 175–184.

25. **Higano, N, Robinson, RW, and Cohen, WD,** Increased Incidence of Cardiovascular Disease in Castrated Women, New Eng J Med 268:1123, 1963.

26. **Ritterband, AB, Jaffe, IA, Densen, PM, Magagna, JF, and Reed, E,** Gonadal Function and The Development of Coronary Heart Disease, Circulation 26:668, 1962.

27. **Rauramo, L,** Effect of Castration and Peripheral Estradiol Valerate and Estriol Succinate Therapy on the Epidermis, in Campbell, S, Editor, *The Management of the Menopause and Postmenopausal Years,* University Park Press, Baltimore, 1976, pp 253–263.

28. **Smith, PJB,** The Effect of Estrogens on Bladder Function in the Female, Campbell, S, Editor, *The Management of the Menopause and Postmenopausal Years,* University Park Press, Baltimore, 1976, pp 291–298.

29. **Hoover, R, Gray, LA, Sr, Cole, P, and MacMahon, B,** Menopausal Estrogens and Breast Cancer, New Eng J Med 295:401, 1976.

30. **Burch, JC, Byrd, BF, and Vaughn, WK,** The Effects of Long-Term Estrogen on Hysterectomized Women, Am J Obstet Gynec 118:778, 1974.

31. **Vellios, F,** Endometrial Hyperplasia and Carcinoma In Situ, Gynec Oncology 2:52, 1974.

32. **Ziel, HG, and Finkle, WD,** Increased Risk of Endometrial Carcinoma Among Users of Conjugated Estrogens, New Eng J Med 293:1167, 1975.

33. **Smith, DC, Prentice, R, Thompson, DJ, and Herrman, WL,** Association of Exogenous Estrogen and Endometrial Carcinoma, New Eng J Med 293:1164, 1975.

34. **Mack, TM, Pike, MC, Henderson, BE, Pfeffer, RI, Gerkins, VR, Arthur, M, and Brown, SE,** Estrogens and Endometrial Cancer in a Retirement Community, New Eng J Med 294:1262, 1976.

35. **Hoover, R, Everson, R, Fraumeni, JF, Jr., and Myers, MH,** Cancer of the Uterine Corpus After Hormonal Treatment for Breast Cancer, Lancet 1:885, 1976.

36. FDA Drug Bulletin 6:19, 1976.

37. **Cramer, DR, Cutler, SJ, and Christine, B,** Trends in the Incidence of Endometrial Cancer in the United States, Gynec Oncology 2:130, 1974.

38. **Weiss, NS, Szekely, DR, and Austin, DF,** Increasing Incidence of Endometrial Cancer in the United States, New Eng J Med 294:1259, 1976.

39. **Hsueh, AJE, Peck, EJ, Jr., and Clark, JG,** Control of Uterine Estrogen Receptor Levels by Progesterone, Endocrinology 98:438, 1976.

40. **Tseng, L, and Gurpide, E,** Effects of Progestins on Estradiol Receptor Levels in Human Endometrium, J Clin Endocrinol Metab 41:402, 1975.

41. **Tseng, L, and Gurpide, E,** Induction of Human Endometrial Estradiol Dehydrogenase by Progestins, Endocrinology 97:825, 1975.

42. **Siiteri, PK, Schwarz, BE, and MacDonald, PC,** Estrogen Receptors and the Estrone Hypothesis in Relation to Endometrial and Breast Cancer, Gynec Oncology 2:228, 1974.

43. **Yen, SSC, Martin, PL, Burnier, AM, Czekala, NM, Gareaney, MO, Jr., and Callantine, MR,** Circulating Estradiol, Estrone, and Gonadotropin Levels Following the Administration of Orally Active 17β-Estradiol in Postmenopausal Women, J Clin Endocrinol Metab 40:518, 1975.

44. **Wise, AJ, Gross, MA, and Schalch, DS,** Quantitative Relationships of the Pituitary-gonadal Axis in Postmenopausal Women, J Lab Clin Med 81:28, 1974.

5   Amenorrhea

Few problems in gynecologic endocrinology are as challenging or taxing to the clinician as amenorrhea. The physician must be concerned with an array of potential diseases and disorders involving, in many instances, unfamiliar organ systems, some carrying morbid and even lethal consequences for the patient. All too often these factors lead to errors of omission and commission in diagnosis and therapeutic management. Not infrequently, the otherwise confident and experienced gynecologist dismisses the problem as too complex for his busy practice and refers the patient to a "specialist" in the field. In doing so, the nonavailability of sophisticated endocrine laboratory techniques is often cited as necessitating the costly and frequently inconvenient transfer of the patient.

The intent of this chapter is to provide a simple mechanism for differential diagnosis of amenorrhea of all types and chronology, utilizing procedures available to all physicians. Strict adherence to this design will unerringly pinpoint the organ system locus of disorder leading to the presenting symptom of amenorrhea. Once this is accomplished, the detailed evidence confirming the diagnosis can be sought and the assistance of appropriate specialists (neurosurgeon, internist, endocrinologist, psychiatrist) confidently chosen. In the end, the patient receives the most reliable diagnosis and therapy at minimum cost and optimum convenience.

The "workup" to be described is not new. With minor modifications, it has been continuously and successfully applied for more than 2 decades. Before presenting the diagnostic workup in detail, it is necessary to provide a definition of amenorrhea designating the appropriate selection of patients. In addition, a brief review of the physiologic mechanisms by which a menstrual flow is produced is included to clarify the logic of the various steps in the diagnostic procedure.

Definition of Amenorrhea

Any patient fulfilling the following criteria should be evaluated as having the clinical problem of amenorrhea

1. No menstruation by age 14 in the absence of growth or development of secondary sexual characteristics.

2. No menstruation by age 16 regardless of the presence of normal growth and development with the appearance of secondary sexual characteristics.

3. In a woman who has been menstruating, the absence of periods for a length of time equivalent to a total of at least three of the previous cycle intervals or 6 months of amenorrhea.

Having affirmed the traditional criteria, let us now point out that strict adherence to these criteria may result in improper management of individual cases. There is no reason to defer the evaluation of a young girl who presents with the obvious and blatant stigmata of Turner's syndrome. Similarly the 14-year-old girl with an absent vagina but who is otherwise completely normal should not be told to return in 2 years. Finally, the possibility of pregnancy should always be considered.

Another tradition has been to categorize amenorrhea as primary or secondary in nature. While these stipulations are inherent in the classic definitions noted above, experience has shown that premature categorization of this sort leads to diagnostic omission in certain instances, and frequently, unnecessary and expensive diagnostic procedures. Because the prescribed workup to be detailed herein applies comprehensively to all amenorrheas, the classical distinctions are not retained.

The clinical presence of menstrual function depends on visible external evidence of the menstrual discharge. This requires an intact outflow tract which connects the internal genital source of flow with the outside. As such, the outflow tract requires patency and continuity of the vaginal orifice, the vaginal canal, and the endocervix with the uterine cavity. The presence of a menstrual flow depends on the existence and development of the endometrium lining the uterine cavity. This tissue is stimulated and regulated by the proper quantity and sequence of the steroid hormones, estrogen and progesterone. The secretion of these hormones originates in the ovary, but more specifically in the evolving spectrum of follicle development, ovulation, and corpus luteum function. This essential maturation of the follicular apparatus is guided by the stimuli provided by the sequence and magnitude of the gonadotropins, follicle-stimulating hormone (FSH) and luteinizing hormone (LH), originating in the anterior pituitary. The secretion of these hormones is in turn directed by a specific peptide releasing hormone produced in the median eminence area of the basal hypothalamus and blood borne via the portal vessels of the stalk to action points within the anterior pituitary. The releasing hormone is regulated by a complex mechanism which integrates biophysical and biochemical information comprised of feedback levels of ovarian steroids and pituitary gonadotropins as well as neurohumors derived from higher hypothalamic and other CNS resources. The releasing hormone responds to both internal and external environmental information.

The basic principles underlying the physiology of menstrual function permit formulation of several discrete compartmental systems on which proper menstruation depends. It is useful to employ a diagnostic evaluation which segregates causes of amenorrhea into the following compartments:

Compartment I:
Disorders of outflow tract or uterine target organ.

Compartment II:
Disorders of the ovary.

Compartment III:
Disorders of the anterior pituitary.

Compartment IV:
Disorders of CNS (hypothalamic) factors.

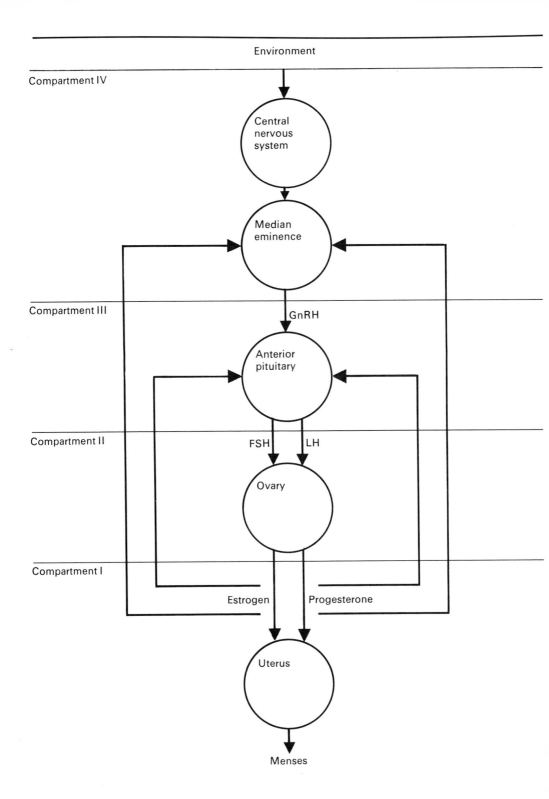

A patient with amenorrhea is exposed to a combined therapeutic and laboratory dissection according to the flow diagrams depicted. Amenorrhea is the sole pertinent initial item of information. Although additional data are undoubtedly available at this time, achieved by history and physical examination and evaluation of other endocrine glands such as the thyroid and adrenal, these items should not be utilized for diagnostic purposes until the entire workup is completed. Experience has shown that premature diagnostic bias at this point, while frequently accurate, not uncommonly leads to erroneous judgments as well as inappropriate, costly, and useless testing patterns.

Step 1

The initial step is to assess the level of endogenous estrogen and the competence of the outflow tract, and to measure the serum prolactin level. In order to test the pituitary-ovarian system, a course of a pure progestational agent totally devoid of estrogenic activity is administered. There are only two choices: progesterone in oil (200 mg intramuscularly) or the orally active compound, medroxyprogesterone acetate (Provera), 10 mg daily for 5 days. The use of an orally active agent avoids an unpleasant intramuscular injection. Other progestins, such as those in birth control pills, are not appropriate since they are metabolized to estrogens within the body, and therefore, do not exert a purely progestational effect.

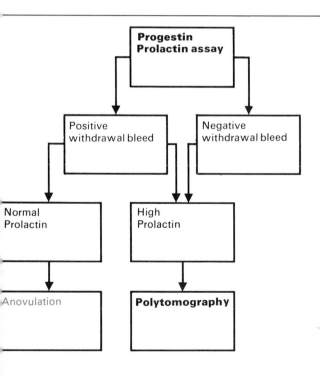

Within 2 to 7 days after the conclusion of progestational medication, the patient will either bleed or not bleed. If the patient bleeds, one has reliably established a diagnosis of anovulation. The presence of a functional outflow tract and a uterus lined by reactive endometrium sufficiently prepared by endogenous estrogen are confirmed. With this demonstration of the presence of estrogen, at least minimal function of the ovary, pituitary, and central nervous system is established. Obviously perfect integration of these systems has not been achieved, the dysfunction resulting in anovulation. At this point all that can be said is that all systems are present and functioning. Systematic analysis of the complex problem of anovulation is the subject of Chapter 6.

In the absence of galactorrhea and if the serum prolactin level is normal (less than 20 ng/ml), further evaluation for the presence of a pituitary tumor is unnecessary. If the serum prolactin level is elevated, polytomography of the sella turcica (discussed below) is essential. The presence of galactorrhea, regardless of the bleeding pattern or the prolactin level, dictates pituitary evaluation. Only a rare patient with a pituitary or nearby tumor will bleed following progestational medication, and the prolactin level serves as an effective screen for these patients. Because of the expense of polytomography, the following statement is a useful clinical rule of thumb: *a positive withdrawal bleeding response to progestational medication, the absence of galactorrhea, and a normal prolactin level together effectively rule out the presence of a pituitary tumor.*

How much bleeding constitutes a positive withdrawal response? The appearance of only a few blood spots following progestational medication implies marginal levels of endogenous estrogen. Such a patient should be followed closely and periodically reevaluated, since the marginally positive response may progress to a clearly negative response, placing the patient in a new diagnostic category. Bleeding in any amount beyond a few spots is considered a positive withdrawal response.

Step 2

If the course of progestational medication does not produce withdrawal flow, either the target organ outflow tract is inoperative or preliminary estrogen preparation of the endometrium has not occurred. Step 2 is designed to clarify this situation. Orally active estrogen is administered in quantity and duration certain to stimulate endometrial proliferation and withdrawal bleeding provided that a completely reactive uterus and patent outflow tract exist. An appropriate dose is 2.5 mg conjugated estrogens daily for 21 days. The terminal addition of an orally active progestational agent (Provera 10 mg daily for the last 5 days) is useful to achieve withdrawal. In this way the capacity of Compartment I is challenged by exogenous estrogen. In the absence of withdrawal flow, a validating second course of estrogen is a wise precaution.

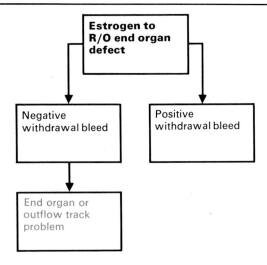

As a result of the pharmacologic test of Step 2, the patient with amenorrhea will either bleed or not bleed. *If there is no withdrawal flow, the diagnosis of a defect in the Compartment I systems (endometrium, outflow tract) can be made with confidence.* If withdrawal bleeding does occur, one can assume that Compartment I systems have normal functional abilities if properly stimulated by estrogen.

In a patient with normal external and internal genitalia by pelvic examination, and in the absence of a history of infection or trauma (such as curettage) Step 2 can be safely omitted. Abnormalities in the systems of Compartment I are not commonly encountered.

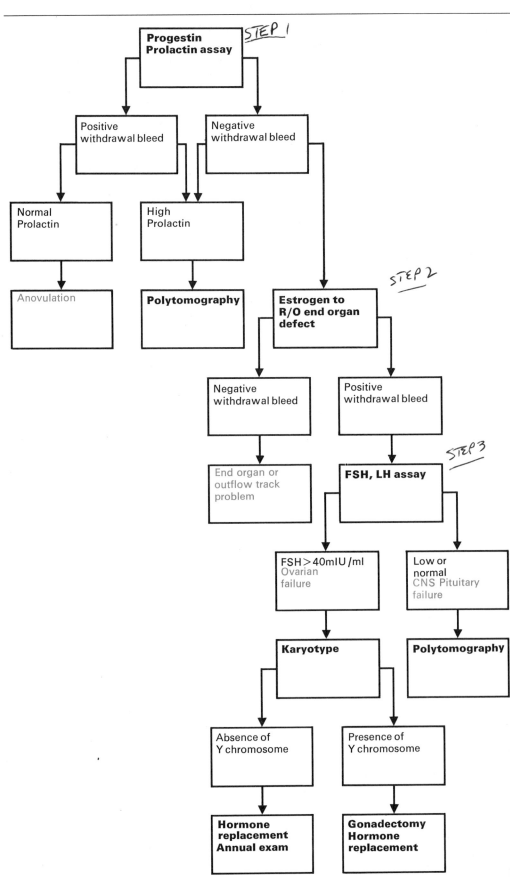

Step 3

With the elucidation of the amenorrheic patient's inability to provide adequate stimulatory amounts of estrogen, the physiologic mechanisms responsible for the elaboration of this steroid must be tested. In order to produce estrogen, gonads containing a normal follicular apparatus and sufficient pituitary gonadotropin as the hormonal means to stimulate that apparatus are required. Step 3 is designed to determine which of these two crucial components (gonadotropins or follicular activity) is functioning improperly.

This step involves an assay of the level of gonadotropins in the patient. Two important points must be made at this step in the workup. Since Step 2 involved administration of exogenous estrogen, endogenous gonadotropin levels may be artificially and temporarily altered from their true baseline concentrations. Hence, a delay of 2 weeks following Step 2 must ensue before doing Step 3, the gonadotropin assay. The second point relates to the type of assay to be done. The total urinary gonadotropin assay performed on a 24-hour urine specimen should be abandoned. Even in a normal patient the urinary assay may return with a zero level or a postmenopausal level. In recent years most physicians have turned to the more precise radioimmunoassay of gonadotropins in serum. The convenience of a single blood specimen is matched by the reliability of the method, and in 2 weeks time one can receive the result from a variety of nationwide commercial or university laboratories. The normal range for LH in serum is 5–25 mIU/ml; under 5 mIU/ml is abnormally low and over 25 mIU/ml is abnormally high. One should keep in mind that the midcycle surge of LH is approximately three times the baseline level. Therefore, if the patient does not bleed 2 weeks after the blood sample was obtained, the high level can be safely interpreted as abnormal. An FSH level below 5 mIU/ml is abnormally low and over 40 mIU is abnormally high.

Step 3 is designed to determine whether the lack of estrogen is due to a fault in the follicle (Compartment II) or in the CNS-pituitary axis (Compartments III and IV). The result of the gonadotropin assay in the amenorrheic woman who does not bleed following a progestational agent will be abnormally high, abnormally low, or in the normal range.

If the FSH is over 40 mIU/ml, the cause of the amenorrhea is gonadal failure. If gonadotropins are abnormally low or in the normal range, pituitary failure or inactivity is diagnosed.

In the presence of normal hypothalamic-pituitary compartments, castration produces peak elevations of FSH and LH secretion. On repletion of steroid feedback, accomplished with estrogen replacement, gonadotropins return to normal noncastrate levels. On the other hand, no matter how high estrogen levels are driven by therapy, gonadotropins cannot be reduced to zero. When the absence of endogenous estrogen causes amenorrhea, extremely low or absent gonadotropins indicate pituitary-CNS failure, whereas high gonadotropins signify gonadal failure.

In practice, a low LH (less than 5 mIU/ml) has been found to be a more reliable indicator of hypogonadotropism, while a high FSH (over 40 mIU/ml) has proved to be a reliable indicator of ovarian failure. FSH values within the normal range (5 to 30 mIU/ml) indicate the presence of ovarian follicles, whereas values over 40 mIU/ml are found only when the supply of ovarian follicles has been exhausted. (1)

Patients with FSH levels over 40 mIU/ml will not respond to ovulatory drugs and should be considered sterile. The association between a high FSH, especially when accompanied by a high LH, and ovarian failure is so reliable that further attempts to document the state of the ovaries are unnecessary and unwarranted. Specifically, laparoscopy in order to visualize the ovaries and to demonstrate the presence of follicles by biopsy only exposes the patient to unessential surgical and anesthetic risks. (2) Because the result of a high FSH has such an immense bearing on the future fertility of the patient, repeat sampling is a wise precaution.

Be aware that high levels of LH by themselves do not reliably establish ovarian failure. Occasionally high peaks of LH may be found in the presence of adequate ovarian follicles. This can be partly explained by the pulsatile secretion pattern associated with LH, producing a marked variation in single measurements taken at random. However, serial determinations of LH and FSH do not yield any additional information and are not worthwhile.

There are conditions in which there is a single gonadotropin deficiency. A patient with an isolated deficiency of FSH would have primary amenorrhea, a high LH level, and undetectable FSH. (3) Other rare conditions which may be associated with high gonadotropins include: the resistant ovary syndrome, the perimenopausal period, gonadotropin-producing tumors, and primary amenorrhea due to 17-hydroxylase deficiency.

High Gonadotropins. Patients with an FSH value over 40 mIU/ml, must have a karyotype in order to rule out the presence of a Y chromosome. The presence of a Y chromosome in an adult carries with it an approximate 25% incidence of malignant tumors within the gonad. Thus all patients who have a Y chromosome in the blood karyotype must have gonadectomy. It is possible that a Y-containing mosaic may be present in the gonad despite the presence of a normal karyotype in the blood. A blood assay for the H-Y antigen (see Chapter 11) may detect the existence of cryptic testicular tissue even in the presence of a normal karyotype. As a precaution, all patients with ovarian failure and normal karyotypes should have an annual pelvic examination. Such preventive care is also indicated in that these patients will be on hormone replacement therapy.

At what age is a karyotype no longer necessary? After the age of 35, an elevated FSH level and amenorrhea are best regarded as premature menopause. Further evaluation is not necessary. Between the ages of 30 and 35, the emergence of a malignant tumor in a heretofore unsuspected Y-containing karyotype is unlikely, but to be safe, a karyotype should be performed. Approximately 30% of Y-containing mosaics will not be associated with signs of masculinization, hence it is unwise to rely on the absence of hirsutism or virilization to establish a normal karyotype.

Normal Gonadotropins. Why is it that hypoestrogenic (negative progestational withdrawal) patients will frequently have normal circulating levels of FSH and LH as measured by the radioimmunoassay? If normal gonadotropins were truly present in the circulation, follicular growth should be maintained and estrogen levels would be adequate to provide a positive withdrawal bleed. The answer to this paradox may lie in the heterogeneity of the glycoprotein hormones.

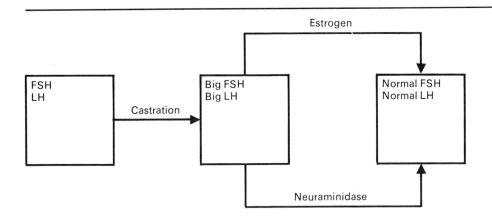

FSH and LH from ovariectomized monkeys are larger in average molecular size. (4) This effect of ovariectomy can be reversed with the administration of estradiol. Thus the hypoestrogenic environment of the pituitary gland results in larger than normal gonadotropins. This phenomenon probably involves changes in the sialic acid content of the gonadotropins because digestion with the enzyme neuraminidase reduces or abolishes the differences in molecular size. Therefore it is probable that the radioimmunoassay recognizes (immunologically) the larger FSH and LH molecules, but these abnormal molecules are not biologically active. The significant clinical point is that FSH and LH levels in the normal range, in a patient with a negative progestational withdrawal test, are consistent with pituitary-CNS failure.

Low Gonadotropins. If the gonadotropin assay is abnormally low or in the normal range, one final localization is required to distinguish between a pituitary (Compartment III) or CNS-hypothalamic (Compartment IV) cause for the amenorrhea. Special skull x-rays (polytomography) should be obtained to examine the sella turcica for signs of abnormal change.

Polytomography consists of tomographic sections (at approximately 1 mm increments) of the sella turcica in the lateral and anteroposterior projections with a hypocycloidal movement which blurs structures not in the plane of section, and gives excellent focal resolution. This technique will detect a microadenoma of 5 to 10 mm in size. With a tumor of this size, a routine skull film will indicate a normal sella turcica. (5, 6) Typical polytomographic findings consistent with a pituitary tumor are: localized bulging of the anteroinferior wall on one side (lateralization is a significant characteristic), and erosion (demineralization) of the anterior or posterior floor of the sella. When the adenoma grows above 10 mm, the diameters of the sella are increased.

Visual field examination is reserved for the evaluation of the patient with abnormal polytomography. We have found that utilization of the visual field examination as a screening procedure is useless. The visual fields have always proved to be normal unless a significant change was already present in the sella turcica.

Laboratory evaluation of thyroid function (including measurement of TSH) is indicated and should be added to the screening procedure.

If amenorrhea is the only presenting symptom in an otherwise normal individual, sella turcica evaluation should be obtained annually as a precaution to rule out an emerging tumor. The patient with an insidiously evolving pituitary tumor may present with amenorrhea years before the tumor becomes evident by sella turcica x-rays. A spectrum beginning with a mildly compromised ovulatory capacity and extending to panhypopituitarism can be encountered. Usually, over the course of time, deterioration in tropic activity is seen, with withdrawal of activity following a fairly predictable pattern: first growth hormone, then FSH and LH, and finally TSH and ACTH. Less commonly, peculiar isolated loss of specific tropic hormones may be found. Only rare cases have been reported of gonadotropin-producing pituitary tumors. (7, 8)

Evaluation of the Abnormal Sella Turcica

Expectations for the utilization of gonadotropin-releasing hormone (GnRH) to discriminate between disorders of the hypothalamus and the anterior pituitary have not been realized. Tremendous variability in response is the rule, even to the degree that the patient with a pituitary tumor may or may not respond to GnRH stimulation. Likewise, maneuvers designed to alter prolactin secretion (L-DOPA, phenothiazine, and ergot alkaloid administration) cannot identify the patient with a pituitary tumor. Therefore the serum prolactin level, and polytomography are the two major screening procedures.

In the presence of a tumor there is a positive correlation between prolactin levels and the size of the sella turcica. (9) However significant tumors may be found in amenorrheic women with normal or slightly elevated prolactin levels. Further sampling is not useful since a random single blood sample appears to be reliable in detecting elevated levels of prolactin. (10)

The physician must also bring his clinical acumen to bear on the problem of amenorrhea. Is there a background of serious emotional disease, or the disruptive intake of psychotropic drugs? Are there the ominous signs of acromegaly or inappropriate lactation? Frequently it is only with meticulous and continued observation and testing over a long period of time that a slowly growing lesion will appear with sufficient clarity to warrant the appropriate therapeutic reaction. If the x-ray of the sella and neurologic scrutiny raise the suspicion of tumor, further evaluation requires an inpatient program along with consultation with expert neurosurgical resources.

Inpatient evaluation of an abnormal sella turcica includes the following schedule of consultations and procedures:

Admission Day

1. Neurosurgical consultation.

2. Ophthalmological consultation for visual field examination.

First Hospital Day

1. Baseline studies: thyroid indices, TSH, FSH, LH, prolactin, growth hormone, AM and PM cortisol.

2. Computerized transverse axial tomography (useful in outlining suprasellar extension and avoids the need for angiography prior to pneumoencephalography).

Second Hospital Day

1. Pneumoencephalogram with tomography (essential to determine suprasellar extension and to rule out the empty sella syndrome).

2. If acromegalic, glucose tolerance test.

Based upon our recent experience with this problem, we have found that the insulin tolerance test and visual field examination are not useful procedures except for establishing a baseline. The insulin tolerance test indicates the pituitary reserve for growth hormone and ACTH. Growth hormone, cortisol, and glucose levels are obtained at time 0, 15, 30, 45, 60, 90, and 120 minutes. Regular insulin (0.15 units/Kg) is given intravenously at time 0. A glucose decrement of 50% or more should be associated with an increment in growth hormone of more than 5 ng/ml. (11)

The assay of pituitary hormones in cerebrospinal fluid removed during pneumoencephalography may be helpful in detecting large tumors. Elevated levels in the CSF indicate suprasellar extension. (12) Evaluation of thyroid function is important in order to detect those patients with elevated prolactin levels due to hypothyroidism. The incidence of empty sella turcia is significant, and pneumoencephalography is essential to avoid unnecessary surgery.

Clinical decisions are largely based upon the results of the prolactin assay, polytomography, and pneumoencephalography.

Specific Disorders Within Compartments	With only modest effort, expense, and time, the amenorrheic problem has been dissected into compartments of dysfunction which positively correlate with specific organ systems. At this point, with the specific anatomic loci of the defect defined, the clinician can now undertake steps to elucidate the specific disorder leading to amenorrhea. Within each anatomic compartment certain diagnostic frequencies are observed.
Compartment I	**Asherman's Syndrome.** Secondary amenorrhea follows destruction of the endometrium (Asherman's Syndrome). This condition generally is the result of an overzealous postpartum curettage resulting in intrauterine scarification and showing a typical pattern of multiple synechiae on a hysterogram. In the presence of normal ovarian function, the basal body temperature over 1 month's time will be biphasic. We treat Asherman's syndrome with a dilatation and curettage to break up the synechiae, and if necessary utilize an on-the-table hysterogram to ensure a free uterine cavity. Current clinical investigation indicates that hysteroscopy with direct lysis of adhesions is a preferred alternative to the "blind" dilatation and curettage (D and C).

At operation, a method should be utilized to prevent the sides of the uterine cavity from adhering. Previously an IUD was used for this purpose, however, a pediatric Foley catheter appears to be a better method. (13) The bag is filled with 3 ml of fluid, and the catheter is removed after 7 days. A broad-spectrum antibiotic is started preoperatively and maintained for 10 days. The patient is treated for 6 months with high stimulatory doses of estrogen (e.g. conjugated estrogens 10 mg daily 3 weeks out of 4 with Provera 10 mg daily added during the 3rd week). When the initial attempt fails to reestablish menstrual flow, repeated attempts are worthwhile. Persistent treatment with repeated procedures may be necessary to regain reproductive potential.

Infectious impairment of the endometrium resulting in amenorrhea is usually attributed to tuberculosis, a rare but still present condition in the United States. Diagnosis is made by culture of the menstrual discharge or endometrial biopsy. Uterine schistosomiasis may be another rare cause of end organ failure and eggs may be found in urine, feces, rectal scrapings, menstrual discharge, or endometrium.

Müllerian Anomalies. In primary amenorrheas, discontinuity by segmental disruptions of the Müllerian tube should be ruled out. Good clinical practice demands a survey which begins distally and works proximally. Thus, imperforate hymen, obliteration of the vaginal orifice, and lapses in continuity of the vaginal canal must be ruled out by direct observation. The cervix or the entire uterus may be absent. Far less common, the uterus may be present, but the cavity absent, or, in the presence of a cavity, the endometrium may be congenitally lacking. With exception of the latter items, the clinical problem of amenorrhea is compounded by the painful distension of hematocolpos, hematometra, or hematoperitoneum. In all instances an effort must be made to incise and drain from below at the points of closure of the Müllerian tube. The unfortunate consequences of operative extirpation of painful masses from above with danger to bladder, ureter, and rectum, as well as irretrievable loss of distended but otherwise healthy, competent tissues are rare but well-remembered. In complicated circumstances reestablishment of Müllerian duct continuity can be surgically achieved. Depending on the type of anomaly, associated lesions of lower genitourinary and gastrointestinal tracts should be ruled out.

Müllerian Agenesis. Lack of Müllerian development (Mayer-Rokitansky-Kuster-Hauser Syndrome) is the diagnosis for the individual with primary amenorrhea and no apparent vagina. (14) This is a relatively common cause of primary amenorrhea, more frequent than testicular feminization, and second only to gonadal dysgensis. These patients have an absence or hypoplasia of the vagina. The uterus may be normal, but lacking a conduit to the introitus, or there may only be rudimentary bicornuate cords present. If a partial endometrial cavity is present, cyclic abdominal pain may be a complaint. Because of the similarity to some types of male pseudohermaphroditism, it is worthwhile to demonstrate the normal female karyotype. Ovarian function is normal, and can be documented with basal body temperatures or peripheral levels of progesterone. Growth and development are normal. Although usually sporadic, occasional occurence may be noted within a family.

Further evaluation should include radiologic studies. Approximately one third have abnormal kidneys and 12% or more have skeletal anomalies, mostly involving the spine. (14). When the presence of a uterine structure is suspected on examination, ultrasound may be utilized to depict the size and symmetry of the structure.

Because of the difficulties and complications experienced in surgical series, we favor abandonment of the surgical construction of an artificial vagina. Instead, we encourage the use of progressive dilatation as first described by

Frank (15) and later by Wabrek, et al (16). Beginning first in a downward, posterior direction, and then after 2 weeks changing upward to the usual line of the vaginal axis, pressure with commercially available glass vaginal dilators is carried out for 20 minutes daily to the point of modest discomfort. Utilizing increasingly larger dilators, a functional vagina can be created in approximately 6 weeks. Operative treatment should be reserved for those cases in which a well-formed uterus is present and fertility might be preserved. The symptoms of retained menstruation should identify these patients.

Reassurance and support are necessary to carry a patient through these procedures. Problems with body image and sexual enjoyment may be avoided and although infertile, a full and normal life as a woman can be achieved.

Testicular Feminization. When a blind vaginal canal is encountered and the uterus is absent, the possibility of testicular feminization must be excluded. The patient with testicular feminization is a male pseudohermaphrodite. The adjective male refers to the gonadal sex, thus the individual has testes and an XY karyotype; pseudohermaphrodite means that the genitalia are opposite of the gonads, thus the individual is phenotypically female, but with absent or meager pubic and axillary hair.

The male pseudohermaphrodite is a genetic and gonadal male with failure of virilization. Failures in male development can be considered as a spectrum with incomplete forms of testicular feminization being represented by some androgen response. Transmission of this disorder is by means of an X-linked recessive gene responsible for the androgen intracellular receptor. (17) Clinically the diagnosis should be considered in: (1) a female child with inguinal hernias, since the testes are frequently partially descended; (2) a patient with primary amenorrhea and an absent uterus; and (3) a patient with absent body hair.

These patients appear normal at birth, except for the possible presence of an inguinal hernia, and most patients are not seen by a physician until puberty. Growth and development are normal, although overall height is usually greater than average and there may be a eunuchoidal tendency (long arms, big hands and feet). The breasts, although large, are abnormal; actual glandular tissue is not abundant and the nipples are small and areolae are pale. More than 50% have an inguinal hernia; the labia minora are usually underdeveloped, and the blind vagina is less deep than normal. Rudimentary Fallopian tubes are composed of fibromuscular tissue with only occasional epithelial lining.

The testes may be intra-abdominal, but often are in the hernia. They are similar to any cryptorchid testis except that they may be nodular. After puberty, the testis has immature tubular development lined by immature germ cells and Sertoli cells. There is no spermatogenesis. The incidence of neoplasia in these gonads is high. In 50 reported cases 30 years old or more, there were 11 malignancies, 15 adenomas, and 10 benign cysts, thus a 22% incidence of malignancy and a 52% incidence of neoplasia. (18) Therefore, once full development is attained after puberty, the gonads should be removed and the patient placed on hormonal replacement therapy. This is the only exception to the rule that gonads with a Y chromosome should be removed prior to puberty. The reason is that development achieved with hormonal replacement does not seem to match the smooth pubertal changes due to endogenous hormones.

When first studied, it was found that the urinary 17-ketosteroids were normal, and it was suggested that there might be a resistance to androgen action rather than an absence of androgens — a congenital androgen insensitivity. Indeed, the plasma levels of testosterone are in the normal to high male range, and the plasma clearance and metabolism of testosterone are normal. Thus, these patients produce testosterone, but they do not respond to androgens, either their own or those given locally or systemically. Therefore, the critical steps in sexual differentiation which require androgens fail to take place and development is totally female.

Cases of incomplete testicular feminization represent individuals with some androgen effect. These cases may have clitoral enlargement or a phallus may even be present. Axillary and pubic hair develop along with breast growth. Gonadectomy should not be deferred in such cases, but would in fact obviate unwanted further virilization. Patients with a deficit in testicular 17-dehydrogenase activity will have impaired testosterone production, and present clinically as incomplete testicular feminization. Since treatment is the same, precise diagnosis is not essential.

Unthinking and needless disclosures of the gonadal and chromosomal sex to a patient with testicular feminization can be disastrous. It should be emphasized that although infertile these patients are completely female in their gender identity, and this should never be challenged, but rather reinforced.

Turner's Syndrome. Turner's syndrome is a well-known and thoroughly discussed entity. The characteristics of short stature, webbed neck, shield chest, and increased carrying angle combined with hypergonadotropic hypoestrogenic amenorrhea make a correct diagnosis usually possible on the most superficial evaluation. However, special attention must be given to the less common variations of this syndrome. Coarctation of the aorta and various renal collecting system anomalies must be ruled out. A karyotype should be performed on all patients with elevated gonadotropins, despite the appearance of a typical case of Turner's. The presence of a pure syndrome, 45, X chromosome single cell line, should be confirmed. This expensive test cannot be viewed just as a step toward academic perfection.

Mosaicism. The presence of mosaicism (multiple cell lines of varying sex chromosome composition) must be ruled out for a very important reason. The presence of a Y chromosome in the karyotype requires laparotomy and excision of the gonadal areas, on the basis that the presence of any medullary (testicular) component within the gonad is a predisposing factor to tumor formation and to heterosexual development (virilization). Only in the patient with the complete form of testicular feminization can laparotomy be deferred until after puberty, since the individual is resistant to androgens. In all other patients with a Y chromosome, gonadectomy should be performed before puberty to avoid virilization. One should be aware that approximately 30% of patients with a Y chromosome will not develop any signs of virilization. Therefore, even the normal appearing adult patient with elevated serum levels of gonadotropins must be karyotyped to detect a silent Y chromosome, so that prophylactic gonadectomy may be performed before neoplastic changes occur.

The impact of mosaicism, even in the absence of a Y-containing line, is significant. With an XX component (e.g. XX/XO), functional cortical (ovarian) tissue can be anticipated to exist within the gonad, leading to a variety of responses, including some degree of female development, and on occasion even menses and reproduction. These individuals may appear normal, attaining normal stature before premature menopause is experienced. The menopause is early, presumably because the number of functioning follicles was limited by an abnormal chromosomal constitution.

This complex array of gonadal dysgenesis variations, from the typical pure form to an otherwise normal appearing and functioning woman with premature menopause, is the result of a variety of mosaicism which produces a complex mixture of cortical and medullary gonadal tissue. The clinical importance of this information justifies obtaining karyotypes in all cases of elevated gonadotropins.

Assays for the H-Y antigen (see Chapter 11) may prove to be more reliable than a karyotype in the effort to detect the presence of testicular tissue.

Gonadal Agenesis. No complicated clinical problems accompany the gonadal failure due to agenesis. Without precise information, only conjecture as to the causes of absent development can be made. Thus, viral and metabolic influences in early gestation are suspected events. Nevertheless, the final result is irretrievable—hypergonadotropic hypogonadism.

The Resistant Ovary Syndrome. There is a rare patient with amenorrhea who has elevated gonadotropins despite the presence of ovarian follicles. (19) These patients require large amounts of exogeneous gonadotropins in order to produce follicular growth and estrogen production. To arrive at a correct diagnosis, laparotomy is necessary to achieve adequate histological evaluation of the ovaries (since laparoscopic biopsy is not representative). (2) Because of the rarity of this condition, and the very low chance of achieving pregnancy even with high doses of exogenous gonadotropins, we do not feel it is worthwhile to perform a laparotomy for the purpose of ovarian biopsy on every patient with amenorrhea, high gonadotropins, and a normal karyotype.

A situation similar to the resistant ovary syndrome may be encountered in the perimenopausal period. In the perimenopausal period (whether it be premature at age 30 to 38, or at the expected time) the remaining few follicles may fail to respond until a high level of gonadotropin is reached. Hence a period of amenorrhea with postmenopausal levels of FSH and LH may very rarely be followed by a pregnancy. (20)

Premature ovarian failure due to antibodies to steroid-producing cells is almost always associated with idiopathic Addison's disease.

Compartment III

Disorders of the hypothalamic-pituitary axis pose the most exacting challenge for the gynecologist. Through the appearance of amenorrhea, the patient with a slowly growing pituitary tumor may present years before the tumor becomes evident by radiologic techniques. Sometimes the suspicion of tumor is increased because of clinical signs of acromegaly, Cushing's syndrome due to excessive secretion of ACTH, or inappropriate lactation, although nonfunctioning tumors must also be considered. Prolactin secreting tumors may be seen in preadolescent and adolescent children, and may be a cause of failure of growth and development.

Not all intrasellar masses are neoplastic. Gummas, tuberculomas, and fat deposits have been reported as causes of pituitary compression leading to hypogonadotropic amenorrhea. Nearby lesions such as internal carotid artery aneurysms and obstruction of the aqueduct of Sylvius may also cause amenorrhea. Pituitary insufficiency may be secondary to ischemia and infarction, and appear as a late sequela to obstetrical hemorrhage — the well-known Sheehan's syndrome.

Pituitary Tumors. With the utilization of the serum prolactin assay and the increased sensitivity of the polytomographic technique, the association of amenorrhea and small pituitary tumors (microadenomas of 5 to 10 mm diameter) is being recognized more frequently. At this time the exact incidence of this clinical problem is unknown. In autopsy series, the number of pituitary glands found to contain adenomas ranges from 9% to 22.5%. (21, 22) The age distribution ranged from 2 to 86, with the greatest incidence in the 6th decade of life. The sex distribution was equal.

Exact statements regarding incidence and frequency will require further accumulation of clinical experience. Preliminary information suggests the following:

1. A high prolactin level may be encountered in 20% of women with no obvious cause of amenorrhea. (23) (It is not surprising that prolactin levels are not elevated in women with obvious causes of amenorrhea, such as genetic problems, anorexia nervosa, and ovarian failure.)

2. Only one third of patients with high prolactin levels will have galactorrhea, probably because the low estrogen environment associated with the amenorrhea prevents a normal response of the breast to prolactin.

3. Possibly as many as one third of patients with secondary amenorrhea will have a pituitary adenoma, (23), and if galactorrhea is present, perhaps one half will have an abnormal sella turcica. (6)

4. In patients with pituitary tumors, the association of amenorrhea and elevated prolactin levels is high. In one series of 62 patients with pituitary tumors (without acromegaly or Cushing's syndrome), 75% of the patients with amenorrhea had elevated prolactin levels. (6)

An important consideration of this problem is the behavior of the adenoma during pregnancy. In the latter half of pregnancy, pituitary and parasellar tumors can expand and lead to optic chiasmal compression, which usually regresses after delivery. This sequence may return in successive pregnancies, eventually leading to complete blindness. (24) In addition to visual disturbances, persistent or worsening headaches are usual symptoms of an enlarging tumor.

113

Fortunately the increased ability to detect pituitary tumors has been accompanied by the development of a surgical technique which very effectively removes the small tumors with a high margin of safety. This technique is the transphenoidal approach to the sella turcica utilizing the operating microscope. (25) The transphenoidal approach is via a sublabial incision (under the upperlip), with dissection under the nasal mucosa, removal of the nasal septum to expose the sphenoidal sinus, and resection of the floor of the sphenoid sinus to expose the sella turcica. The operating microscope adds magnification to allow direct visualization. Tumor tissue is usually distinguishable from the yellow-orange, firm tissue of the normal anterior pituitary. However since pituitary adenomas do not have a capsule, the borderline between tumor and normal tissue is often doubtful. The ideal time for excision is when the adenoma is a small nodule. When enlarged it becomes difficult to distinguish normal from pathological tissue. Once the adenoma grows beyond the sella, total removal is essentially impossible. The need for postoperative irradiation is determined by histologic examination of the edges of the resected tissue, and postoperative prolactin levels. Visual impairment due to suprasellar extension improves immediately with operative relief of pressure on the optic nerves.

These considerations have led to the following guidelines (which may change as clinical experience and data accumulate):

1. *Abnormal Polytomography and Elevated Prolactin.*
Admit for inpatient evaluation as outlined previously in Step 3.

If pneumoencephalography indicates the presence of a tumor, perform surgery, transphenoidal microsurgery if possible.

If pneumoencephalography is normal, but the prolactin level is very high, or anterior pituitary function other than gonadotropin secretion is also impaired: perform transphenoidal microsurgery.

If pneumoencephalography is normal, and the prolactin level is only moderately elevated (20–50 ng/ml), the decision is difficult. If the patient desires pregnancy and treatment with ergot alkaloids is not available, microsurgery is appropriate. If the polytomogram is only minimally abnormal, medical treatment with ergot alkaloids (with close follow-up) is also appropriate. Because it is currently impossible to determine which tumors will grow and which will persist with little, if any, change over the years, it is reasonable to adopt a conservative approach as long as close surveillance is maintained.

2. *Abnormal Polytomography and Normal Prolactin.*
Admit for inpatient evaluation.

If the pneumoencephalogram is normal, and there is no other impairment of anterior pituitary function, follow closely. Evidence of growth may appear within 6 months, or not for 10–20 years. If pregnancy is achieved, frequent visual field evaluation is indicated.

If pneumoencephalography is consistent with a significant tumor or if there is impaired pituitary function in addition to amenorrhea, perform transphenoidal microsurgery.

If polytomography is only minimally abnormal, it is appropriate to consider postponing inpatient evaluation, and following the patient with repeat prolactin measurements and periodic polytomography (perhaps of limited scope, utilizing only a few views).

3. *Normal Polytomography and Elevated Prolactin.*
If the prolactin level is very high, admit for inpatient evaluation. If further evaluation is negative, or the prolactin level is 20–50 ng/ml, the patient may be followed closely, or treated with ergot alkaloids. A tumor may be present, but it may be too small to have produced changes which can be detected.

4. *Normal Polytomography and Normal Prolactin.*
Annual evaluation (polytomography of limited scope and prolactin assay) is necessary because the nature of these tumors is to grow slowly. Meanwhile the patient should be given hormone replacement therapy, or induction of ovulation should be pursued if pregnancy is desired. An initial program of ergot alkaloids may be considered because even anovulatory patients with normal levels of prolactin have responded with ovulation. (26)

The reason for the amenorrhea associated with elevated prolactin levels is not exactly clear. Prolactin may interfere with ovarian response to gonadotropins as well as the pituitary response to GnRH. Regardless of the mechanism, treatment which lowers the circulating levels of prolactin restores ovarian responsiveness and menstrual function. This is true whether the treatment consists of removal of a prolactin-secreting tumor or suppression of prolactin secretion. Because ergot alkaloids inhibit both prolactin secretion and growth of tumor cells (9, 27), surgical treatment may not be necessary for all patients, especially those patients with only minimal radiologic evidence for a tumor. Final decisions regarding this problem await the knowledge to be gained from acquired clinical experience.

The Empty Sella Syndrome. A patient may have an abnormal sella turcica, but rather than a tumor, she may have the empty sella syndrome. This is a condition in which there is a congenital incompleteness of the sellar diaphragm, allowing an extension of the subarachnoid space into the pituitary fossa. The pituitary gland is flattened, and the sella floor may be demineralized due to pressure from the cerebrospinal fluid. The empty sella syndrome may also occur secondary to surgery or radiotherapy.

An empty sella is found in approximately 5% of autopsies and approximately 85% are in women, mostly middle aged and obese. (28) (Obesity may lead to an elevation in CSF pressure.) The most common endocrine problem found in approximately one third of cases is decreased gonadotropins and a reduced response of growth hormone to hypoglycemia. Adrenal and thyroid function are rarely affected. Occasionally, rhinorrhea may develop.

This condition is benign; it does not progress to pituitary failure. The chief hazard to the patient is inadvertent treatment for a pituitary tumor. Even though enlargement of the sella turcica with a normal shape is more likely an empty sella than a tumor (29), *all patients should have pneumoencephalography prior to surgical intervention.*

Compartment IV

Hypothalamic Amenorrhea. Compartment IV (hypothalamic) problems are usually diagnosed by exclusion of pituitary lesions, and are the most common category of hypogonadotropic amenorrheas. Frequently there is an association with a stressful situation. In a study of the total female population aged 18–35 years of Uppsala, Sweden, pronounced psychologic stress was more frequent in women with secondary amenorrhea than in their age-matched controls. (30) There was also a higher proportion of underweight women and a higher occurrence of previous menstrual irregularity. Nevertheless, the physician is obliged to go through the process of excluding other causes of amenorrhea prior to prescribing hormone replacement therapy or attempting induction of ovulation in order to achieve pregnancy. A good practice is to evaluate such patients annually after a 2 month period without hormone medication. Returning function will thus be detected by rising gonadotropins and the demonstration of a positive withdrawal response to a progestational agent. Even though a patient may not be currently interested in pursuing pregnancy, it is important to assure these patients that at the appropriate time, treatment for induction of ovulation will be available and that fertility can be achieved. Concern with potential fertility is often an unspoken fear, especially in the younger patients. On the other hand, induction of ovulation with clomiphene or Pergonal should be carried out only for the purpose of producing a pregnancy. There is no evidence that cyclic hormone administration or induction of ovulation will stimulate the return of normal function.

Anorexia. A special example of hypothalamic amenorrhea is that associated with weight loss. It is true that obesity may be associated with amenorrhea, but amenorrhea in an obese patient is usually due to anovulation, and a hypogonadotropic state is not encountered unless

116

the patient also has a severe emotional disorder. Acute weight loss, on the other hand, in some unknown way, may lead to the hypogonadotropic state. Again the physician must exclude the presence of a tumor, and the diagnosis is made by exclusion.

Clinically, a spectrum is encountered from a limited period of amenorrhea associated with a crash diet to the severely ill patient with the life-threatening attrition of anorexia nervosa. It is a common experience for the gynecologist to be the first to recognize anorexia nervosa in a patient presenting with the complaint of amenorrhea. It is also not infrequent that a gynecologist will evaluate and manage an infertility problem due to hypogonadotropism and not be aware of a developing case of anorexia. It is important that attention be directed to this syndrome which is associated with a mortality rate of approximately 7%. (31)

The serious case of anorexia nervosa is seen more often by an internist. However the borderline anorexic frequently presents to the gynecologist as a teenager characterized by low body weight, amenorrhea, and hyperactivity (excellent grades and many extracurricular activities). The amenorrhea can precede, follow, or appear coincidentally with the weight loss. Endocrine studies can be summarized as follows (31, 32, 33): The FSH level is normal. The LH level is low. 17-ketosteroids and 17-hydroxysteroids may be low and plasma cortisol levels are elevated. Thyroid studies are normal, except for low T_3 levels, suggesting an impaired peripheral conversion of T_4 to T_3. Prolactin levels are normal.

There is a decreased response to GnRH in anorexia nervosa. The central origin for the amenorrhea is suggested by the demonstration that the response to GnRH is regained at approximately 15% below the ideal weight, and this return to normal responsiveness occurs before the resumption of menses. (34) This change in pituitary responsiveness is not seen in women with secondary amenorrhea which is not assocated with self-imposed weight loss.

Extensive laboratory testing in these patients is not necessary. Adherence to our scheme for the evaluation of amenorrhea is indicated to rule out other pathological processes, however further endocrine assessment is not essential for patient management. It is believed that because of a fear of the responsibilities and consequences of sexual maturation, these patients avoid development during adolescence by avoiding weight gain. (35) A careful and gentle revelation to the patient of the relationship between the amenorrhea and the low body weight is often all that is necessary to stimulate the patient to return to normal weight and normal menstrual function. Occasionally it is necessary to see the patient frequently and become involved in a program of daily calorie counting (a minimum intake of 2600 calories) in order to break the patient's established eating habits. If progress

117

is slow, hormone replacement therapy should be initiated. In an adult weighing less than 100 pounds, continued weight loss requires psychiatric consultation.

Amenorrhea and Anosmia. A rare condition in females is the syndrome of hypogonadotropic hypogonadism associated with anosmia. A similar syndrome in the male is hereditary and known as Kallman's Syndrome. In the female, this problem is characterized by primary amenorrhea, infantile sexual development, low gonadotropins, a normal female karyotype, and the inability to perceive odors, e.g. coffee grounds or perfume. (36) The gonads can respond to gonadotropins, therefore induction of ovulation with exogenous gonadotropins has been successful. However clomiphene is ineffective.

Postpill Amenorrhea. It has been assumed that amenorrhea may reflect persistent suppressive effects of oral contraceptive medication or the use of the intramuscular depot form of medroxyprogesterone acetate. Recently it has been appreciated that the fertility rate is normal following discontinuance of either of these forms of contraception (Chapter 14). Therefore amenorrhea following the use of steroids for contraception requires investigation as described in order to avoid missing a pituitary tumor.

Hormone Replacement Therapy

The patient who is hypoestrogenic and is not a candidate for induction of ovulation deserves hormone replacement therapy (discussed in Chapter 4). This includes patients appropriately evaluated and diagnosed as gonadal failure, patients with hypothalamic amenorrhea, and postgonadectomy patients. A good schedule is the following: on days 1 through 24 of each month, take 1.25 mg of conjugated estrogens; on days 20 through 24, add 10 mg of medroxyprogesterone acetate (Provera). Beginning medication on the first of every month establishes an easily remembered routine. Menstruation generally occurs 3 days after the last medication, the 27th of each month. In a few individuals the estrogen dose must be reduced because of bothersome estrogenic effects such as fluid retention. In individuals who have not developed secondary sexual characteristics, it is best to start with higher doses of estrogen (10 mg conjugated estrogens) in an effort to achieve breast development and a more feminine appearance.

Since many of these patients are in school, it is useful to adopt the academic year schedule for the annual re-evaluation process. Hormone replacement therapy can be discontinued in June and re-evaluation scheduled for August. If there is no change in status, hormone replacement therapy can begin again in September.

Patients with hypothalamic amenorrhea must be cautioned that replacement therapy will not protect against pregnancy in the event that normal function unknowingly returns. In the occasional patient who must have the

118

most effective contraception possible, it is reasonable to utilize a low dose oral contraceptive to provide the missing estrogen.

The importance of monthly menstruation to a young girl cannot be overemphasized. Regular and visible menstrual bleeding is often a gratifying experience in the young patient with gonadal dysgenesis, and serves to reinforce the patient's identification with a feminine gender role.

References

1. **Goldenberg, RL, Grodin, JM, Rodbard, D, and Ross, GT,** Gonadotropins in Women with Amenorrhea: The Use of Plasma Follicle-Stimulating Hormone to Differentiate Women With and Without Ovarian Follicles, Am J Obstet Gynec 116:1003, 1973.

2. **Sutton, C,** The Limitations of Laparoscopic Ovarian Biopsy, J Obstet Gynec Br Commonwlth 81:317, 1974.

3. **Rabin, D, Spitz, I, Bercovici, B, Bell, J, Laufer, A, Benveniste, R, and Polishuk, W,** Isolated Deficiency of Follicle-Stimulating Hormone, New Eng J Med 287:1313, 1972.

4. **Peckham, WD, and Knobil, ED,** The Effects of Ovariectomy, Estrogen Replacement, and Neuraminidase Treatment on the Properties of the Adenohypophysial Glycoprotein Hormones of the Rhesus Monkey, Endocrinology 98:1054, 1976.

5. **Vezina, JL, and Sutton, TJ,** Prolactin-Secreting Pituitary Microadenomas, Am J Roentgenology 120:46, 1974.

6. **Nader, S, Mashiter, K, Doyle, FH, and Joplin, GF,** Galactorrhea, Hyperprolactinemia and Pituitary Tumors in the Female, Clin Endocrinol 5:245, 1976.

7. **Woolf, PD, and Schenk, EA,** An FSH-Producing Pituitary Tumor in a Patient with Hypogonadism, J Clin Endocrinol Metab 38:561, 1974.

8. **Snyder, PJ, and Sterling, FH,** Hypersecretion of LH and FSH by a Pituitary Adenoma, J Clin Endocrinol Metab 42:544, 1976.

9. **Child, DG, Nader, S, Mashiter, K, Kjeld, M, Banks, L, and Russell Fraser, T,** Prolactin Studies in "Functionless" Pituitary Tumors, Brit Med J 1:604, 1975.

10. **Boyar, RM, Kapen, S, Weitzman, ED, and Hellman, L,** Pituitary Microadenoma and Hyperprolactinemia, New Eng J Med 294:263, 1976.

11. **Eddy, RL, Gilliland, PF, Ibarra, JD, McMurry, JF, and Thompson, JQ,** Human Growth Hormone Release, Am J Med 56:179, 1974.

12. **Jordan, RM, Kendall, JW, Seaich, JL, Allen, JM, Paulsen, A, Kerber, CW, and Vanderlaan, WP,** Cerebrospinal Fluid Hormone Concentration in the Evaluation of Pituitary Tumors, Ann Int Med 85:49, 1976.

13. **Klein, SM, and Garcia, CR,** Asherman's Syndrome: A Critique and Current Review, Fertil Steril 24:722, 1973.

14. **Griffin, JE, Edwards, C, Madden, JD, Harrod, MJ, and Wilson, JD,** Congenital Absence of the Vagina, Ann Int Med 85:224, 1976.

15. **Frank, RT,** Formation of Artificial Vagina Without Operation, Am J Obstet Gynec 35:1053, 1938.

16. **Wabrek, AJ, Millard, PR, Wilson, WB, Jr., and Pion, RJ,** Creation of a Neovagina by the Frank Nonoperative Method, Obstet Gynec 37:408, 1971.

17. **Meyer, WJ, Migeon, BR, and Migeon, CJ,** Locus on Human X Chromosome for Dihydrotestosterone Receptor and Androgen Insensitivity, Proc Nat Acad Sci 72:1469, 1975.

18. **Morris, JM, and Mahesh, VB,** Further Observations on the Syndrome "Testicular Feminization," Am J Obstet Gynec 87:731, 1963.

19. **Jones, GS, and De Moraes-Ruehsen, M,** A New Syndrome of Amenorrhea in Association with Hypergonadotropism and Apparently Normal Ovarian Follicular Apparatus, Am J Obstet Gynec 104:597, 1969.

20. **Polansky, S, and De Papp, EW,** Pregnancy Associated with Hypergonadotropic Hypogonadism, Obstet Gynec 47:47, 1976.

21. **McCormick, WF, and Halmi, NS,** Absence of Chromophobe Adenomas from a Large Series of Pituitary Tumors, Arch Path 92:231, 1971.

22. **Costello, RT,** Subclinical Adenoma of the Pituitary Gland, Am J Path 12:205, 1936.

23. **Franks, S, Murray, MAF, Jequier, AM, Steele, SJ, Nabarro, JDN, and Jacobs, HS,** Incidence and Significance of Hyperprolactinemia in Women with Amenorrhea, Clin Endocrinol 4:597, 1975.

24. **Falconer, MA, and Stafford-Bell, MA,** Visual Failure from Pituitary and Parasellar Tumors Occuring with Favourable Outcome in Pregnant Women, J Neurol, Neurosurg, and Psychiatry 38:919, 1975.

25. **Hardy, J,** Transphenoidal Hypophysectomy, J Neurosurg 34:581, 1971.

26. **Seppala, M, Hirvonen, E, and Ranta, T,** Bromocriptine Treatment of Secondary Amenorrhea, Lancet 1:1154, 1976.

27. **MacLeod, RM, and Lehmeyer, JE,** Suppression of Pituitary Tumor Growth and Function by Ergot Alkaloids, Cancer Res 33:849, 1973.

28. **Hodgson, SF, Randall, RV, Holman, CB, and MacCarty, CS,** Empty Sella Syndrome, Med Clinics of No America 56:897, 1972.

29. **Neelon, FA, Goree, JA, and Lebovitz, HE,** The Primary Empty Sella: Clinical and Radiographic Characteristics and Endocrine Function, Medicine 52:73, 1973.

30. **Fries, H, Nillius, SJ, and Pettersson, F,** Epidemiology of Secondary Amenorrhea, Am J Obstet Gynec 118:473, 1974.

31. **Warren, MP, and Vande Wiele, RL,** Clinical and Metabolic Features of Anorexia Nervosa, Am J Obstet Gynec 117:435, 1973.

32. **Beumont, PJV, Griesen, HG, Gelder, MG, and Kolakowska, T,** Plasma Prolactin and Luteinizing Hormone Levels in Anorexia Nervosa, Psychological Med 4:219, 1974.

33. **Moshang, T, Jr., Parks, JS, Baker, L, Vaidya, V, Utiger, RD, Bongiovanni, AM and Snyder, PJ,** Low Serum Triiodothronine in Patients With Anorexia Nervosa, J Clin Endocrinol Metab 40:470, 1975.

34. **Warren, MP, Jewelewicz, R, Dyrenfurth, I, Ans, R, Khalaf, S, and Vande Wiele, RL,** The Significance of Weight Loss in the Evaluation of Pituitary Response to LH-RH in Women With Secondary Amenorrhea, J Clin Endocrinol Metab 40:601, 1975.

35. **Crips, AH,** Primary Anorexia Nervosa, Gut 9:370, 1968.

36. **Tagatz, G, Fialkow, PJ, Smith, D, and Spadoni, L,** Hypogonadotropic Hypogonadism Associated with Anosmia in the Female, New Eng J Med 282:1326, 1970.

6 Anovulation

Anovulation is a very common problem which presents itself in a variety of clinical manifestations, ranging from amenorrhea to irregular menses and hirsutism. Serious consequences of chronic anovulation include infertility, and a greater risk for developing carcinoma of the endometrium and the breast. The physician must appreciate the clinical impact of anovulation and undertake therapeutic management of all anovulatory patients to avoid these unwanted consequences.

Normal ovulation requires coordination of the menstrual system at all levels: the central hypothalamic-pituitary axis, the feedback signals, and local responses within the ovary. The loss of ovulation may be due to any one of a variety of factors operating at each of these levels. The end result is a dysfunctional state: anovulation. *In this chapter, we will discuss the variety of mechanisms by which dysfunction of the ovulatory cycle can occur and how the clinical expressions of the resulting abnormal menstrual function are produced.*

Pathogenesis of Anovulation

During menses, the hypothalamus responds to the low levels of estradiol with the production of a releasing hormone to stimulate gonadotropin secretion from the anterior pituitary. This initial increase in gonadotropins is essential for follicular growth and steroidogenesis. With continued growth of the follicle, estradiol production within the follicle maintains follicular sensitivity to FSH by inducing FSH receptors. The combined action of FSH and estradiol increases the number of LH receptors, allowing the responses of luteinization and ovulation. Ovulation is triggered by the rapid rise in circulating levels of estradiol, a positive feedback response within the hypothalamus which results in the midcycle surge of gonadotropins necessary for expulsion of the egg and formation of the corpus luteum. A rise in progesterone follows ovulation along with a second rise in estradiol, forming the well-known 14 day luteal phase characterized by low FSH and LH levels. The demise of the corpus luteum, with a fall in hormone levels, allows the gonadotropins to increase again, initiating a new cycle.

This recycling mechanism is regulated largely by estradiol. The negative feedback relationship of estradiol with FSH results in the critical initial rise in that gonadotropin during menses, and the positive feedback relationship with LH is the ovulatory stimulus. Within the ovary, estradiol induces follicular receptor responses necessary for growth and function. Estradiol may therefore be viewed as the critical agent for appropriate hypothalamic-pituitary-ovarian responses in this system. Dysfunction in the cycle may be due to an abnormality in one of the various roles for estradiol. Problems in normal function may be conveniently organized into: central defects, abnormalities in the feedback signals, and abnormal function within the ovary itself.

Central Defects

Given adequate and appropriately timed feedback signals, the hypothalamic-pituitary axis may be unable to respond. A pituitary tumor represents the obvious example of a central defect in menstrual function, and is discussed in Chapter 5, Amenorrhea.

Although difficult to demonstrate definitively, malfunction within the hypothalamus is both a likely as well as a favorite explanation for ovulatory failure. A variety of problems, such as stress and anxiety, borderline anorexia nervosa, acute weight loss after a crash diet, and perhaps increased levels of circulating androgens, can inhibit function of the anterior hypothalamic "cyclic" area, such that only the "tonic" medial area of the hypothalamus operates. With this disability, the gonadotropin surge is not possible, and only homeostatic pituitary-ovarian function is maintained. In addition to inadequate releasing hormone synthesis and release, central dysfunction may take the form of a failure to sustain releasing hormone stimulation over a sufficient time period, or it can involve functional pituitary refractoriness to releasing hormone.

124

Abnormal feedback can be due to failures within the system or due to the introduction of confounding factors. It is instructive to focus on the blood estradiol concentration as the critical signal for the machinery of the ovulatory cycle. In order to achieve the appropriate changes within the cycle, estradiol levels must rise and fall in synchrony with morphologic events. Therefore, two possible signal failures may occur: (1) estradiol levels may not fall low enough to allow sufficient FSH response for the initial growth stimulus, and (2) levels of estradiol may be inadequate to produce the positive stimulatory effects necessary to induce the ovulatory surge of LH.

1. **Loss of FSH Stimulation.** In order to achieve recycling, a nadir in blood sex steroid levels must occur so that the initial event in the cycle, the rise in FSH, may take place. Sustained estradiol levels at such a key moment would not permit FSH stimulation of follicular growth and maturation, and recycling would be thwarted. The necessary decline in blood estradiol requires cessation of secretion, appropriate clearance and metabolism, and the absence of a significant contribution of estrogen to the circulation by extragonadal sources.

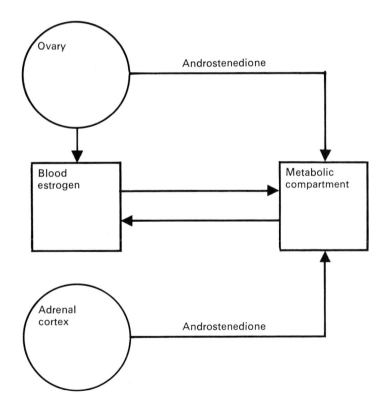

The clearance and metabolism of estradiol can be impaired by other pathologic conditions, such as hypothyroidism or hepatic disease. It is for this reason that a careful history and physical examination are important elements in the differential diagnosis of anovulation.

Extragonadal contribution to the blood estrogen level can reach significant proportions. While the adrenal gland does not secrete appreciable amounts of estrogen into the circulation, it indirectly contributes to the total estrogen level. This is accomplished by the extragonadal peripheral conversion of C-19 androgenic precursors, mainly androstenedione, to estrogen. In this manner, psychologic or physical stress may increase the adrenal contribution of estrogenic precursor, and subsequent conversion to estrogen may sustain the blood level of estrogen at a time when a decline is necessary for successful recycling of the menstrual system. In addition, adipose tissue is capable of converting androstenedione to estrogen, hence the percent conversion increases with increasing body weight. (1) This could be the mechanism for the well-known association between obesity and anovulation.

2. **Loss of LH Stimulation.** A failure in gonadal production of estrogen need not be absolute. Obviously the patient with gonadal dysgenesis and ovarian failure will present with amenorrhea and infertility because of a total lack of estrogen secretion. More commonly, the clinician is concerned with the patient who has gonadotropin and estrogen production, but does not ovulate. The failure to achieve a critical midcycle level of estradiol necessary to trigger the gonadotropin surge may be due to a relative deficiency in steroid production, perhaps associated with asynchrony in follicular growth and maturation.

The teenager between menarche and the onset of ovulation cannot generate an adequate estradiol signal and response until a certain degree of coordination of the hypothalamic-pituitary-ovarian axis is accomplished. The perimenopausal woman undergoes a terminal period of anovulation which may represent a steroidogenic refractoriness within the remaining elderly follicles.

These inadequacies may be due to intrinsic follicular weaknesses or an impairment in the follicular-gonadotropin interaction, due to immaturity, aging or local steroid effects. In any case, the end result is the same — a failure to achieve critical signal levels of estradiol at appropriate times in the cycle.

**Local
Ovarian
Effects**

An understanding of the critical role for estradiol within the follicle indicates possible points of failure which may lead to anovulation. Estradiol prevents atresia despite declining FSH levels by increasing the number of FSH receptors within the follicle, thus increasing follicular sensitivity to FSH. In addition, estradiol enhances the induction of LH receptors by FSH, making it possible for the follicle to respond to the LH surge at midcycle. A follicle can fail to grow and ovulate either because of inadequate estradiol production within the follicle, or because of interference with the action of estradiol.

The factors which control follicular production of estradiol are poorly understood. Surely a very precise coordination is necessary between morphologic development and hormonal stimulation. Perturbations may arise in an infectious process, from the presence of endometriosis, or the necessary biologic effects may be blocked by an improper molecular constitution of the gonadotropins (heterogenity of the glycopeptide hormones) or by abnormal qualitative or quantitative changes in tropic hormone receptors (ovarian insensitivity).

Local androgens may induce follicular atresia (see Chapter 3). While this action in the normal cycle may be important in ensuring that the proper number of follicles reaches the point of ovulation, an excessive concentration of androgens may prevent normal cycling. This effect of androgens may be mediated by interference with estradiol action, perhaps by reducing the concentration of cytoplasmic estradiol receptors. Thus the important effects of estradiol on gonadotropin receptors will be impeded, and premature atresia may result, leading to chronic anovulation.

**Precise
Etiology**

In considering abnormal menstrual function, except in severe disease states such as pituitary tumors, anorexia nervosa, gonadal dysgenesis, and perhaps, obesity, it is usually impossible to reduce the issue of etiology to a single factor. The normal ovulatory function of the menstrual system relies on a dynamic coordination of complex actions. Abnormal function may represent discordance at all of the levels reviewed in the above paragraphs. Thus a minor deficiency in the estradiol signal will be associated with a subnormal hypothalamic response, and inappropriate pituitary production of gonadotropins, and an impaired or inappropriate degree of follicular growth and function. Dysfunction is sustained, therefore, by the internal feedback mechanisms within the system, and anovulation may become a chronic problem.

Regardless of the nature of the initial cause of the problem, the final clinical statement of the dysfunction is predictable and easily diagnosed. In patients who have abnormal or absent menstrual function, but are otherwise medically well, the diagnosis will fall into one of three categories:

1. **Ovarian Failure.** Hypergonadotropic hypogonadism, the inability of the ovary to respond to any gonadotropic stimulation, generally due to the absence of follicular tissue on a genetic basis. (Discussed in Chapter 5).

2. **Central Failure.** Hypogonadotropic hypogonadism, hypothalamic or pituitary unresponsiveness as expressed in abnormally low or normal serum gonadotropins. (Discussed in Chapter 5).

3. **Anovulatory Dysfunction.** The patient who has asynchronous gonadotropin and estrogen production, and does not ovulate, presents with a variety of clinical problems. The major morphologic characteristic of this problem is the polycystic ovary.

Anovulation-Clinical Presentation

The associated clinical manifestations depend upon the level of gonadal function preserved, and fall into the following principal categories:

1. Amenorrhea (Chapter 5)

2. Hirsutism (Chapter 7)

3. Dysfunctional Uterine Bleeding (Chapter 8)

4. Infertility (Chapter 19)

5. Endometrial Hyperplasia and Cancer (Chapter 4)

6. Breast Disease (Chapter 9)

7. The Polycystic Ovary (this chapter)

The Polycystic Ovary

In contrast to the characteristic picture of fluctuating estradiol levels in the normal cycle, a "steady state" of tonic gonadotropin and estrogen function, associated with persistent anovulation, can be depicted. This steady state is only relative, and is being exaggerated here to present a concept of this clinical syndrome.

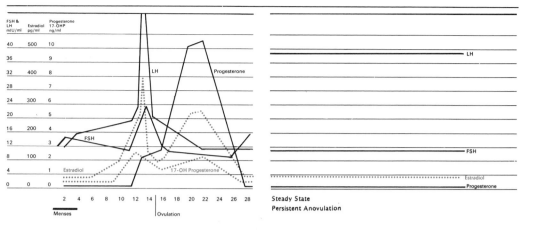

FSH & LH mIU/ml	Estradiol pg/ml	Progesterone 17-OHP ng/ml							
40	500	10							
36		9							
32	400	8			LH		Progesterone		
28		7							
24	300	6							
20		5							
16	200	4							
12		3		FSH					
8	100	2							
4		1	Estradiol			17-OH Progesterone			
0	0	0							

2   4   6   8   10   12   14 | 16   18   20   22   24   26   28

Menses   Ovulation

LH

FSH

Estradiol

Progesterone

Steady State
Persistent Anovulation

In patients with chronic anovulation, the average daily production of estrogen and androgens is increased. This is reflected in higher circulating levels of testosterone and androstenedione, and higher levels of estrogen, largely estrone derived from the peripheral conversion of androstenedione. (2) When compared to levels found in normal women, patients with this syndrome have higher mean concentrations of LH, but low or low-normal levels of FSH. (2, 3, 4) The elevated levels of LH may be in the range of the midcycle surge or equivalent to postmenopausal values. Evidence (an augmented response to GnRH) suggests that the elevated LH levels are due to an increased sensitivity of the pituitary to releasing hormone stimulation. (4) This increased sensitivity is probably the effect of the increased estrone levels since a correlation exists between the estrogen and the LH levels. It is possible that the elevated androgens contribute to the increased LH in another fashion. The hypothalamus aromatizes androgens to estrogens (5), and this local change may sufficiently raise estrogen levels in the anterior hypothalamus to stimulate the positive feedback mechanism. The lower FSH levels probably represent the sensitivity of the FSH negative feedback system to the elevated levels of estrone.

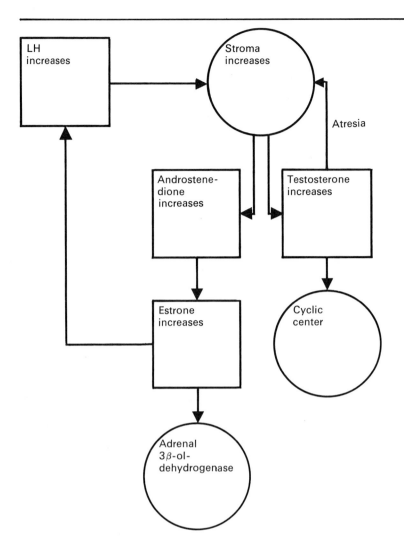

Because the FSH levels are not totally depressed, new follicular growth is continuously stimulated, but not to the point of full maturation and ovulation. Despite the fact that full growth potential is not realized, follicular lifespan may extend several months in the form of multiple follicular cysts, 2–6 mm in diameter. These follicles are surrounded by hyperplastic theca cells, often luteinized in response to the high LH levels. The accumulation of follicular tissue in various stages of development allows an increased and relatively constant production of steroids in response to the gonadotropin stimulation. This condition is self-sustaining. As various follicles undergo atresia, they are immediately replaced by new follicles of similar limited growth potential.

The tissue derived from follicular atresia is also sustained by the steady state, and now contributes to the stromal compartment of the ovary. This functioning stromal tissue secretes significant amounts of androstenedione and testosterone. In response to the elevated LH levels, the androgen production rate is increased. In turn, the elevated androgen levels, through the process of extraglandular conversion, result in elevated estrogen levels (principally estrone). This steady elevated estrogen level is a major factor in sustaining this condition by depressing FSH levels and elevating LH secretion by augmenting the pituitary response to GnRH. The elevated androgens may also contribute to the morphologic effect within the ovary by blocking the actions of estradiol on the granulosa cells and inducing premature atresia. Indeed the ovulatory response to wedge resection appears to follow a sustained reduction in testosterone levels, suggesting that the intraovarian androgen effect is the major obstacle to complete follicular maturation and normal cycling. (6)

In this manner the classic picture of the polycystic ovary is attained, displaying numerous follicles in all stages of development and atresia, and dense stromal tissue. The loss of recycling has resulted in a hormonal steady state causing persistent anovulation which may be associated with the increased production of androgens. This condition has been referred to by many eponyms, most commonly the Stein-Leventhal Syndrome, polycystic ovary disease, or sclerocystic ovaries.

The polycystic ovary is palpably enlarged (up to 2 times) and is characterized by a smooth pearly white capsule. For years, it was erroneously believed that the thick sclerotic capsule acted as a mechanical barrier to ovulation. A more accurate concept is that the polycystic ovary is a consequence of the loss of ovulation and the achievement of a steady state of persistent anovulation. The histologic characteristics reflect this dysfunctional state. An accumulation of atretic tissue along with the constant and elevated LH stimulation results in stromal hyperplasia. It is doubtful that hyperthecosis represents a separate syndrome. Hyperthecosis refers to patches of luteinized theca-like cells scattered throughout the ovarian stroma, and it is characterized by the same clinical, histologic, and endocrine findings as seen with polycystic ovaries. (7) It is likely that both are morphologic manifestations of the same process, anovulation.

One group of investigators has indicated that high LH levels in anovulatory patients are associated with big ovaries, while low LH levels are found in association with small ovaries. (8) Another group has failed to find a relationship between the size of polycystic ovaries and the levels of LH. (4) There is a spectrum of time involved in the development of this clinical syndrome, and it is useful to view the attainment of high LH levels and large ovaries as a stage of maximal effect of persistent anovulation. However the key to understanding this clinical problem is an appreciation for the disruption in ovulatory recycling function. The size of the ovaries is not a critical feature, nor is it necessary to assign a specific etiology. The polycystic ovary may be associated with a variety of disorders in the hypothalamic-pituitary-ovarian axis, as well as extragonadal sources of androgens (9), or with ovarian androgen-producing tumors (10).

It appears that at least one group of patients with this condition inherits the disorder, possibly by means of an X-linked dominant transmission or an autosomal dominant. Studies of families have indicated that there is a twofold higher incidence of hirsutism and oligomenorrhea, with paternal transmission, but with marked variability of phenotypic expression. (11)

The adrenal gland is involved in this syndrome. Higher circulating levels of dehydroepiandrosterone sulfate (DS), almost exclusively an adrenal product, testify to adrenal participation. (2) The mechanism involving the 3β-ol-dehydrogenase enzyme and the clinical importance of this involvement will be discussed in Chapter 7, Hirsutism.

Clinical Effects and Treatment

Anovulation is the key feature of this syndrome and presents as amenorrhea in approximately 55% of cases, and with irregular, heavy bleeding in 28%. (12) True virilization is rare, but 70% of anovulatory patients complain of cosmetically disturbing hirsutism. (12) Obesity has been classically regarded as a common feature, but its presence is extremely variable and has no diagnostic value.

While an elevated LH value in the presence of a low or low-normal FSH may be diagnostic, the diagnosis is easily made by the clinical presentation alone. The symptoms are a consequence of the loss of ovulation: dysfunctional bleeding, amenorrhea, hirsutism, and infertility. These presentations each require a specific diagnostic and therapeutic approach, as discussed in separate chapters in this book.

There are potentially severe clinical consequences of the steady state of hormone secretion. Besides the problems of infertility, hirsutism, amenorrhea, and bleeding, the effect of the unopposed and uninterrupted estrogen is to place the patient in considerable risk for cancer of the endometrium and cancer of the breast. If left unattended, patients with persistent anovulation develop clinical problems, and therefore, appropriate therapeutic management is essential for all anovulatory patients.

The typical patient presents with anovulation and irregular menses. If there is no hirsutism or virilism, evaluation of androgen production is not necessary. There is no need for urinary 17-ketosteroids, plasma testosterone, or any other laboratory procedures. In the patient whose only problem is long-standing anovulation, and especially if the patient is over 35, an endometrial biopsy (with extensive sampling) is a wise precaution. The well-known association between this syndrome and abnormal endometrial changes must be kept in mind. Documentation of anovulation is usually unnecessary, especially in view of menstrual irregularity with periods of amenorrhea.

Therapy of most anovulatory patients can be planned at the first visit. If the patient desires pregnancy, she is a candidate for the medical induction of ovulation (Chapter 19). If the patient presents with amenorrhea, an investigation must be pursued as outlined in Chapter 5. The management of significant dysfunctional uterine bleeding is discussed in Chapter 8, and hirsutism in Chapter 7.

For the patient who does not wish to become pregnant and does not complain of hirsutism, but is anovulatory and has irregular bleeding, therapy is directed toward interruption of the steady state effect on the endometrium. The use of Provera (10 mg daily for 5 days, every 2 months) is favored to ensure complete withdrawal bleeding, and to prevent endometrial hyperplasia and atypia. Spacing of the progestational medication in this fashion (every 2 months) will allow the patient to be aware of spontaneous bleeding due to the onset of ovulatory cycles. The use of oral contraception medication for therapy in these patients requires individual patient judgment. In our opinion, when reliable contraception is essential, the use of low dose combination oral contraception in the usual cyclic fashion is appropriate.

References

1. **Siiteri, PK, and MacDonald, PC,** Role of Extraglandular Estrogen in Human Endocrinology, in Geyer, SR, Astwood, EB and Greep, RO, Eds, *Handbook of Physiology, Section 7, Endocrinology*, American Physiology Society, Washington DC, 1973, pp 615–629.

2. **DeVane, GW, Czekala, NM, Judd, HL, and Yen, SSC,** Circulating Gonadotropins, Estrogen and Androgens in Polycystic Ovarian Disease, Am J Obstet Gynec 121:496, 1975.

3. **Kletzky, OA, Davajan, V, Nakamura, RM, Thorneycroft, IH, and Mishell, DR, Jr.,** Clinical Categorization of Patients with Secondary Amenorrhea Using Progesterone Induced Uterine Bleeding and Measurement of Serum Gonadotropin Levels, Am J Obstet Gynec 121:695, 1975.

4. **Rebar, R, Judd, HL, Yen, SSC, Rakoff, J, Vandenberg, G, and Naftolin, F,** Characterization of the Inappropriate

Gonadotropin Secretion in Polycystic Ovary Syndrome, J Clin Invest 57:1320, 1976.

5. **Naftolin, F, and Ryan, KJ,** The Metabolism of Androgens in Central Neuroendocrine Tissues, J Steroid Biochem 6:993, 1975.

6. **Judd, HL, Rigg, LA, Anderson, DC, and Yen, SSC,** The Effects of Ovarian Wedge Resection on Circulating Gonadotropin and Ovarian Steroid Levels in Patients with Polycystic Ovary Syndrome, J Clin Endocrinol Metab 43:347, 1976.

7. **Judd, HL, Scully, RE, Herbst, AL, Yen, SSC, Ingersol, FM, and Kliman, B,** Familial Hyperthecosis: Comparison of Endocrinologic and Histologic Findings with Polycystic Ovarian Disease, Am J Obstet Gynec 117:976, 1973.

8. **Berger, MJ, Taymor, ML, and Patton, WC,** Gonadotropin Levels and Secretory Patterns in Patients with Typical and Atypical Polycystic Ovarian Disease, Fertil Steril 26:619, 1975.

9. **Kase, N, Kowal, J, Perloff, W, and Soffer, LJ,** In vitro Production of Androgens by a Virilizing Adenoma and Associated Polycystic Ovaries, Acta Endocrinol 44:15, 1963.

10. **Zourlas, PA, and Jones, HW, Jr.,** Stein-Leventhal Syndrome with Masculinizing Ovarian Tumors, Obstet Gynec 34:861, 1969.

11. **Givens, JR,** Hirsutism and Hyperandrogenism, Adv Int Med 21:221, 1976.

12. **Prunty, FTG,** Hirsutism, Virilism, and Apparent Virilism, and Their Gonadal Relationships, J Endocrinol 38:203, 1967.

7 Hirsutism

Excessive facial and body hair usually is associated with loss of cyclic menstrual function. The more severe states of virilism (clitoromegaly, deepening of the voice, balding, and changes in body habitus) are rarely seen and usually are associated with adrenal hyperplasia or androgen-producing tumors of adrenal or ovarian origin. Although the most common cause of hirsutism is excess androgen production by non-cycling ovaries, diagnostic evaluation is required. Furthermore, a concerned and sympathetic approach must be offered to the patient. The responsible physician must view hirsutism both as an endocrine problem and as a cosmetic problem. To the affected woman, hair growth over the face, abdomen, or breasts is disturbing on several levels: is there disease? is sexuality changing? is social acceptance altered? is fertility impaired?

This chapter will review the biology of hair growth and the endocrine possibilities which may yield hirsutism. An uncomplicated, effective program for diagnostic evaluation and therapeutic management will be offered.

Biology of Hair Growth

Embryology

Each hair follicle develops at about 8 weeks gestation as a derivative of the epidermis. It is composed initially of a solid column of cells which proliferates from the basal layers of the epidermis and protrudes downward into the dermis. As the column elongates it encounters a cluster of mesodermal cells (the dermal papilla) which it envelops at its bulbous tip (bulb). The solid epithelial column then hollows out to form a hair canal and the pilosebaceous apparatus is laid down.

Hair growth begins with proliferation of the epithelial cells at the base of the column in contact with the dermal papilla. The lanugo hair present at this stage is lightly pigmented, thin in diameter, short in length and fragile in attachment. Important to note here is the fact that the total endowment of hair follicles is made at an early gestational stage, and that no new hair follicles will be produced de novo. Furthermore, the concentration of hair follicles laid down per unit area of facial skin does not differ materially between sexes but does differ between races and ethnic groups (caucasian > oriental; mediterranean > nordic).

Structure and Growth

Hair does not grow continuously, but rather in a cyclic fashion with alternating phases of activity and inactivity. The cycles are referred to in the following terms:

Anagen — the growing phase
Catagen — rapid involution phase
Telogen — quiescent phase

In the resting phase (telogen), the hair is short and loosely attached to the base of the epithelial canal. The bulb is formed around the dermal papilla. As growth begins (anagen), epithelial matrix cells at the base begin to proliferate and extend downward into the dermis. The bulb is reformed and the epithelial column elongates some 4–6 times from the resting state. Once downward extension is completed, continued rapid growth of the matrix cells pushes upward to the skin surface. The tenuous contact of the previous hair is broken, and that hair is shed. The superficial matrix cells differentiate forming a keratinized column. Growth continues as long as active mitoses persist in the basal matrix cells. When finished (categen), the column shrinks, the bulb shrivels, and the resting state is reachieved (telogen).

The length of hair is primarily determined by duration of the growth phase (anagen). Scalp hair remains in anagen for 2–6 years and has only a relatively short resting phase. Elsewhere (forearm) a short anagen and long telogen will lead to short hair of stable nongrowing length. The appearance of continuous growth (or periodic shedding) is determined by the degree to which individual hair follicles act asynchronously with their neighbors. Scalp hair is asynchronous and therefore always seems to be growing. The resting phase that some hairs are in is not apparent. If marked synchrony is achieved, then all hairs may undergo telogen at the same time leading to the appearance of shedding. Occasionally women will complain of marked hair loss from the scalp, but this time period of shedding is usually limited, and normal growth resumes.

Factors Which Influence Hair Growth

The dermal papilla is the director of the events which control hair growth. Despite major injury to the epithelial component of the follicle (such as freezing, x-rays, or a skin graft), if the dermal papilla survives, the hair follicle will regenerate and regrow hair. Injury to or degeneration of the dermal papilla are the crucial factors in permanent hair loss.

Sexual hair can be defined as that hair which responds to the sex steroids. Sexual hair grows on the face, lower abdomen, anterior thighs, the chest, the breasts, and in the axillae and pubic area. From animal studies and human disease patterns, the following list of hormonal effects can be compiled:

1. Androgens, particularly testosterone, initiate growth, increase the diameter and pigmentation of the keratin column, and probably increase the rate of matrix cell mitoses, in all but scalp hair.

2. Estrogens act essentially opposite from androgens, retarding the rate and initiation of growth, and leading to finer, less pigmented and slower growing hair.

3. Progestins have minimal effect on hair.

4. Pregnancy (high estrogen and progesterone) may increase the synchrony of hair growth, leading to periods of growth or shedding.

An important clinical characteristic of hair growth can be understood from studies of the effects of castration. If castration occurs before puberty, the male will not grow a beard. If castration occurs after puberty with beard and sexual hair distribution fully developed, then these hairs continue to grow albeit more slowly and with finer caliber. Clearly androgen stimulates sexual hair follicle conversion from lanugo to adult hair growth patterns, but *once established, these patterns persist despite withdrawal of androgen.*

Other hormone dependencies are displayed by all hair (sexual and nonsexual). In hypopituitarism, there is marked reduction of hair growth. Acromegaly will be associated with hirsutism in 10–15% of patients. While the impact of thyroid hormone is not clear, hypothyroid individuals sometimes display less axillary, pubic, and curiously, lateral eyebrow hair.

Hair growth may be influenced by nonhormonal factors, such as local skin temperature, blood flow, edema, and stasis. Hair growth may be seen with CNS problems such as encephalitis, cranial trauma, multiple sclerosis, and with drugs such as Dilantin.

Evaluation of Hirsutism

Cosmetically disfiguring hirsutism is the end result of a number of factors:

1. The number of hair follicles present (Japanese women bearing androgen-producing tumors rarely achieve hirsutism because of the low concentration of hair follicles per unit skin area).

2. The degree to which androgen has converted resting lanugo hair to adult independent hair.

3. The ratio of the growth to resting phases in the affected hair follicles.

4. The asynchrony of growth cycles in aggregates of hair follicles.

5. The thickness and degree of pigmentation of individual hairs.

The primary factor is an increase in androgen levels (primarily testosterone) which produces an initial growth stimulus and then acts to sustain continued growth. If studied with sophisticated techniques, essentially every woman with hirsutism will be found to have an increased production rate of testosterone and androstenedione. (1) Although anovulatory ovaries are usually the source for these androgens, a minimal workup is necessary to rule out adrenal sources and tumors. It should be emphasized that it is rarely necessary to hospitalize patients for extensive evaluation of hirsutism.

The Diagnostic Workup

The initial laboratory tests in the evaluation of hirsutism are a 24 hour urine collection for measurement of 17-ketosteroids and 17-hydroxysteroids, and a blood sample for testosterone. Ovarian production of androgens may result in slight or moderate elevations of 17-ketosteroids. *If the initial value of 17-ketosteroids is less than 20 mg/24 hours, adrenal disease is most unlikely, and the diagnosis of excess androgen production by the ovaries is established.* There are only rare cases of adrenal tumors with normal 17-ketosteroids (2, 3, 4), and further evaluation of such cases would be indicated by the presence of markedly elevated blood levels of testosterone. These rare tumors are responsive to LH, suggesting that they are derived from embryonic rest cells.

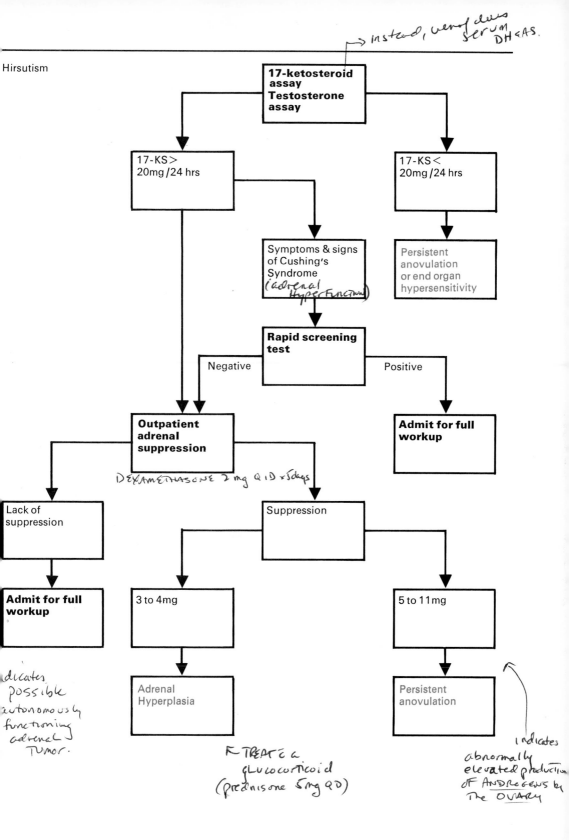

Hirsutism

17-ketosteroid assay
Testosterone assay

→ Instead, use of does serum DHEAS.

17-KS >
20mg /24 hrs

17-KS <
20mg /24 hrs

Symptoms & signs
of Cushing's
Syndrome
(adrenal Hyperfunction)

Persistent
anovulation
or end organ
hypersensitivity

Rapid screening test

Negative   Positive

Outpatient adrenal suppression

DEXAMETHASONE 2 mg QID × 5days

Admit for full workup

Lack of
suppression

Suppression

Admit for full workup

Indicates possible autonomously functioning adrenal Tumor.

3 to 4mg

5 to 11mg

Adrenal
Hyperplasia

Persistent
anovulation

← TREAT c̄ a glucocorticoid (prednisone 5mg QD)

Indicates abnormally elevated production of ANDROGENS by the OVARY

If the 17-ketosteroid value is 20 mg/24 hours or more, along with an elevated 17-hydroxysteroid excretion, and the patient has signs and symptoms suggestive of Cushing's syndrome (a rare occurrence), a rapid screening test can be utilized to indicate whether the patient should be admitted to the hospital for full evaluation. Dexamethasone (1 mg) is given orally at 11 PM and blood is drawn at 8 AM the next morning for a plasma cortisol. A value less than 6 μg% rules out Cushing's syndrome; Cushing's syndrome is unlikely with intermediate values between 6 and 10 μg%; while a value of 10 μg% or higher is indicative of adrenal hyperfunction.

If the patient does not have signs and symptoms of Cushing's syndrome, but the 17-ketosteroids are over 20 mg/24 hours, suppression of adrenal function with dexamethasone will reveal the nature and extent of the adrenal androgen contribution. Suppression may be carried out on an outpatient basis with 2.0 mg dexamethasone q.i.d. for 5 days. On the last day of suppression a repeat 24 hour urine is collected for 17-ketosteroids. Adrenal suppression requires a minimum of 4 days. (5)

The reliability of this test requires that dexamethasone suppress only adrenal steroidogenesis, and not affect ovarian function. Estradiol, progesterone, and 17-hydroxyprogesterone levels are not affected by dexamethasone administered to normally cycling women. (5) Similarly androstenedione, testosterone, and 17-hydroxyprogesterone are not suppressed by dexamethasone when given to patients with polycystic ovaries. (6) These findings indicate that dexamethasone suppression reliably separates the adrenal contribution from the ovarian contribution to 17-ketosteroid excretion.

A lack of adrenal suppression may be due to an autonomously functioning adrenal tumor, and hospital admission with consultation is indicated. If suppression is to a level of 3–4 mg/24 hours, a value consistent with normal ovarian function, the etiology of the hirsutism and menstrual irregularity is diagnosed as adrenal hyperplasia and treated with a glucocorticoid to maintain 17-ketosteroid excretion in the normal range (e.g. start with prednisone, 5 mg daily). This infrequently encountered problem is the only one in which the patients should be treated with cortisol derivatives. Suppression to a level of 5–11 mg/24 hours indicates an abnormally elevated production of androgens by the ovary, a finding consistent with persistent anovulation. Any uncertainty in response requires hospitalization and consultation.

The Testosterone Level

Plasma testosterone levels (normal 0.2–0.8 ng/ml) are elevated in the majority of women (70%) with anovulation and hirsutism, but individual variation is great. The reason for this variation should be appreciated by the clinician; it is directly related to changes in the testosterone binding capacity in the blood.

The testosterone binding capacity is decreased by androgen and increased by estrogen. Hence, the binding capacity in men is lower than that in normal women, and the binding globulin level in women with increased androgen production is also depressed. Routine assays determine the total hormone concentration, bound plus free. Thus a total testosterone concentration may be in the normal range in a woman who is hirsute or virilized, but because the binding globulin levels are depressed by the androgenic effects, the percent free and active testosterone is elevated. Indeed, the unbound or free testosterone is approximately twice normal (an increase from 1% to 2%) in women with anovulation and polycystic ovaries. (7) Therefore a normal testosterone level in a hirsute woman is still consistent with elevated androgen production rates.

If the testosterone level exceeds 2.0 ng/ml, an androgen-producing tumor must be suspected. Stimulation and suppression tests (as outlined at the end of this chapter) have been utilized in the attempt to establish the presence of adrenal and ovarian tumors. Because of the variability in such tests, the evaluation of high testosterone levels is better performed with retrograde catheterization studies of the androgen levels in the adrenal and ovarian venous effluence. This will be discussed below.

The measurement of androstenedione levels is complicated by a significant circadian variation (synchronous with cortisol), with as much as a 50% change during a 24 hour period. (8) The normal range of androstenedione is 1.5–2.5 ng/ml. If this assay is to be utilized, care should be taken to control the time of sampling, and multiple samples are necessary. Testosterone is more useful, having the advantage of no significant circadian rhythm.

The urinary 17-ketosteroid evaluation may be replaced by the measurement of blood levels of dehydroepiandrosterone sulfate (DS). (9) DS is the most abundant adrenal steroid in the blood (1500–2500 ng/ml), (8, 10), and only a minimal amount of blood is required for the assay. There is little daily variability and a lack of significant diurnal variation.

Treatment of Hirsutism

Almost all patients presenting to a gynecologist with hirsutism represent excess androgen production in association with the steady state of persistent anovulation. Treatment is directed toward interruption of the steady state. Two treatment regimens are available. In those patients who wish to become pregnant, ovulation can be induced with clomiphene. (See Chapter 19.) In patients in whom pregnancy is not desired, the steady state can be interrupted by suppression of ovarian steroidogensis with a combination birth control pill.

Androgen production in hirsute women is usually an LH-dependent process (11), and suppression of ovarian steroidogensis depends upon adequate LH suppression. (Remember that steroidogensis in all compartments of the ovary requires LH support and stimulation.) The use of estrogen to suppress LH is not recommended since estrogen has both a positive and a negative feedback effect on LH, and in pharmacologic doses, the positive effect prevails. LH suppression with estrogen has been demonstrated to be unreliable despite long-term treatment. (12) The combination birth control pill, on the other hand, has a potent negative feedback effect. We have found that plasma testosterone levels are effectively suppressed with any combination type birth control pill, even including the new low estrogen dose pills (containing 30 μg ethinyl estradiol). The testosterone value in hirsute patients shows a decrease within 1 to 3 months of treatment. This reduction has been associated with a gratifying clinical improvement in the progression of hirsutism.

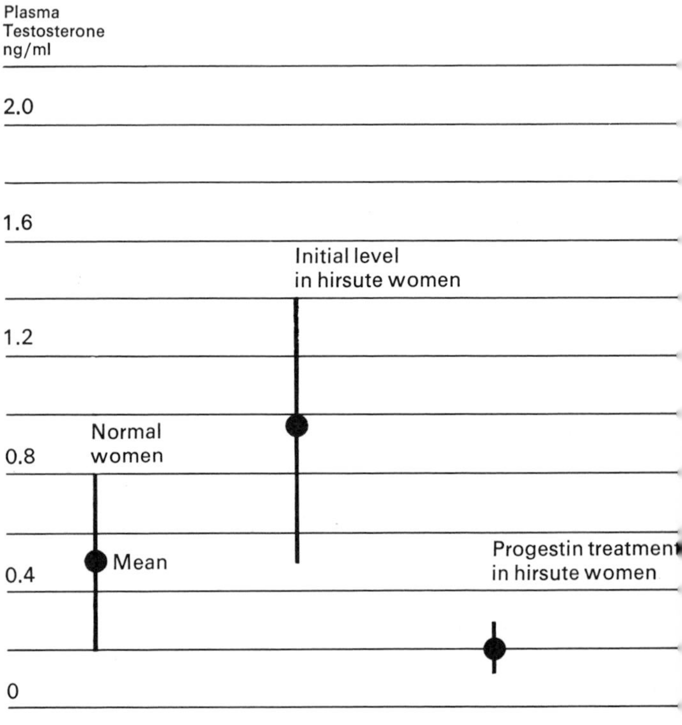

Plasma
Testosterone
ng/ml

2.0

1.6

Initial level
in hirsute women

1.2

Normal
women

0.8

Mean

0.4

Progestin treatment
in hirsute women

0

In the patient in whom oral contraceptive pills are contraindicated, good results can be achieved with the use of Depo-Provera, 150 mg intramuscularly every 3 months. The mechanism of action of Depo-Provera is slightly different from that of the birth control pill. Suppression of gonadotropins is less intense, hence ovarian follicular activity continues. Even though LH suppression is not as great, some reduction in LH results in a decreased testosterone production rate. In addition, testosterone clearance from the circulation is increased. (13) This latter effect may be due to an induction of liver enzyme activity. The overall effect (decreased production and increased clearance) yields a clinical result comparable to that achieved with the birth control pill (where the mechanism is principally decreased androgen production with a minor contribution from an elevation in binding globulin capacity).

Cyproterone acetate is an antiandrogen with progestational behavior. This agent has been only moderately successful in treating hirsutism, requiring high doses, and it is associated with loss of libido. (14)

A noteworthy feature of this clinical problem is the slow response to treatment. The average patient should be cautioned that treatment with a combination oral contraceptive will be necessary for 6 months to 1 year before an observable diminution in hair growth occurs. Combined treatment with electrolysis is not recommended, therefore, until hormone suppression has been used at least 6 months (except with extreme hirsutism).

New hair follicles will no longer be stimulated to grow, but hair growth which has been previously established will not disappear with hormone treatment alone. This may be affected temporarily by shaving, tweezing, waxing, or the use of depilatories. None of these tactics alters the inherent growth of the hair, therefore they must be reapplied at frequent intervals. Permanent removal of hair can be accomplished only by electrocoagulation of dermal papillae. Some patients return after a period of treatment expressing disappointment because hair is still present. The effect of the treatment (prevention of new hair growth) may not be apparent unless the previously established hair is removed. The combination of ovarian suppression preventing new hair growth and electrolysis removing the old hair yields the most complete and effective treatment of hirsutism.

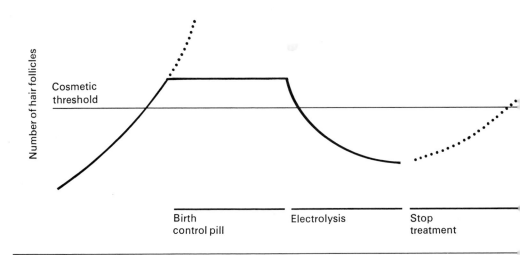

Adrenal Gland Participation

Adrenal involvement in this syndrome of persistent anovulation and hirsutism has long been recognized. Adrenal suppression, for example, will induce regular menses and ovulation in some patients, and empiric treatment with glucocorticoid has been advocated in the past.

The excessive androstenedione production seen in hirsute women is significantly dependent upon ACTH. In contrast testosterone production is (not) related to ACTH stimulation. (15) Occasionally high 17-ketosteroid excretion (30–40 mg/24 hours) is seen in an anovulatory patient, and treatment with a birth control pill returns the 17-ketosteroids to normal.

The adrenal involvement can be explained by the presence of a relative enzyme block within the adrenal cortex in association with the steady state of persistent anovulation. Estrogen administration to postmenopausal women results in increased levels of pregnenolone, dehydroepiandrosterone, and dehydroepiandrosterone sulfate. (16) There is no effect on cortisol, testosterone, or androstenedione. Elevation of these steroids by exogenous estrogen is consistent with an estrogen-induced 3β-ol-dehydrogenase block. Similar results were obtained when patients with gonadal dysgenesis were treated with estrogen, and in addition, growth of pubic and axillary hair is significant after estrogen therapy of such patients. (17)

Thus the elevated estrogen levels in anovulatory patients with polycystic ovaries (see Chapter 6) may induce a relative enzyme insufficiency within the adrenal cortex, resulting in excessive 17-ketosteroid production. Since the birth control pill is not associated with an increase in 17-ketosteroids, ethinyl estradiol and mestranol may not affect this enzyme.

Androgens inhibit 11β-hydroxylase activity within adrenal tissue; however there is no evidence that excessive ovarian androgens are responsible for an induced enzyme insufficiency within the adrenal.

The empiric use of cortisol and its derivatives to achieve adrenal suppression is not indicated in patients presenting with irregular menses and hirsutism. Not only is the long-term use of these drugs hazardous, it is also an indirect attack on the basic problem. In the absence of specific adrenal disease, the more reasonable approach is direct treatment of the menstrual dysfunction, either by medical induction of ovulation or progestin suppression of ovarian steroidogensis.

Androgen-producing tumors

There are two findings which should stimulate the clinician to suspect the presence of an androgen-producing tumor. One is a history of rapidly progressive masculinization. Hirsutism associated with anovulation is generally slow to develop, often covering a time period of at least several years. Tumors are associated with a short time course, measured in months. The second finding which should arouse suspicion is a testosterone level greater than 2.0 ng/ml. A high level of testosterone is even more worrisome in the presence of normal or only slightly elevated 17-ketosteroids.

Retrograde venous catheterization studies are indicated when the clinical presentation strongly indicates the presence of a tumor, and the pelvic examination is normal. When the ovary is the source of the high testosterone, catheterization studies are quite reliable; however adrenal values may be difficult to interpret because of pulsatile secretions and responses to stress. (18, 19) The adminis-

145

tration of human chorionic gonadotropin (2000 IU intra
venously) may be useful; an ovarian response is see
within 10 minutes in the ovarian veins and in 30 minute
peripherally. (19) The technique of venous catheteriza
tion should be reserved for patients in whom an androger
producing tumor is strongly suspected. The risks involved
the technical difficulty in achieving bilateral catheteriza
tion, episodic adrenal secretion, dissimilar hormonal ou
put by the ovaries, and the radiation exposure—all argu
against the use of this procedure in the evaluation of th
routine patient with hirsutism. (20)

Regardless of what the initial testosterone levels are, on
should expect a significant decrease after 6 months
treatment with suppression of LH. An elevated testoste
one and a lack of clinical response after at least 6 month
of treatment indicate a need for further evaluation, pe
haps with retrograde catheterization studies.

**End-Organ
Hypersensitivity
(Idiopathic
Hirsutism)**

There are some patients who present with hirsutism, bu
ovulate regularly. This category of patients has in th
past been labeled idiopathic or familial hirsutism, and
more pronounced in certain geographic areas and amon
certain ethnic groups. The only satisfactory explanatic
for this distressing problem is hypersensitivity of th
skin's hair apparatus to normal levels of androgen
Because of this excessive sensitivity, normal levels
androgen stimulate hair growth. Even in these case
hirsutism responds to ovarian suppression with a comb
nation birth control pill. Suppression of normal femal
androgen levels to subnormal concentrations diminishe
the stimulus to the hair follicles, yielding the same stabili
ing results seen in other hirsute women. While hirsutis
due to an endocrine disorder requires control, end orga
hypersensitivity is treated only for the purpose of cosmet
improvement. Electrolysis is a useful adjunct in this grou
of patients.

**Patients
Requiring
Hospitalization
for Evaluation**

Under the following circumstances, the patient require
full diagnostic evaluation as an inpatient:

1. A testosterone level greater than 2.0 ng/ml.

2. Signs and symptoms of Cushing's syndrome with a
   abnormally elevated plasma cortisol following dexameth
   asone.

3. Failure to suppress 17-ketosteroid excretion with dexa
   methasone.

4. Hirsutism with a unilaterally enlarged ovary.

5. In the absence of adrenal disease, failure of treatment t
   suppress plasma testosterone after 6 months.

146

Hospital Orders for Diagnostic Differentiation of Excess Androgen Production

Day 1: Baseline: Plasma 17-hydroxyprogesterone (normal: <2 ng/ml); Plasma cortisol at 8 AM and 4 PM (normal: 8 AM—12-24 μg%, 4 PM—usually 50% less than 8 AM value); 24 hour urine for 17-ketosteroids (17-KS) (normal: 7-13 mg), 17-hydroxysteroids (17-OHC) (normal: 4-10 mg), pregnanetriol (normal: 2-4 mg, depending upon the laboratory), creatinine. Routine studies: electrolytes, blood urea nitrogen, Ca, P, fasting blood sugar, thyroid indices.

Day 2: Repeat baseline.

Day 3: ACTH stimulation: 0.5 mg Cortrosyn in 1000 ml normal saline in by 4 PM (500 ml in by 1 PM) ; at 8 AM, 1 PM, and 5 PM: plasma cortisol; 24 hour urine for 17-KS, 17-OHC, pregnanetriol, and creatinine (normal response: 3-5 fold increase in plasma cortisol, but not greater than 70 μg%; less than 2 fold increase in 17-KS and 17-OHC).

Days 4, 5, and 6: Low dose dexamethasone suppression: 0.5 mg every 6 hours; on days 5 and 6: Plasma cortisol in AM: 24 hour urine for 17-KS, 17-OHC, creatinine, pregnanetriol (normal response: decrease in plasma cortisol to less than 6 μg%; 17-OHC to less than 4 mg; 17-KS to less than 6 mg).

Days 7, 8, 9: High dose dexamethasone suppression: 2.0 mg every 6 hours. Days 8 and 9: plasma cortisol in AM; 24 hour urine for 17-KS, 17-OHC, pregnanetriol, and creatinine (normal response: plasma cortisol to less than 3 μg%; 17-OHC to less than 2 mg; 17-KS to less than 4 mg).

In Cushing's syndrome due to adrenal hyperplasia, there may be little suppression of 17-OHC with low dose dexamethasone, but a decrease to less than 50% of baseline 17-OHC is to be expected on high dose dexamethasome. In excess androgen production due to adrenal hyperplasia, 17-KS excretion is suppressed to less than 4 mg on high dose dexamethasone. With an androgen-producing adrenal or ovarian tumor, there is no significant suppression. Occasionally high dose dexamethasone will suppress an androgen-producing adrenal tumor, and therefore a lack of suppression with low dose dexamethasone will be helpful in the diagnosis.

We and others have utilized human chorionic gonadotropin stimulation (10,000 IU intramuscularly daily) while continuing the high dose dexamethasone adrenal suppression. An increase (2 fold) in 17-ketosteroid excretion due to this gonadotropic stimulation of the ovary is thought to delineate an ovarian source for excess androgens. We now feel that this response is highly variable, frequently difficult to interpret, and almost always unnecessary.

When a high degree of clinical indication exists for the presence of an androgen-producing tumor, retrograde catheterization studies are useful prior to surgical exploration.

References

1. **Bardin, CW, and Lipsett, M,** Testosterone and Androstenedione Blood Production Rates in Normal Women and Women with Idiopathic Hirsutism and Polycystic Ovaries, J Clin Invest 46:891, 1967.

2. **Larson, BA, Vanderlaan, WP, Judd, HL, and McCullough, DL,** A Testosterone-producing Adrenal Cortical Adenoma in an Elderly Woman, J Clin Endocrinol Metab 42:882, 1976.

3. **Werk, EE, Jr., Sholiton, LJ, and Kalejs, L,** Testosterone-secreting Adrenal Adenoma Under Gonadotropin Control, New Eng J Med 289:767, 1973.

4. **Givens, JR, Andersen, RN, Wiser, WL, Coleman, SA, and Fish, SA,** A Gonadotropin-responsive Adrenocortical Adenoma, J Clin Endocrinol Metab 38:126, 1974.

5. **Abraham, GE,** Ovarian and Adrenal Contribution to Peripheral Androgens During the Menstrual Cycle, J Clin Endocrinol Metab 39:340, 1974.

6. **Judd, HL, Anderson, DC, and Yen, SSC,** Delineation of Abnormal Adrenal Function in Polycystic Ovary Syndrome, Gynec Invest 7:76, 1976.

7. **Easterling, WE, Jr., Talbert, LM, and Potter, HD,** Serum Testosterone Levels in the Polycystic Ovary Syndrome, Am J Obstet Gynec 120:385, 1974.

8. **Givens, JR,** Hirsutism and Hyperandrogenism, Adv In Med 21:221, 1976.

9. **Korth-Schutz, S, Levine, LS, and New, MI,** Dehydroepiandrosterone Sulfate (DS) Levels, a Rapid Test for Abnormal Adrenal Androgen Secretion, J, Clin Endocrinol Metab 42:1005, 1976.

10. **Abraham, GE, Chakmakjian, ZH, Buster, JE, and Marshall, JR,** Ovarian and Adrenal Contributions to Peripheral Androgens in Hirsute Women, Obstet Gynec 46:169, 1975.

11. **Givens, JR, Andersen, RN, Wiser, WL, Umstot, ES, and Fish, SA,** The Effectiveness of Two Oral Contraceptives in Suppressing Plasma Androstenedione, Testosterone, LH, and FSH, and in Stimulating Plasma Testosterone-binding Capacity in Hirsute Women, Am J Obstet Gynec 124:333, 1976.

12. **Kirschner, MA, Bardin, CW, Hembree, WC, and Ross, GT,** Effect of Estrogen Administration on Androgen Production and Plasma Luteinizing Hormone in Hirsute Women, J Clin Endocrinol Metab 30:727, 1970.

13. **Gordon, GG, Southren, AL, Tochimoto, S, Olivo, J, Altman, K, Rand, J, and Lemberger, L,** Effect of Medroxyprogesterone Acetate (Provera) on the Metabolism and Biological Activity of Testosterone, J Clin Endocrinol Metab 30:449, 1970.

14. **Hammerstein, J, Mickies, J, Leo-Rossberg, I, Moltz, L, and Zielske, F,** Use of Cyproterone Acetate in the Treatment of Acne, Hirsutism, and Virilism, J Steroid Biochem 6:827, 1975.

15. **Givens, JR, Andersen, RN, Ragland, JB, Wiser, WL, and Umstot, ES,** Adrenal Function in Hirsutism. II. Diurinal Change and Response of Plasma Androstenedione, Testosterone, 17-Hydroxyprogesterone, Cortisol, LH and FSH to Dexamethasone and 12 Units of ACTH, J Clin Endocrinol Metab 40:988, 1975.

16. **Abraham, GE, and Maroulis, GB,** Effect of Exogenous Estrogen on Serum Pregnenolone, Cortisol, and Androgens in Postmenopausal Women, Obstet Gynec 45:271, 1975.

17. **Sobrinho, LG, Kase, NG, and Grunt, JA,** Changes in Adrenocortical Function of Patients with Gonadal Dysgensis After Treatment with Estrogen. J Clin Endocrinol Metab 33:110, 1971.

18. **Stahl, NL, Teeslink, CR, and Greenblatt, RB,** Ovarian, Adrenal, and Peripheral Testosterone Levels in the Polycystic Ovary Syndrome, Am J Obstet Gynec 117:194, 1973.

19. **Parker, CR, Bruneteau, DW, Greenblatt, RB, and Mahesh, VB,** Peripheral Ovarian and Adrenal Vein Steroids in Hirsute Women: Acute Effects of HCG and ACTH, Fertil Steril 26:877, 1975.

20. **Wentz, AC, White, RI, Jr., Migeon, CJ, Hsu, TH, Barnes, HV, and Jones, GS,** Differential Ovarian and Adrenal Vein Catheterization, Am J Obstet Gynec 125:1000, 1976.

3

Dysfunctional Uterine Bleeding

The thesis advanced in this chapter is that dysfunctional uterine bleeding, defined as a variety of bleeding manifestations of anovulatory cycles, can be confidently managed without surgical intervention, by therapeutic regimens founded on sound physiologic principles. This formulation is based on knowledge of how the postovulatory menstrual function is naturally controlled, and utilizes pharmacologic application of sex steroids to reverse the abnormal tissue factors which lead to the excessive and prolonged flow typical of anovulatory cycles.

Three major categories of dysfunctional endometrial bleeding are dealt with:

1. estrogen breakthrough bleeding;

2. estrogen withdrawal bleeding; and

3. progesterone breakthrough bleeding.

In each instance the manner in which the endometrium deviates from the norm is depicted and specific steroid therapy is recommended to counter the difficulties each situation presents.

This mode of clinical management has been in regular u
for many years and *failure to control vaginal bleeding wi
this therapy, despite appropriate application and utiliz
tion, excludes the diagnosis of dysfunctional uterine blee
ing. If this occurs, attention is directed to a patholog
entity within the reproductive tract as the cause of abnorm
bleeding.*

In the following pages, we will substantiate our thesis in
more detailed fashion. First, a review of the endometri
changes associated with an ovulatory cycle will be offere
Second, endometrial-sex steroid interactions will I
listed. Finally, typical clinical situations will be presente
and specific acute and long-term management progran
will be itemized.

Histologic Changes in Endometrium during an Ovulatory Cycle

The sequence of endometrial changes associated with a
ovulatory cycle has been carefully studied by Noyes in tl
human and Bartelmez and Markee in the subhuma
primate. (1, 2, 3) From these data a theory of menstru
physiology has developed based upon specific anatom
and functional changes within glandular, vascular, ar
stromal components of the endometrium. These chang
will be discussed in five phases: (1) menstrual endom
trium; (2) the proliferative phase; (3) the secretory phas
(4) preparation for implantation; and finally (5) the pha:
of endometrial breakdown. While these distinctions a
not entirely arbitrary, it must be recalled that the enti
process is an integrated evolutionary cycle of endometri
growth and regression, which is repeated some 300–4C
times during the adult life of the human female.

Menstrual Endometrium

The menstrual endometrium is a relatively thin but den:
tissue. It is composed of the stable nonfunctioning basal
component and a variable amount of residual stratu
spongiosum. At menstruation this latter tissue displays
variety of functional states including disarray and brea
age of glands, fragmentation of vessels and stroma wi
persisting evidence of necrosis, white cell infiltration, ar
red cell interstitial diapedesis. Even as the remnants
menstrual shedding dominate the overall appearance
this tissue, evidence of repair in all tissue components ca
be detected. The menstrual endometrium is a transition.
state bridging the more dramatic exfoliative and prolife
ative phases of the cycle. Its density implies that tr
shortness of height is not entirely due to desquamatio
Collapse of the supporting matrix also contributes signif
cantly to the shallowness. Reticular stains in rhesus end
metrium confirm this "deflated" state.

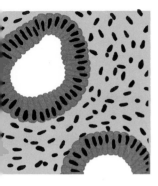 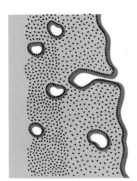

The proliferative phase is associated with ovarian follicle growth and increased estrogen secretion. Undoubtedly as a result of this steroidal action, reconstruction and growth of the endometrium are achieved. The glands are most notable in this response. At first they are narrowed and tubular, lined by low columnar epithelium cells. Mitoses become prominent and pseudostratification is observed. As a result, the glandular epithelium extends peripherally and links one gland segment with its immediate neighbor. A continuous epithelial lining is formed facing the endometrial cavity. The stromal component evolves from its dense cellular menstrual condition through a brief period of edema to a final loose syncytial-like status. Coursing through the stroma, spiral vessels extend unbranched to a point immediately below the epithelial binding membrane. Here they form a loose capillary network.

During proliferation, the endometrium has grown from approximately 0.5 mm to 3.5–5.0 mm in height. Restoration of tissue constituents has been achieved by estrogen-induced new growth as well as incorporation of salt, water, and amino acids. The stromal ground substance has re-expanded from its menstrual collapse. While true tissue growth has occurred, a major element in achievement of endometrial height is "reinflation" of the stroma.

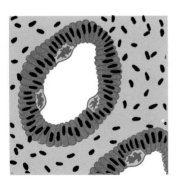 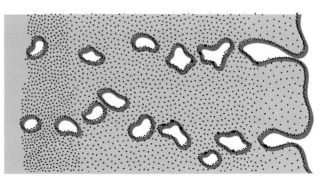

Secretory
Phase

The endometrium now demonstrates a combined reactio to estrogen and progesterone activity. More impressive that total endometrial height is fixed at roughly its pro ovulatory extent despite continued availability of estroger This restraint or inhibition is believed to be induced b progesterone. Individual components of the tissue con tinue to display growth, but confinement in a fixe structure leads to progressive tortuosity of glands an intensified coiling of the spiral vessels. The secretor events within the glandular cells, with progression c vacuoles from intracellular to intraluminal appearance are well-known and take place approximately over a 7 day postovulatory interval. At the conclusion of thes events, the glands appear exhausted, the tortuous lumin variably distended, and individual cell surfaces frag mented and lost (sawtooth appearance). Stroma is in creasingly edematous and spiral vessels are prominen and densely coiled.

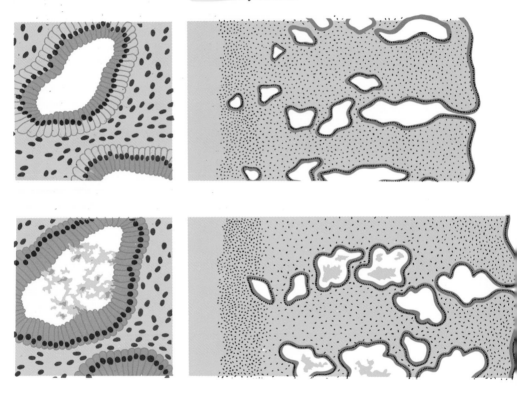

From the 8th to 14th day postovulation, significant changes occur within the endometrium. At the onset of this period, the distended tortuous secretory glands have been most prominent with little intervening stroma. By 13 days postovulation, the endometrium has differentiated into three distinct zones. Something less than one-fourth of the tissue is the unchanged basalis fed by its straight vessels and surrounded by indifferent spindle-shaped stroma. The mid-portion of the endometrium (approximately 50% of the total) is lace-like stratum spongiosa, composed of loose edematous stroma with tightly coiled but ubiquitous spiral vessels and exhausted dilated glandular ribbons. Overlying the spongiosa is the superficial layer of the endometrium (about 25% of the height) called the stratum compacta. Here the prominent histologic feature is the stromal cell, which has become large and polyhedral. In its cytoplasmic expansion one cell abuts the other forming a compact, structurally sturdy layer. The necks of the glands transversing this segment are compressed and less prominent. The subepithelial capillaries and spiral vessels are engorged.

In the absence of fertilization, implantation, and the consequent lack of sustaining quantities of human chorionic gonadotropin from the trophoblast, the otherwise fixed lifespan of the corpus luteum is completed and estrogen and progesterone levels wane. The most prominent immediate effect of this hormone withdrawal is a modest shrinking of the tissue height and remarkable spiral arteriole vasomotor responses. From direct observations of rhesus endometrium, the following vascular sequence has been constructed. With shrinkage of height, blood flow within the spiral vessels diminishes, venous drainage is decreased, and vasodilatation ensues. Thereafter, the spiral arterioles undergo rhythmic vasoconstriction and relaxation. Each successive spasm is more prolonged and profound, leading eventually to endometrial blanching. Within the 24 hours immediately preceding menstruation, these reactions lead to endometrial ischemia and stasis. White cells migrate through capillary walls, at first remaining adjacent to vessels, but then extending throughout the stroma. During arteriolar vasomotor changes, red blood cells escape into the interstitial space.

Eventually considerable leakage occurs as a result of diapedesis and finally interstitial hemorrhage occurs due to breaks in superficial arterioles and capillaries. As ischemia and weakening progress, the continuous binding membrane is fragmented and intercellular blood is extruded into the endometrial cavity. With further tissue disorganization, the endometrium shrinks further and coiled arterioles are buckled. Additional ischemic breakdown ensues with necrosis of cells and defects in vessels adding to the menstrual effluvium. A natural cleavage point exists between basalis and spongiosa and once breached the loose vascular edematous stroma of the

spongiosa desquamates and collapses. In the end, th
typical deflated shallow dense menstrual endometriu
results. Menstrual flow stops as a result of the combine
effects of prolonged vasoconstriction, tissue collapse, an
total vascular stasis. Resumption of estrogen secretic
with its "healing" effects leads to clot formation over th
decapitated stumps of endometrial vessels.

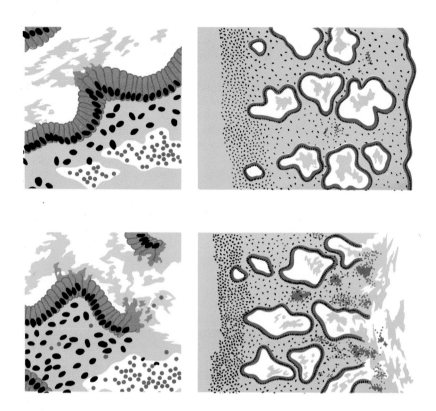

Teleologic Theory of Endometrial – Menstrual Events

An unabashedly teleologic view of the events just d
scribed has been offered by Rock, Garcia and Menk
(4). The basic premise of this thesis is that every end
metrial cycle has as its only goal support of an ear
embryo. Failure to accomplish this objective is followe
by orderly elimination of unutilized tissue and prom
renewal to achieve a more successful cycle.

The ovum must be fertilized within 12–24 hours
ovulation. Over the next 2 days, it remains unattache
within the tubal lumen utilizing tubal fluids and residu
cumulus cells to sustain nutrition and energy for ear
cellular segmentation. After this stay, the solid ball
cells which is the embryo leaves the tube and enters th
uterine cavity. Here the embryo undergoes another 2-
days of unattached but active existence. Fortunately b
this time endometrial gland secretions have filled th

rifices on surface

capillary plexus

lake

ar capillary plexus

rtery

trium

artery

rium

rtery

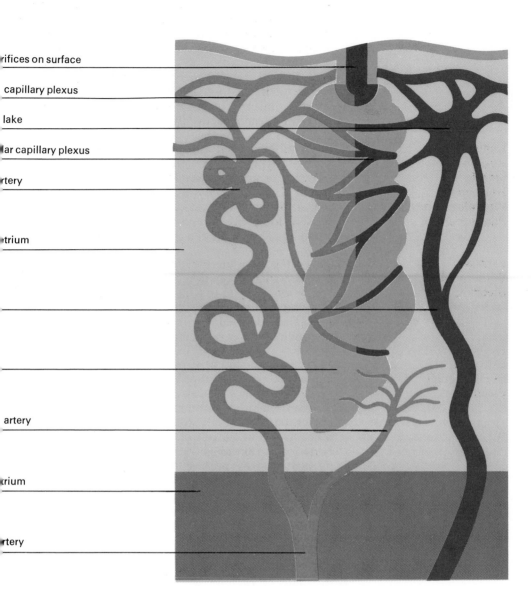

cavity and they bathe the embryo in nutrients. This is the first of many neatly synchronized events that mark the egg-endometrial relationship. By 6 days after ovulation the embryo (now a blastocyst) is ready to attach and implant. It finds by this time an endometrial lining of sufficient depth, vascularity, and nutritional richness to sustain the important events of early placentation to follow. Just below the epithelial lining, a rich capillary plexus has been formed and is available for creation of the trophoblast-maternal blood interface.

Failure of the appearance of human chorionic gonadotro pin (HCG), despite otherwise appropriate tissue reac tions, leads to the vasomotor changes associated wit estrogen-progesterone withdrawal and menstrual desqua mation. However, not all the tissue is lost, and in an event a residual basalis is always available, making re sumption of growth with estrogen a relatively rapid pro cess. Indeed, even as menses persists, early regeneration can be seen. As soon as follicle maturation occurs (in a short a time as 10 days), the endometrium is ready t perform its reproductive function.

Endometrial Responses to Steroid Hormones — Physiologic and Pharmacologic

Obviously estrogen and progesterone withdrawal is no the only type of endometrial bleeding provoked by th presence of sex steroids and their effects on the endome trium. There are clinical examples for estrogen with drawal bleeding and estrogen breakthrough bleeding, a well as for progesterone withdrawal and breakthroug bleeding. The events can be summarized.

Estrogen Withdrawal Bleeding

This category of uterine bleeding can occur after bilatera oophorectomy, radiation of mature follicles, or adminis tration of estrogen to a castrate and then discontinuatio of therapy. Similarly the bleeding which occurs postcastra tion can be delayed by concomitant estrogen therapy. O discontinuation of exogenous estrogen flow will occur.

Estrogen Breakthrough Bleeding

Here a semiquantitative relationship exists between th amount of estrogen stimulating the endometrium and th type of bleeding which can ensue. Relatively low doses o estrogen yield intermittent spotting which may be pro longed but is generally light in quantity of flow. On th other hand, high levels of estrogen and sustained availa bility lead to prolonged periods of amenorrhea followe by acute, often profuse bleeds with excessive loss o blood.

Progesterone Withdrawal Bleeding

Removal of the corpus luteum will lead to endometria desquamation. Pharmacologically, a similar event can b achieved by administration and discontinuation of proges terone or a nonestrogenic progestin derivative. Progester one withdrawal bleeding occurs only if the endometrium is initially proliferated by endogenous or exogenous estro gen. If estrogen therapy is continued as progesterone i withdrawn, the progesterone withdrawal bleeding stil occurs. Only if estrogen levels are increased 10–20 fol will progesterone withdrawal bleeding be delayed.

Progesterone Breakthrough Bleeding

Progesterone breakthrough occurs only in the presence o an unfavorably high ratio of progesterone to estrogen. I the absence of sufficient estrogen, continuous progester one therapy will yield intermittent bleeding of variabl duration, similar to low dose estrogen breakthrough note above.

Of all the types of hormonal-endometrial relationships, the most stable endometrium and the most reproducible menstrual function in terms of quantity and duration is the postovulatory estrogen-progesterone withdrawal bleeding response. It is so controlling that many women over the years come to expect a certain characteristic flow pattern. Any slight deviations, such as plus or minus 1 day in duration or minor deviation from expected napkin or tampon utilization, are causes for major concern in the patient. So ingrained is the expected flow that considerable physician reassurance may be required in some instances. The usual duration of flow is 4–6 days, but many women flow as little as 2 days, and as much as 8 days. While the postovulatory phase averages 14 days, greater variability in the proliferative phase produces a distribution in the duration of a menstrual cycle.

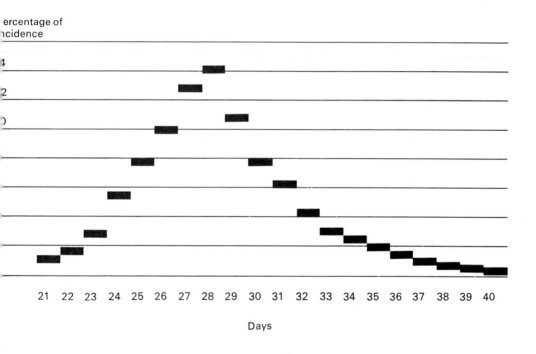

There are three reasons for the self-limited character of estrogen-progesterone withdrawal bleeding:

1. It is a universal endometrial event. Because the onset and conclusion of menses are related to a precise sequence of hormonal events, the initiation of menstrual changes occurs almost simultaneously in all segments of the uterine endometrium.

2. The endometrial tissue which has responded to an appro priate sequence of estrogen and progesterone is structu ally stable. Furthermore, the events leading to ischemi disintegration of the endometrium are orderly and pro gressive, being related to rhythmic waves of vasoconstric tion of increasing duration.

3. Inherent in the events that start menstrual function fo lowing estrogen-progesterone are the factors involved i stopping menstrual flow. Just as waves of vasoconstrictio initiate the ischemic events provoking menses, so wi prolonged vasoconstriction abetted by the stasis assoc ated with endometrial collapse enable clotting factors t seal off the exposed bleeding sites. Additional and signif cant effects are obtained by resumed estrogen activity.

Suggestions as to Why Anovulatory Bleeding is Excessive

Most instances of anovulatory bleeding are examples c estrogen withdrawal or estrogen breakthrough bleeding Furthermore, the most virulent type of bleeding is second ary to high sustained levels of estrogen associated with th polycystic ovary syndrome, obesity, immaturity of th hypothalamic-pituitary-ovarian axis as in postpuberta teenagers, and late anovulation, usually involving wome in their late thirties and early forties. Unopposed estroge induces a progression of endometrial responses in th following pattern: proliferative hyperplasia, adenomatou hyperplasia, and in some, over the course of many years atypia and carcinoma. In the absence of growth limitin progesterone and periodic desquamation, the endome trium attains an abnormal height without concomitan structural support. The tissue increasingly displays intens vascularity, back to back glandularity but without a intervening stromal support matrix. This tissue is fragile and will suffer spontaneous superficial breakage an bleeding. As one site heals, another, and yet another ne site of breakdown will appear. The typical clinical pictur is that of a pale frightened teenager who has bled fo weeks. Also frequently encountered is the older woma with prolonged bleeding who is deeply concerned ove this experience as a manifestation of neoplasia.

In these instances the usual endometrial control mecha nisms are missing. This bleeding is *not a universal even* but rather it involves random portions of the endome trium at variable times and in asynchronous sequences The fragility of the vascular adenomatous hyperplasti tissue is responsible for this experience, in part because o excessive growth, but mostly because of irregular stimu lation in which the *structural rigidity of a well-developed stroma or stratum compactum does not occur.* Finally, th flow is prolonged and excessive not only because there i a large quantity of tissue available for bleeding but mor importantly because there is a disorderly, abrupt, ran dom, accidental breakdown of tissue with consequen opening of multiple vascular channels. There is *no vaso constrictive rhythmicity,* no tight coiling of spiral vessels no orderly collapse to induce stasis. The anovulatory tissue can only rely on the "healing" effects of endogenous estrogen to stop local bleeds. However, this is a vicious cycle in that this healing is only temporary, and leads to certain repeat breakdown in the near future.

Alternate Hypothesis

Another explanation for the control of postovulatory endometrial bleeding and regeneration has recently been presented. (5) Based on light and scanning electron microscopy of hysterectomy specimens, this thesis favors non-hormone related regeneration of surface epithelium from basal glands and cornual area residual tissue with restoration of the continuous binding membrane as the critical events in cessation of blood flow. By this account, estrogen withdrawal or breakthrough bleeding is uncontrolled because insufficient stimulus (loss of tissue) for binding surface restoration occurs. Furthermore, curettage is effective in this condition by reachieving sufficient basal glandular denudation (as is seen in combined estrogen and progestin withdrawal) which stimulates regeneration of surface integrity and thus controls blood flow.

Additional studies are needed to clarify the difference of opinion concerning the pathophysiology of dysfunctional uterine bleeding. The therapeutic approach favored in this book utilizes hormonal control of endometrial events and rarely finds it necessary to resort to surgery.

Treatment Program for Anovulatory Bleeding

The immediate objective of medical therapy in anovulatory bleeding is to retrieve the natural controlling influences missing in this tissue: universal, synchronous endometrial events, structural stability, and vasomotor rhythmicity.

This is accomplished rapidly and easily (but sometimes with considerable symptomatology) with oral high dose progestin-estrogen combination birth control pills. Any of the oral combination tablets are useful. Whatever dose is available or chosen, therapy is administered as one pill 4 times a day for 5–7 days. This 4 pills a day therapy is prolonged over this duration despite the anticipated cessation of flow within 12–24 hours. If flow does not clearly abate, other diagnostic possibilities (pathologic causes such as polyps, incomplete abortion, and neoplasia) should be re-evaluated by examination under anesthesia and dilatation and curettage (D and C). If flow does diminish rapidly, the remainder of the week of treatment can be given over to the evaluation of causes of anovulation, hemorrhagic tendencies, and iron or blood replacement. In addition, the week provides time to prepare the patient for the progestin-estrogen withdrawal flow that will soon be induced.

161

For the moment, this therapy has induced the structural rigidity intrinsic to the compact pseudodecidual reaction. As a result, continued random breakdown of formerly fragile tissue is avoided and blood loss stopped. However, a relatively huge amount of tissue remains to react to progestin-estrogen withdrawal. Consequently the patient must be warned to anticipate a heavy and severely cramping flow 2–4 days after stopping therapy. If not prepared in this way, it is certain that the patient will view the problem as recurrent disease or failure of hormonal therapy, and will surely wind up on the operative D and C treadmill.

Therapy   P/E × 7 days   P/E × 21 days   P/E × 21 days   P/E × 21 days

P/E = Progestin-Estrogen combination

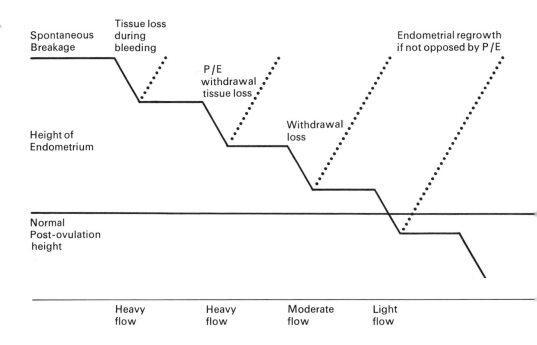

Spontaneous Breakage

Tissue loss during bleeding

Endometrial regrowth if not opposed by P/E

P/E withdrawal tissue loss

Withdrawal loss

Height of Endometrium

Normal Post-ovulation height

Heavy flow   Heavy flow   Moderate flow   Light flow

162

Even more reassuring than the anticipation of difficulty is the confident prophesy that this withdrawal bleed, despite the pain and volume, will be self-limited (as a result of the induced vasomotor rhythmicity). However, to ensure success in this regard, on the 5th day of flow, a low dose cyclic combination birth control medication is initiated with three 3-week treatments, punctuated by 1-week withdrawal flow intervals. Not only does the decreasing volume and pain with each successive cycle reaffirm confidence in control mechanisms, but it also serves to prevent any unopposed estrogen regrowth that might occur. Early application of the progestin-estrogen combination limits growth and allows orderly regression of excessive endometrial height to normal controllable levels. If the progestin-estrogen combination is not applied, abnormal endometrial height and persistent excessive flow would recur.

In the patient not exposed to potential pregnancy, in whom cyclic progestin-estrogen for 3 months has reduced endometrial tissue reservoirs to normal height, the pill may be discontinued and unopposed endogenous estrogen permitted to reactivate the endometrium. At 2-month intervals in the absence of spontaneous (possibly post-ovulatory) menses, the recurrence of the anovulatory status is suspected, sustained estrogen stimulation of the endometrium is assumed, and, before overstimulation of the endometrium is permitted to occur, a brief course of an orally active progestin derivative is administered. Our favorite is Provera, 10 mg orally daily for 5 days. Restrained reasonable flow (progesterone withdrawal flow) will occur 2–7 days after the last pill. With this therapy, excessive endometrial buildup is avoided. Spontaneous ovulation is given a chance to occur and is not impeded as it might be by chronic birth control pill utilization.

Exceptions to Use of Progestin Therapy

Certain exceptions apply in the medical control of dysfunctional uterine bleeding with progestin therapy. Obviously in the age group over 35 years, an initial endometrial biopsy (with multiple sampling) is required to seek worrisome pathology which requires specific therapy. This is especially true in the older woman in the 4th or 5th decade, where adenocarcinoma of the endometrium is a significant problem.

Bleeding manifestations are frequently associated with *minimal (low) estrogen stimulation,* and a partially stimulated endometrial proliferation (see Estrogen Breakthrough Bleeding above) yielding intermittent vaginal spotting. In this circumstance, where minimal endometrium exists, the beneficial effect of progestin treatment is of no avail since a tissue base is lacking on which the progestin can exert its organizational, strengthening action. A similar circumstance also exists in the younger anovulatory patient in whom *prolonged hemorrhagic desquamation* leaves little residual tissue. In these instances the appropriate therapeutic reaction is *not* the traditional operative D and C, which, although it frequently manage the acute problem, does not improve but, in fact, compounds the long-range difficulty by denuding the endometrial reserve even further.

We recommend high dose estrogen therapy using Premarin, 25 mg intravenously every 4 hours until bleeding abates (up to 6 doses can be given). This is the sign that the "healing" events are initiated to a sufficient degree Progestin treatment can be started at the same time.

Progestin therapy is not always a positive controlling factor. Two examples in clinical medicine are evidence of the problems associated with progestin breakthrough bleeding. These are the breakthrough bleeding episode occurring with prolonged use of birth control pills or with depot forms of progesterone derivatives. In the absence of sufficient endogenous and exogenous estrogen, the endometrium shrinks to a shallow height. Furthermore, it is composed almost exclusively of pseudodecidual stroma and blood vessels with minimal glands. Peculiarly, experience has shown that this type of endometrium also yields to the fragility bleeding more typical of pure estrogen stimulation. The clinical story is often that of oral contraception of longstanding, with marked diminution of withdrawal flow. Frequently no bleeding occurs in the nontreatment interval. This is associated with intermittent variable vaginal spotting during the month. The clinical reflex is to double therapy, but this only rarely succeed because the effect is to intensify the progestin atrophic effect. The more appropriate reaction in view of the endometrial condition is estrogen therapy (ethinyl estradiol 20 μg or conjugated estrogens 2.5 mg daily for 1 days) during and in addition to the birth control pill administration. This rejuvenates the endometrium, intermenstrual flow stops, and appropriate withdrawal resumes.

One problem frequently encountered is the progestin breakthrough bleeding experienced in chronic depot administration of progestin. This therapy is used not only for nonwithdrawal contraception, but also in certain situations for chemotherapy. In 75% of cases, continuous therapy provides control without menstrual bleeding. In the remainder, breakthrough progestin bleeding occurs Judicious use of estrogen is the appropriate and effective therapy.

Summary of Key Points in Therapy of Anovulatory (Dysfunctional) Bleeding	Teenager	Adult
	Preliminary: Pelvic or rectal examination	*Preliminary:* Pelvic examination PAP smear Endometrial biopsy

1. Intense progestin-estrogen therapy for 7 days

2. Cyclic low dose oral contraceptive for 3 months

3. If exposed to pregnancy, continue oral contraception

4. If not exposed to pregnancy, Provera, 10 mg daily × 5 every 2 months

---

If bleeding has been prolonged:
If biopsy yields minimal tissue:
If patient is on progestin medication:
If follow-up is uncertain:
Premarin, 25 mg intravenously every 4 hours until bleeding stops, then proceed to step 1 above. If no response in 12–24 hours, proceed with D and C.

The clinical problem of dysfunctional bleeding is associated with either anovulation and estrogen withdrawal or breakthrough bleeding, or with anovulation due to exogenous progestin medication, and therefore bleeding due to progestational endometrial breakthrough. Both categories of bleeding lack the three important characteristics of normal estrogen-progesterone withdrawal bleeding:

1. universal, simultaneous change in all segments of the endometrium;

2. an orderly progression of events involving a rigid, compact structure, and;

3. vasomotor rhythmicity with vasoconstriction, structural collapse, and clotting.

After evaluation and examination, including biopsies where appropriate, therapy involves an initial choice between intensive progestin-estrogen combination medication or high doses of estrogen. The progestin-estrogen combination will be ineffective unless endometrium of sufficient quantity and responsiveness to allow the formation of pseudodecidual tissue is present. Therefore, the initial choice of therapy should be high doses of estrogen (Premarin, 25 mg intravenously every 4 hours until bleeding stops or for 24 hours) in the following situations:

1. when bleeding has been heavy for many days and it is likely that the uterine cavity is now lined only by a raw basalis layer;

165

2. when the endometrial curet yields minimal tissue;

3. when the patient has been on progestin medication (oral contraceptives, intramuscular progestins) and the endometrium is shallow and atrophic; and

4. when follow-up is uncertain, because estrogen therapy will temporarily stop all categories of dysfunctional bleeding.

If high dose estrogen therapy does not significantly abate flow within 12–24 hours, re-evaluation is mandatory, and the need for curettage is likely.

Once the acute bleeding episode in an anovulatory patient is under control, the patient should not be forgotten. With persistent anovulation, recurrent hemorrhage is a common pattern, and more importantly, chronic unopposed estrogen stimulation to the endometrium will eventually lead to atypical tissue changes. It is absolutely necessary that the patient undergo periodic progestational withdrawal, either with a routine oral contraceptive regimen, or if exposure to pregnancy is not a consideration, a progestational agent (Provera, 10 mg daily for 5 days) should be administered every 2 months.

Curettage is *Not* the first line of defense, but rather the last. The utilization of appropriate steroids for the clinical management of dysfunctional bleeding is based upon a physiologic understanding of the endometrium and its response to hormones. Adherence to this program will avoid dilatation and curettage except in a rare case of dysfunctional bleeding, and except in those cases where bleeding is due to a pathologic entity within the reproductive tract where D and C is truly indicated and necessary.

References

1. **Noyes, RW, Hertig, AW, and Rock, J,** Dating the Endometrial Biopsy, Fertil Steril 1:3, 1950.

2. **Bartlemez, GW,** The Phases of the Menstrual Cycle and Their Interpretation in Terms of the Pregnancy Cycle, Am J Obstet Gynec 74:931, 1957.

3. **Markee, JE,** Morphological Basis for Menstrual Bleeding, Bull NY Acad Med 24:253, 1948.

4. **Rock, J, Garcia, CR, and Menkin, M,** A Theory of Menstruation, Ann NY Acad Sci 75:830, 1959.

5. **Ferenczy, A,** Studies on the Cytodynamics of Human Endometrial Regeneration. I. Scanning Electron Microscopy. Am J Obstet Gynec 124:64, 1976.

9   **The Breast**

As mammals, breasts define our biological class. Breast function nourishes and sustains us, while breast contours occupy our attention. As obstetricians, we seek to enhance or diminish function, and as gynecologists, the appearance of inappropriate lactation (galactorrhea) is of grave concern. Cancer of the breast is a leading cause of death in women.

In this chapter, the factors involved in normal growth and development of the breast will be reviewed, including the physiology of normal lactation. A description of the numerous factors leading to inappropriate lactation will follow, and finally, the endocrine aspects of breast cancer will be considered.

Growth and Development

The basic component of the breast lobule is the hollow alveolus or milk gland lined by a single layer of milk-secreting epithelial cells, derived from an ingrowth of epidermis into the underlying mesenchyme at 10–12 weeks of gestation. Each alveolus is encased in a criss-crossing mantle of contractile myoepithelial strands. Also surrounding the milk gland is a rich capillary network. The lumen of the alveolus connects to a collecting intralobar duct by means of a thin nonmuscular duct. Contractile muscle cells encase the intralobular ducts that eventually reach the exterior via the apertures in the areola.

Growth of this milk-producing system is dependent on numerous hormonal factors which occur in two sequences, at puberty and then in pregnancy. Although there is considerable overlapping of hormonal influences, the differences in quantities of the stimuli in each circumstance and the availability of entirely unique inciting factors (HPL and prolactin) during pregnancy permit this chronologic distinction.

Overall the major influence to breast growth at puberty is estrogen. In most girls the first response to the increasing levels of estrogen is an increase in size and pigmentation of the areola, and the formation of a mass of breast tissue just underneath the areola. Breast tissue binds estrogen in a manner similar to events in the uterus and vagina. The primary effect of this steroid, in subprimate mammals, is to stimulate growth of the ductal portion of the gland system. Progesterone in similar systems appears to influence growth of the alveolar components of the lobule. However, neither hormone alone or in combination is capable of yielding optimum breast growth and development. Full differentiation of the gland requires the availability of insulin, cortisol, thyroxine, prolactin, and growth hormone.

The estrogen-induced impetus to mammary epithelial stem cell division requires the presence of insulin. Final differentiation of the alveolar epithelial cell into a mature milk cell is accomplished in the presence of prolactin, but only after prior exposure to cortisol and insulin. The complete reaction depends on the availability of minimal quantities of thyroid hormone. Thus the endocrinologically intact organism in which estrogen, progesterone, thyroxine, cortisol, insulin, prolactin, and growth hormone are available can have appropriate breast growth. Mild deficiencies in any of the prerequisites, short of severe restrictions or total absence, can be compensated for by excess prolactin. Furthermore, the growth of the breast and breast function can be incited by an excess of prolactin.

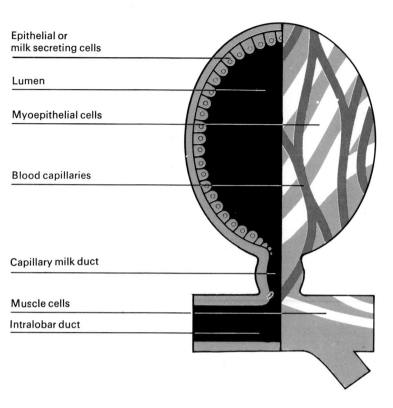

Epithelial or
milk secreting cells

Lumen

Myoepithelial cells

Blood capillaries

Capillary milk duct

Muscle cells

Intralobar duct

Abnormal Shapes and Sizes

Early differentiation of the mammary gland anlage is under fetal hormonal control. Abnormalities in adult size or shape may reflect the impact of hormones (especially the presence or absence of testosterone) during this early period of development. Occasionally the breast bud will begin to develop on one side first. Similarly one breast may grow faster than the other. These inequalities usually disappear by the time development is complete. However exact equalness in size is usually never attained. Significant asymmetry is only correctable by the plastic surgeon. Likewise hypoplasia and hypertrophy can only be treated by corrective surgery. Hormone therapy is totally ineffective in producing a permanent change in breast shape or size. Of course in patients with primary amenorrhea secondary to deficient ovarian function, estrogen replacement will induce significant and gratifying breast growth.

Pregnancy and Milk Secretion

During pregnancy, in addition to huge increments in estrogen and progesterone, prolactin levels rise to high levels, reaching a peak at parturition. Elevated blood levels of prolactin first appear at about 8 weeks gestation, and reach a mean level of 200 ng/ml at term. (1, 2)

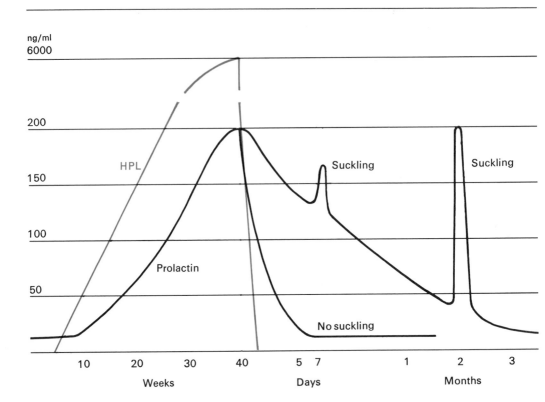

The amniotic fluid content of prolactin is extremely high. Early in pregnancy the concentration is about 2500 ng/ml, declining to 350 ng/ml near term. (1) Maternal prolactin does not pass to the fetus in significant amounts. Therefore the origin of the prolactin in amniotic fluid must be either the fetal pituitary gland or trophoblastic tissue. It has been speculated that chorionic tissue may synthesize prolactin, and prolactin in this tissue may play a role similar to its regulation of sodium transport and water movement across the gills in fish. (2)

There is marked variability in prolactin levels in pregnancy, with a diurnal variation as is also found in nonpregnant persons. The peak level occurs 4–5 hours after the onset of sleep. (3) The initial rise at 7–8 weeks gestation correlates with the rising levels of estradiol (4), which appears to act at the hypothalamic level to increase prolactin secretion. (5)

Pregnancy is also characterized by increased availability of free cortisol, hyperinsulinemia, and production of HPL. Made by the placenta and actively secreted into the maternal circulation from the 6th week of pregnancy, HPL levels rise progressively reaching approximately

6000 ng/ml at term. Though displaying less activity than prolactin, HPL is produced in such large amounts that the overall effect is marked breast growth stimulation.

Although all the hormones necessary for growth are available in pregnancy, only non-milk colostrum (composed of desquamated epithelium and transudate) is produced during the gestation. Full lactation is believed to be inhibited by a restraining effect on prolactin action at the target tissue by estrogen. The increasing levels of estrogen are responsible for the rising level of prolactin secretion, but at the same time, they prevent the full effects of prolactin. (3, 6)

Breast engorgement occurs on the 3rd or 4th day postpartum, when estrogen and progesterone levels have waned. The clearance of prolactin is slower, requiring 7 days in non-breast-feeding women to reach non-pregnant levels following delivery. (1) After delivery the rapid decrease in estrogen levels results in the removal of estrogen interference with prolactin action upon the breast.

Therefore maintenance of this interference by the administration of estrogen will prevent breast engorgement and lactation. Ergot alkaloids (e.g. bromergocriptine, 5 mg bid) which directly inhibit pituitary secretion of prolactin are even more effective in preventing milk secretion postpartum. (7)

In the first postpartum week, prolactin levels in breast-feeding women decline approximately 50% (to about 100 ng/ml). Suckling elicits transient increases in prolactin, which are probably important to initiate milk production. Until 2–3 months postpartum, basal levels are approximately 40–50 ng/ml, and there are large (about 10–20 fold) increases after suckling. After 3–4 months, the basal levels are normal, and suckling may or may not produce an increase. It is not understood why the prolactin response to suckling is lost after 4 months.

Once produced, milk is secreted into the lumen of the alveolus. Maintenance of milk production at high levels is dependent on the joint action of both anterior and posterior pituitary factors. By mechanisms to be described in detail shortly, suckling causes continued release of both prolactin and oxytocin. The former sustains milk protein, casein, fatty acids, lactose, and volume of secretion, while the latter, by contracting myoepithelial cells and emptying the alveolar lumen, enhances further milk secretion and alveolar refilling. Again the optimum quantity and quality of milk are dependent upon the availability of thyroid, insulin, cortisol, and the dietary intake of nutrients and fluids. Frequent emptying of the lumen is an important feature in maintaining an adequate level of secretion. Indeed, after the 4th postpartum month, suckling appears to be the only stimulant required, but environmental and

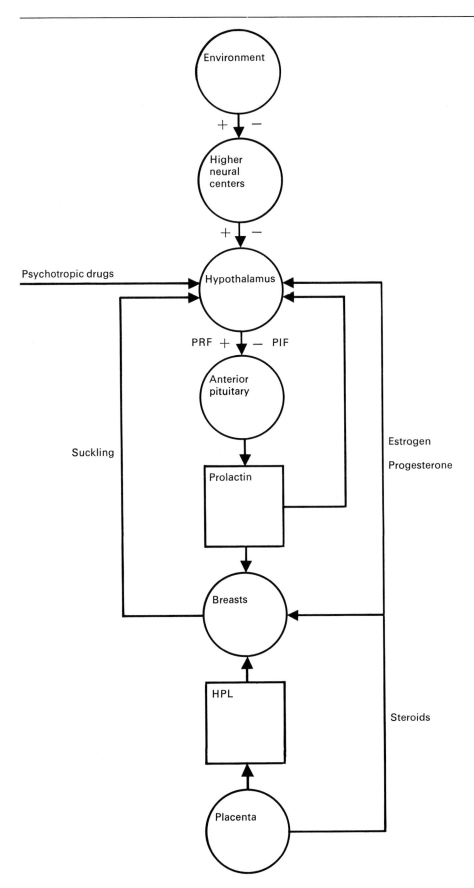

emotional states also are important for continued alveolar activity. The failure to lactate within the first 7 days postpartum may be the first sign of Sheehan's syndrome (hypopituitarism following intrapartum infarction of the pituitary gland).

The ejection of milk from the breast does not occur as the result of a mechanically induced negative pressure produced by suckling. Tactile sensors concentrated in the areola activate an afferent sensory neural arc which stimulates the paraventricular and supraoptic nuclei of the hypothalamus to synthesize and transport oxytocin to the posterior pituitary, and to release oxytocin from the posterior pituitary. The efferent arc (oxytocin) is blood-borne to the breast alveolus ductal systems to contract myoepithelial cells and empty the alveolar lumen. Milk contained in major ductal repositories is ejected from openings in the areola. This rapid release of milk is called "letdown." In many instances the activation of oxytocin release leading to letdown does not require initiation by tactile stimuli. The central nervous system can be conditioned to respond to the presence of the infant, or to the sound of the infant's cry to induce activation of the efferent arc.

The oxytocin effect is a release phenomenon acting on secreted and stored milk. For continued secretory replacement of ejected milk, at least in the first months of breast-feeding, prolactin must be available in sufficient quantities. As previously noted, suckling ensures adequate prolactin availability until the 4th postpartum month, after which elevated prolactin levels are no longer necessary.

Prolactin Inhibiting Factor (PIF)

Suckling suppresses the formation of a hypothalamic substance, prolactin inhibiting factor (PIF). This intrahypothalamic effect is either mediated by dopamine, or in contrast to the peptide nature of other hypothalamic hormones, PIF may be dopamine itself. (8) PIF is secreted by the basal hypothalamus into the portal system and conducted to the anterior pituitary. PIF suppresses secretion of prolactin into the general circulation. In the absence of PIF, prolactin is secreted. Suckling, therefore, acts to refill the breast with milk by activating both portions of the pituitary (anterior and posterior) to cause the breast to eject milk and to replace milk by production.

Prolactin Releasing Factor (PRF)

Prolactin may also be influenced by a positive hypothalamic factor (prolactin releasing factor, PRF). PRF does exist in various fowl (e.g. pigeon, chicken, duck, turkey, and the tricolored blackbird). While the identity of this material has not been elucidated or its function substantiated in normal human physiology, it is possible that thyroid releasing hormone (TRH) may be active as a PRF. Synthetic TRH is a potent stimulant of prolactin secretion in man. The smallest doses of TRH which are capable of producing an increase in TSH, also increase prolactin levels, a finding which supports a physiologic role for TRH in the control of prolactin secretion. (9) However normal physiologic changes as well as abnormal prolactin secretion are best explained and understood in terms of variations in the inhibiting factor, PIF, except in hypothyroidism.

Contraceptive Effect of Lactation

A moderate contraceptive effect accompanies lactation. It is well-known that this is a temporary and at best a contraceptive effect of low reliability. Approximately 40–75% of breast-feeding women resume menstrual function while still nursing. The mechanism of this contraceptive effect is of interest in that similar interference with normal pituitary-gonadal function is seen in association with elevated prolactin levels in non-pregnant women, e.g. in the syndrome of galactorrhea and amenorrhea.

Experimental evidence suggests that the ovaries may be refractory to gonadotropin stimulation during lactation, and in addition, the pituitary may be less responsive to GnRH stimulation. (10, 11) However other studies indicate that the pituitary as well as the ovaries in the postpartum period are responsive to tropic hormone stimulation. (12, 13) Elevated prolactin levels are associated with decreased gonadal function, but the mechanism of action remains unclear and requires further investigation.

Cessation of Lactation

Lactation can be concluded by specifically stopping suckling. The primary effect of this cessation is loss of milk letdown via the neural evocation of oxytocin. With passage of a few days, the swollen alveoli depress milk formation, probably via a local pressure effect. Furthermore, the absence of suckling reactivates PIF production so that less prolactin stimulation of milk secretion is available. However after approximately 4 months of breast-feeding, prolactin probably serves only a permissive role, as levels gradually decline and response to suckling diminishes. With resorption of fluid and solute, the swollen engorged breast diminishes in size in a few days.

Inappropriate Lactation – Galactorrheic Syndromes

Galactorrhea refers to the mammary secretion of a milky fluid which is nonphysiologic in that it is inappropriate (not immediately related to pregnancy or the needs of a child), persistent, and sometimes excessive. Although usually white or clear, the color may be yellow or even green. In the latter circumstances local breast disease should also be considered. To elicit breast secretion, pressure should be applied to all sections of the breast, beginning at the base of the breast, and working up towards the nipple. The quantity of secretion is not an important criterion. Any galactorrhea demands evaluation in a nulliparous woman, and if at least 12 months have ensued since the last pregnancy, in a parous woman. Galactorrhea can involve both breasts, or just one breast.

Amenorrhea does not necessarily accompany galactor-rhea, even in the most serious provocative disorders.

Differential
Diagnosis

The differential diagnosis of galactorrhea syndromes is a difficult and complex clinical challenge. The difficulty arises from the multiple factors involved in the control of prolactin release. Before proceeding, it would be proper to re-emphasize the mechanisms controlling prolactin secretion. In most pathophysiologic systems the final common pathway leading to galactorrhea is an inappropriate augmentation of prolactin release. Prolactin is under a chronic tonic inhibition due to the hypothalamic secretion into the pituitary portal system of PIF, prolactin inhibiting factor. The following considerations are important:

1. Excessive estrogen (e.g. birth control pills) can lead to milk secretion via hypothalamic suppression, causing reduction of PIF and release of pituitary prolactin. Galactorrhea developing during birth control pill administration may be most noticeable during the days free of medication (when the steroids are cleared from the body and the prolactin interfering action of estrogen wanes). Galactorrhea caused by excessive estrogen disappears within 3 to 6 months after discontinuing medication.

2. Prolonged intensive suckling can also release prolactin, via the same process of hypothalamic reduction of PIF. Similarly, thoracotomy scars, cervical spinal lesions, and herpes zoster can induce prolactin release by activating the afferent sensory neural arc, thereby simulating suckling.

3. A variety of drugs can also inhibit hypothalamic PIF. (14) There are nearly 100 phenothiazine derivatives with indirect mammotropic activity of this type. In addition, there are many phenothizine-like compounds, reserpine derivatives, amphetamines, and an unknown variety of other drugs which can initiate galactorrhea via hypothalamic suppression (opiates, diazepines, butyrophenones, α-methyldopa, and tricyclic anti-depressants such as Elavil and Tofranil). The final action of these compounds is either to deplete dopamine levels or to block dopamine receptors. Chemical features common to many of these materials are an aromatic ring with a polar substituent as in estrogen, and at least two additional rings or structural attributes making spatial arrangements similar to two rings possible. Thus these compounds may act in a manner similar to estrogens to decrease PIF. In support of this conclusion, it has been demonstrated that estrogen and phenothiazine derivatives compete for the same receptors in the median eminence. Prolactin is uniformly elevated in patients on therapeutic amounts of phenothiazines. Approximately 30–50% will exhibit galactorrhea, which should not persist beyond 3 to 6 months after drug treatment is discontinued.

4. Stresses (capable of *increasing* hypothalamic PIF and diminishing prolactin) can also *inhibit* hypothalamic PIF and induce prolactin secretion and galactorrhea. Trauma, surgical procedures, and anesthesia can be seen in temporal relation to the onset of galactorrhea.

5. Hypothalamic lesions, stalk lesions, or stalk compression (events that physically reduce production or delivery of PIF to the pituitary) can release excess prolactin leading to galactorrhea.

6. Hypothyroidism (juvenile or adult) can be associated with galactorrhea. With diminished circulating levels of thyroid hormone, hypothalamic TRH is produced in excess and may act as a PRF to release prolactin from the pituitary. Juvenile hypothyroidism in association with breast development, and galactorrhea may be seen. Reversal with thyroid is strong circumstantial evidence to support the conclusion that TRH stimulates prolactin.

7. Increased prolactin release may be the consequence of prolactin elaboration and secretion from pituitary tumors which function independently of the otherwise appropriate restraints exerted by PIF from a normally functioning hypothalamus. This potentially dangerous tumor, which has endocrine, neurologic, and ophthalmologic liabilities that are potentially disabling, makes the differential diagnosis of persistent galactorrhea a major clinical challenge. Beyond producing prolactin, the tumor may also suppress pituitary parenchyma by expansion and compression interfering with the secretion of other tropic hormones.

Clinical Problem of Galactorrhea	A variety of eponymic designations have been applied to variants of the lactation syndromes. These are based on the association of galactorrhea with intrasellar tumor (Forbes, Henneman, Griswold, and Albright, 1951), antecedent pregnancy with inappropriate persistence of galactorrhea (independently reported by Chiari and Frommel in 1852), and the absence of previous pregnancy (Argonz and del Castillo, 1953). In all, the association of galactorrhea with eventual amenorrhea was noted.

On the basis of currently available information, categorization of individual cases according to these eponymic guidelines is neither helpful nor does it permit discrimination of patients who have serious intrasellar or suprasellar pathology.

Symptoms of galactorrhea can antedate the recognition of intrasellar tumors by many years. It is recognized that 10–12 years of galactorrhea and amenorrhea may precede the radiologic demonstration of a pituitary adenoma by routine skull films. With the use of the new technique of polytomography (described in Chapter 5) this interval may be shortened. Nevertheless, follow-up must be prolonged and zealous. Furthermore, the criterion of antecedent pregnancy does not necessarily suggest a different pathophysiologic process involved in the galactorrhea. Cases of pituitary adenoma which did not alter competent gonadotropin secretion are known, and conception has occurred in some of these patients.

Galactorrheic women with pituitary tumors shown by x-ray can demonstrate withdrawal from progestin administration and even have menses and ovulate, as noted above. However, a single lesion is usually sufficiently extensive or critically placed to impair menstrual function, and on rare occasions, other tropic hormones (growth hormone, TSH, ACTH). In many patients the amenorrhea or anovulation is directly due to elevated prolactin levels interfering at either the ovarian or pituitary level (or both).

Regardless of the clinical circumstances, when galactorrhea has been present 6 months to 1 year, a pituitary tumor must be considered.

Methods of
Differential
Diagnosis

Clinical Data. Is there historical, physical, or laboratory evidence for other tropic hormone loss (hypothyroidism, hypoadrenalism, hypogonadism) in addition to galactorrhea? Is there neurologic, or ophthalmologic evidence of tumor compression, erosion, or extension? Is there excessive suckling precoitally, or drug intake? Is there a lung tumor, or a chest wall lesion? Turkington has reported ectopic production of prolactin in one patient without galactorrhea and with a bronchogenic carcinoma, and in one patient with galactorrhea and with a hypernephroma. (15) An occult carcinoma, although a remote possibility, should be a consideration in the diagnostic workup. Abnormal lactation may be associated with acromegaly. An association has been noted between elevated prolactin levels and elevated 17-ketosteroid excretion (16). Therefore hirsutism may be noted with inappropriate lactation. These are clinical considerations to be reviewed when confronting a patient with galactorrhea. However the two essential procedures which are not to be avoided are the prolactin assay and polytomography of the sella turcica.

The Prolactin Assay. Almost all patients with galactorrhea have an elevated prolactin level (greater than 20 ng/ml). Measurement of the prolactin level serves two purposes: (1) the basal level will be helpful in following response to treatment, and (2) extremely elevated levels are more likely to be associated with pituitary tumors. A single random blood sample is reliable in detecting elevated levels. (17) If the prolactin level is greater than 50 ng/ml, the patient should be admitted for in-patient evaluation as outlined in Chapter 5.

Polytomography. Regardless of bleeding history or demonstration of withdrawal to progestin, all patients with galactorrhea require polytomography for evaluation of the sella turcica. The technique and findings with polytomography are described in Chapter 5. If x-ray polytomography detects an abnormality in the sella turcica, the patient should be admitted for evaluation as described in Chapter 5.

Treatment of Galactorrhea

Treatment of galactorrhea follows the same guidelines as outlined in Chapter 5 for the treatment of amenorrhea. Even with a normal prolactin level and normal polytomography, if the galactorrhea is disturbing or if pregnancy is desired and the patient is anovulatory, treatment with ergot alkaloids is indicated. (18)

In patients with amenorrhea, treatment with ergot alkaloids leads to the onset of menses in about 30 days. (19) The usual dose is 2.5 mg b.i.d. or t.i.d. Side effects include mild nausea, and slight dizziness. Though only a few cases have been reported, there appear to be no teratogenic effects when taken early in pregnancy. (19) The ergot alkaloids stimulate dopaminergic receptors in the brain and appear to act directly on the pituitary gland. (8, 20) Functional galactorrhea as well as tumor secretion of prolactin (and tumor growth) can be suppressed; therefore the ergot alkaloids are not helpful in demonstrating the presence of a tumor. (21, 22) Unfortunately, galactorrhea and hypogonadism return when treatment ceases. (23) Nevertheless, this method of treatment currently offers the best prospect of achieving pregnancy, short of surgical intervention or extensive efforts to induce ovulation with clomiphene or gonadotropins.

Pyridoxine (Vitamin B_6) has been used to treat galactorrhea (200–600 mg/day). (24) However its effectiveness has not been confirmed in a large series of patients. Pyridoxine is a precursor of the compound, pyridoxal phosphate, which functions as a coenzyme in the decarboxylation and transamination of amino acids. Thus pyridoxine probably increases the conversion of DOPA to dopamine in the hypothalamus.

L-DOPA has proved to be ineffective because large doses are necessary to overcome the short half-life of the drug and gastrointestinal side effects limit the amount that can be given.

The earlier a tumor is diagnosed the better the treatment result. Early diagnosis and extirpation avoid unnecessary progressive endocrine, neurologic, and ophthalmologic complications. Optimal therapy is possible if tumors are small and completely intrasellar. In this favorable circumstance, a transphenoidal approach is possible with direct visualization of the sella contents. Removal of the tumor, good hemostasis, and preservation of residual pituitary tissue can be achieved. Finally, early diagnosis and specific therapy avoid the hazards of induction of ovulation and pregnancy in the presence of an occult tumor. If pregnancy ensues following medical treatment of a patient with an elevated prolactin and with a normal or only a suspicious polytomogram, careful follow-up is required to detect intragestational tumor expansion. This can lead to acute hemorrhage with abrupt hypopituitarism, optic tract or chiasma compression, or hypothalamic disruption.

Despite the above considerations, it is impossible to assume a dogmatic position regarding surgical treatment of small pituitary adenomas. Patients with galactorrhea and amenorrhea have been followed for many years without evidence of tumor enlargement. Pregnancy has been successfully achieved and completed in such patients without problems. Further clinical experience with this situation will be necessary before a definitive judgment can be reached. In the meantime, when surgical intervention is not elected, annual surveillance is necessary to detect early changes. As a minimum, polytomography and the measurement of prolactin levels and thyroid function should be obtained. In severe hypogonadism, hormone replacement is appropriate as outlined in Chapter 5. Fertility can be achieved with the use of ergot alkaloids, or with clomiphene or human menopausal gonadotropins (Chapter 19).

Cancer of The Breast

Scope of the Problem

One of every 15 women will develop breast cancer during her lifetime. The breast is the leading site of cancer in women (28% of all cancers), and the leading cause of death from cancer in women is breast cancer (20% of cancer deaths). Over the years breast cancer has continued this deadly impact despite advances in surgical and diagnostic techniques. Recently a growing appreciation for the hormonal influences on breast cancer has kindled a new hope for better therapeutic management.

Risk Factors

A constellation of factors influences the risk for breast cancer. (25) These include: reproductive experience, ovarian activity, benign breast disease, familial tendency, genetic differences, and specific endocrine factors.

Reproductive Experience. The risk of breast cancer increases with the increase in age at which a woman bears her first full term child. A woman pregnant before the age of 18 has about one third the risk of one who first delivers after the age of 35. To be protective pregnancy must occur before the age of 30. Births after the first convey little or no additional protection.

The fact that pregnancy early in life is associated with reduced breast cancer implies that etiologic factors are operating during that period of life. The protection afforded only by the first pregnancy and not substantially modified by subsequent births suggests that the first full term pregnancy has a trigger effect which either produces a permanent change in the factors responsible for breast cancer or changes the breast tissue and makes it less susceptible to malignant transformation. Lactation is not significant in this mechanism. Whether a patient breast feeds or not has little if any effect on risk.

Ovarian Activity. Women who have an oophorectomy have a lower risk and the lowered risk is greater the younger a woman is when ovariectomized. There is a 70% risk reduction in women who have surgery before age 35. This implies that ovarian activity plays a role in at least two thirds of breast cancer patients. There is a small increase in risk with early menarche and with late natural menopause, indicating that ovarian activity plays a continuing role throughout reproductive life.

Benign Breast Disease. Women with cystic mastitis have about 4 times the breast cancer rate of comparable normal women. Despite their risk, women with prior benign breast disease form only a small proportion of breast cancer patients—approximately 5%.

Familial Tendency. Female relatives of women with breast cancer have 2 to 3 times the rate of the general population. There is an excess of bilateral disease among patients with a family history of breast cancer. Relatives of women with bilateral disease have about a 45% lifetime chance of developing breast cancer.

Specific Endocrine Factors.

1. *Adrenal Steroids.* Subnormal levels of etiocholanolone (a urinary excretion product of androstenedione) have been found from 5 months to 9 years before the diagnosis of breast cancer in women living on the island of Guernsey, off the English coast. (26) A subnormal excretion of this 17-ketosteroid was also found in sisters of patients with breast cancer. A sixfold increase in the incidence of breast cancer was found between women excreting less than 0.4 mg of etiocholanolone and those excreting over 1 mg/24 hours. Since about 25% of the population excretes less than 1 mg/24 hours, measurement of this 17-ketosteroid might be a useful screening procedure to detect a high risk group of patients, if these results are confirmed in additional studies.

2. *Endogenous Estrogen.* Estriol has generally failed to produce breast cancer in rodents, and in fact, estriol protects the rat against breast tumors induced by various chemical carcinogens. The hypothesis is that a higher estriol level protects against the more potent effects of estrone and estradiol. This might explain the protective effect of early pregnancies. Women having had an early pregnancy continue to excrete more estriol than nulliparous women. (27) Premenopausal healthy Asiatic women have a lower breast cancer risk than Caucasians, and also

have a higher rate of urinary estriol excretion. (28) Lemon has suggested that impaired estriol production is due to an autosomal mutant recessive gene, prevalent in Caucasians. (29) However when Asiatic women migrate to the United States, their rate of breast cancer increases, and their urinary excretion of estriol decreases.

3. *Exogenous Estrogen.* Retrospective and prospective studies have not indicated an increased risk of breast cancer in premenopausal women taking birth control pills, except for the suggestion that women with pre-existing benign disease may have an increased risk after prolonged use (Chapter 14). Long-term follow-up of postmenopausal women on replacement estrogen has suggested a small increase in risk. (30) However this observation was only of borderline statistical significance, and a similar study has been negative. (31) The long-term effect remains to be determined.

4. *Thyroid.* In hospitalized patients with breast cancer, there is a lower level of thyroid function, primary to the thyroid and therefore associated with elevated levels of TSH. (32) In addition, a higher incidence of breast cancer has been reported in patients receiving thyroid medication for hypothyroidism. (33) The level of thyroid hormone in the blood may affect the metabolism of steroids or the degree of effect of hormones on the breast. The geographic differences in estriol excretion noted above may be related to thyroid function differences as influenced by iodine intake in the different populations.

5. *Prolactin.* Carcinogen-induced tumor growth in rats is dependent upon prolactin. However there is no increase in prolactin levels in women with breast cancer, nor is there a difference in response to TRH. (34) In countries where prolonged lactation is common, the incidence of breast cancer is low.

Breast tumors appear to be modified in their growth by their hormonal environment. No clear cut etiologic factor has emerged, and rather than a stimulating or initiating role, the endocrine background of a patient may serve a permissive role. The implication is that determination of **the hormonal environment may delineate a high risk group**, while alteration of the endocrine environment may aid favorable treatment.

Treatment of
Breast Cancer

The classical treatment of breast cancer has involved surgical excision followed by irradiation and either hormonal treatment or ablation of endocrine resources. The endocrinologic approach has been largely empiric, resulting in approximately a one third rate of remission. This "blind" approach is now being replaced with decisions based upon the demonstration and measurement of estrogen receptors in the tumor tissue.

Tumors which do not contain estrogen receptors respond very poorly to steroid therapy or endocrine ablation. The percentage of tumors which contain estrogen receptors is approximately 50%. (35) However not all estrogen receptor-containing tumors respond well to such treatment. Approximately 40% of tumors which contain receptors are resistant to endocrine therapy. (36) The presence of the binder does not guarantee that the tissue is responsive to estrogen action. Because the presence of the progesterone receptor is dependent upon estrogen action, it has been suggested that the presence of progesterone receptors within tumor tissue indicates that the tumor is responsive to estrogen, and hence the tissue would respond to a change in the endocrine environment. (36)

As these methods are explored further and become standardized, and positive and negative tests become strictly defined, accuracy in predicting response of tumors to therapy should increase.

References

1. **Tyson, JE, Hwang, P, Guyda, H, and Friesen, HG,** Studies of Prolactin Secretion in Human Pregnancy, Am J Obstet Gynec 113:14, 1972.

2. **Friesen, HG, Fournier, P, and Desjardins, P,** Pituitary Prolactin in Pregnancy and Normal and Abnormal Lactation, Clin Obstet Gynec 16:25, 1973.

3. **Tyson, JE, and Friesen, HG,** Factors Influencing the Secretion of Human Prolactin and Growth Hormone in Menstrual and Gestational Women, Am J Obstet Gynec 116:377, 1973.

4. **Barberia, JM, Abu-Fadil, S, Kletzky, OA, Nakamura, RM, and Mishell, DR, Jr.,** Serum Prolactin Patterns in Early Human Gestation, Am J Obstet Gynec 121:1107, 1975.

5. **Ehara, Y, Siler, TM, and Yen, SSC,** Effects of Large Doses of Estrogen on Prolactin and Growth Hormone Release, Am J Obstet Gynec 125:455, 1976.

6. **Bruce, JO, and Ramirez, VD,** Site of Action of the Inhibitory Effect of Estrogen Upon Lactation, Neuroendocrinology 6:19, 1970.

7. **Varga, L, Latterbech, PM, Pryor, JS, Wenier, R, and Erb, H,** Suppression of Puerperal Lactation with an Ergot Alkaloid—A Double Blind Study, Brit Med J 2:273, 1972.

8. **Macleod, RM, and Lehmeyer, JE,** Studies on the Mechanism of the Dopamine-Mediated Inhibition of Prolactin Secretion, Endocrinology 94:1077, 1974.

9. **Noel, GL, Dimond, RC, Wartofsky, L, Earll, JM, and Frantz, AG,** Studies of Prolactin and TSH Secretion by Continuous Infusion of Small Amounts of Thyrotropin-Releasing Hormone (TRH), J Clin Endocrinol Metab 39:6, 1974.

10. **Zarate, A, Canales, ES, Soria, J, Ruiz, F, and MacGregor, C,** Ovarian Refractoriness During Lactation in Women: Effect of Gonadotropin Stimulation, Am J Obstet Gynec 112:1130, 1972.

11. **Maneckjee, R, Srinath, BR, and Moudgal, NR,** Prolactin Suppresses Release of Luteinizing Hormone During Lactation in the Monkey, Nature 262:507, 1976.

12. **Andreassen, B, and Tyson, JE,** Role of the Hypothalamic-Pituitary-Ovarian Axis in Puerperal Infertility, J Clin Endocrinol Metab 42:1114, 1976.

13. **Archer, DF, and Josimovich, JB,** Ovarian Response to Exogenous Gonadotropins in Women with Elevated Serum Prolactin, Obstet Gynec 48:115, 1976.

14. **Dickey, RP, and Stone, SC,** Drugs that Affect the Breast and Lactation, Clin Obstet Gynec 18:95, 1975.

15. **Turkington, RW,** Ectopic Production of Prolactin, New Eng J Med 285:1455, 1971.

16. **Donabedian, RK, May, PB, and Tan, SY,** Abnormal Adrenal Steroidogenesis in Patients with Hyperprolactinemia, Galactorrhea, or Both, Program, 58th Meeting, The Endocrine Society, 1976, Abstract No. 372.

17. **Boyar, RM, Kapen, S, Weitzman, ED, and Hellman, L,** Pituitary Microadenoma and Hyperprolactinemia, New Eng J Med 294:263, 1976.

18. **Seppala, M, Hirvonen, E, and Ranta, T,** Bromocriptine Treatment of Secondary Amenorrhea, Lancet 1:1154, 1976.

19. **Tyson, JE, Andreassen, B, Huth, F, Smith, B, and Zacur, H,** Neuro-Endocrine Dysfunction with Psychogenic Implications in Postpill Galactorrhea-Amenorrhea, Obstet Gynec 46:1, 1975.

20. **Stone, TW,** Further Evidence for a Dopamine Receptor Stimulating Action of an Ergot Alkaloid, Brain Res 72:177, 1974.

21. **MacLeod, RM, and Lehmeyer, JE,** Suppression of Pituitary Tumor Growth and Function by Ergot Alkaloids, Cancer Res 33:849, 1973.

22. **Lloyd, HM, Meares, JD, and Jacobi, J,** Effects of Estrogen and Bromocryptine on In Vivo Secretion and Mitosis in Prolactin Cells, Nature 255:497, 1975.

23. **Thorner, MO, McNeilly, AS, Hagan, C, and Besser, GM,** Long-Term Treatment of Galactorrhea and Hypogonadism with Bromocryptine, Brit Med J 2:419, 1974.

24. **McIntosh, EN,** Treatment of Women with Galactorrhea-Amenorrhea Syndrome with Pryridoxine (Vitamin B_6), J Clin Endocrinol Metab 42:1192, 1976.

25. **MacMahon, B, Cole, P, and Brown, J,** Etiology of Human Breast Cancer: A Review, J Natl Cancer Inst 50:21, 1973.

26. **Bulbrook, RD,** Urinary Androgen Excretion and the Etiology of Breast Cancer, J Natl Cancer Inst 48:1039, 1972.

27. **Cole, P, Brown, JB, and MacMahon, B,** Oestrogen Profiles of Parous and Nulliparous Women, Lancet 2:596, 1976.

28. **Dickinson, LE, MacMahon, B, Cole, P, and Brown, JB,** Estrogen Profiles of Oriental and Caucasian Women in Hawaii, New Eng J Med 291:1211, 1974.

29. **Lemon, HM,** Oestriol and Prevention of Breast Cancer, Lancet 1:546, 1973.

30. **Hoover, R, Gray, LA, Sr., Cole, P, and MacMahon, B,** Menopausal Estrogen and Breast Cancer, New Eng J Med 295:401, 1976.

31. **Burch, JC, Byrd, BF, and Vaughn, WK,** The Effects of Long-term Estrogen Administration to Women Following Hysterectomy, in van Keep, PA, and Lauritzen, C, eds., *Estrogens in the Post-Menopause*, S. Karger, Basal, 1975, pp. 208–214.

32. **Mittra, I, Hayward, JL, and McNeilly, AS,** Hypothalamic-Pituitary-Prolactin Axis in Breast Cancer, Lancet 1:889, 1974.

33. **Kapdi, CC, and Wolfe, JN,** Breast Cancer, Relationship to Thyroid Supplements for Hypothyroidism, JAMA 236:1124, 1976.

34. **Mittra, I, and Hayward, JL,** Hypothalamic-Pituitary-Thyroid Axis in Breast Cancer, Lancet 1:885, 1974.

35. **McGuire, WL, Carbone, PP, Sears, ME, and Escher GC,** Estrogen Receptors in Human Breast Cancer: An Overview, in McGuire, WL, Carbone, PP, and Vollmer EP, eds, *Estrogen Receptors in Human Breast Cancer* Raven Press, New York, 1975, p. 1.

36. **Horwitz, KB, McGuire, WL, Pearson, OH, and Segaloff A,** Predicting Response to Endocrine Therapy in Human Breast Cancer: A Hypothesis, Science 189:726, 1975.

0 The Endocrinology of Pregnancy

Impairment of growth and development during intrauterine life leaves its impact in terms of handicaps to adult function and capabilities. It is not surprising that there should exist mechanisms by which a growing fetus can exert some influence or control over its environment. Hormonal messages from the conceptus can affect metabolic processes, uteroplacental blood flow, and cellular differentiation. *This chapter will review steroid and protein hormones of pregnancy, including their assay for clinical utilization. In addition the endocrinology of parturition will be described as an example of the fetal influence on human pregnancy.*

Steroid Hormones in Pregnancy

Steroidogenesis in the fetal-placental unit does not follow the conventional mechanisms of hormone production within a single organ. Rather, the final products result from critical interactions and interdependence of separate organ systems which individually do not possess the necessary enzymatic capabilities. It is helpful to view the process as consisting of a fetal compartment, a placental compartment, and a maternal compartment. The fetal and placental compartments separately lack certain steroidogenic activities; however together they are complementary and form a complete unit, which utilizes the maternal compartment as a source of basic building materials and as a resource for clearance of steroids.

Progesterone

In its key location as a way station between mother and fetus, the placenta may utilize precursors from either mother or fetus to circumvent its own deficiencies in enzyme activity. The placental converts little, if any, acetate to cholesterol or its precursors. Cholesterol as well as pregnenolone are obtained from the maternal blood stream for progesterone synthesis. The fetal contribution is negligible since progesterone levels remain high after fetal demise. Thus the massive amount of progesterone produced in pregnancy depends upon placental-maternal cooperation.

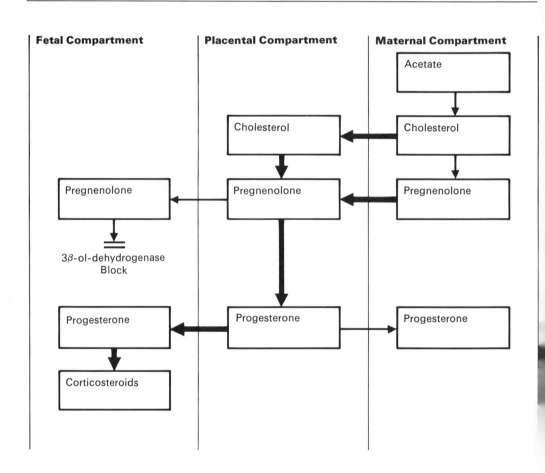

Progesterone is largely produced by the corpus luteum until about 10 weeks of gestation. Indeed until approximately the 7th week, the pregnancy is dependent upon the presence of the corpus luteum. (1) After a transition period of shared function between the 7th week to the 12th week the placenta emerges as the major source of progesterone. At term, progesterone levels range from 100 to 300 ng/ml. However, a measurement of the progesterone level or of its metabolites (e.g. pregnanediol in the urine) is presently of no clinical usefulness.

In early pregnancy the levels of 17-hydroxyprogesterone rise, marking the activity of the corpus luteum. By the 10th week of gestation this compound has returned to baseline levels, indicating that the placenta has little 17-hydroxylase activity. However, beginning about the 32nd week there is a second, more gradual rise in 17-hydroxyprogesterone, due to placental utilization of fetal precursors. (2)

Little is known about specific functions for the various steroids produced throughout pregnancy. Progesterone appears to have a role in parturition as will be discussed later in this chapter. Recent studies also suggest that progesterone may be important in suppressing the maternal immunological response to the fetus. (3) Perhaps the most important role for progesterone is to serve as the principal substrate pool for fetal adrenal gland production of gluco-and mineralocorticoids.

The fetal adrenal gland is extremely active, but produces steroids with a 3β-hydroxy-Δ^5 configuration like pregnenolone and dehydroepiandrosterone, rather than 3-keto-Δ^4 products such as progesterone. The fetus therefore lacks significant activity of the 3β-hydroxysteroid dehydrogenase, Δ^{4-5} isomerase system. Thus the fetus must borrow progesterone from the placenta to circumvent this lack, in order to synthesize the biologically important corticosteroids. In return the fetus supplies what the placenta lacks, 19 carbon compounds to serve as precursors for estrogens.

Estrogens

The basic precursors of estrogens are 19 carbon andro gens. However, there is a virtual absence of 17-hydroxy ation and 17–20 desmolase activity in the human pla centa. As a result, 21 carbon products (progesterone an pregnenolone) cannot be converted to 19 carbon steroid (androstenedione and dehydroepiandrosterone). Lik progesterone, estrogen produced by the placenta mu also derive its precursors outside of the placenta itself.

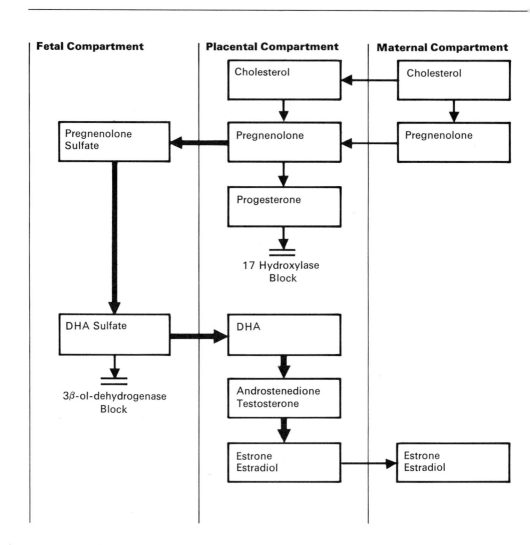

The androgen compounds utilized for estrogen synthesis in human pregnancy are, in the early months of gestation, derived from the maternal blood stream. By the 20th week of pregnancy, the vast majority of estrogen excreted in the maternal urine is derived from fetal androgens. In particular, approximately 90% of estriol excretion can be accounted for by dehydroepiandrosterone sulfate (DS) production by the fetal adrenal gland.

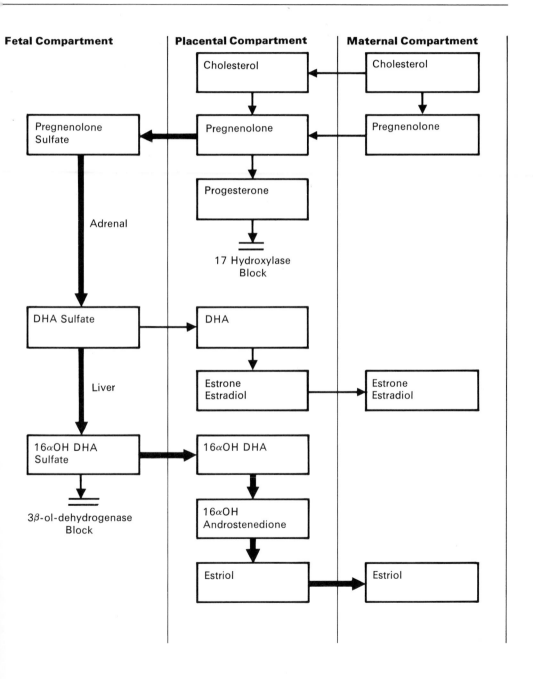

The fetal endocrine compartment is also characterized b
rapid and extensive conjugation of steroids with sulfate
Perhaps this is a protective mechanism, blocking th
biologic effects of potent steroids present in such grea
quantities during pregnancy. In order to utilize feta
precursors, the placenta must be extremely efficient i
cleaving the sulfate conjugates brought to it via the feta
bloodstream. Indeed the sulfatase activity in the placent
is rapid and quantitatively very significant. It is clinicall
recognized that a deficiency in placental sulfatase
associated with low estriol excretion giving reality to th
importance of this metabolic step. This syndrome will b
discussed in greater detail later in this chapter.

The placenta also lacks 16α-hydroxylation ability, an
estriol with its 16α-hydroxyl group must therefore b
derived from an immediate fetal precursor. The fetus
very active in 16-hydroxylation, especially in the feta
liver. Therefore the fetal adrenal provides dehydroepia
drosterone sulfate as precursor for placental productio
of estrone and estradiol, while the fetal adrenal with th
aid of 16α-hydroxylation in the fetal liver provides th
16α-hydroxydehydropepiandrosterone sulfate for placer
tal estriol formation. After birth neonatal 16-hydroxy
ation activity rapidly disappears. The maternal contribu
tion of dehydroepiandrosterone sulfate to total estroge
synthesis must be negligible because in the absence c
normal fetal adrenal glands (as in an anencephalic infant
maternal estrogen levels and excretion are extremely low

The concentrations of the unconjugated compounds i
the maternal compartment for the 3 major estrogens i
pregnancy are as follows: (2) The rise in estrone begin
at 6 to 10 weeks and reaches 2 to 30 ng/ml at term. Thi
wide range in normal values precludes the use of estron
measurements in clinical applications. Estradiol varie
between 6 to 40 ng/ml at 36 weeks of gestation, and the
undergoes an accelerated rate of increase. At term a
equal amount of estradiol arises from maternal DS an
fetal DS and its importance in fetal monitoring is minima
Estriol is first detectable at 9 weeks when the feta
adrenal gland secretion of precursor becomes active
Estriol concentrations plateau at 31–35 weeks, then in
crease again at 35–36 weeks. (4) During pregnancy
estrone and estradiol excretion is increased about 10
times over nonpregnant levels. However, the increase i
maternal estriol excretion is about a thousand-fold. Thi
enormous rise coupled with its dependence on fetal pre
cursor is the basis of its utility in fetal monitoring.

The estrogens presented to the maternal blood strean
are rapidly metabolized by the maternal liver prior t
excretion into the maternal urine as a variety of mor
than 20 products. The bulk of these maternal urinar
estrogens are composed of glucosiduronates conjugate
at the 16-position. Significant amounts of the 3-glucosi
duronate and the 3-sulfate-16-glucosiduronate are als

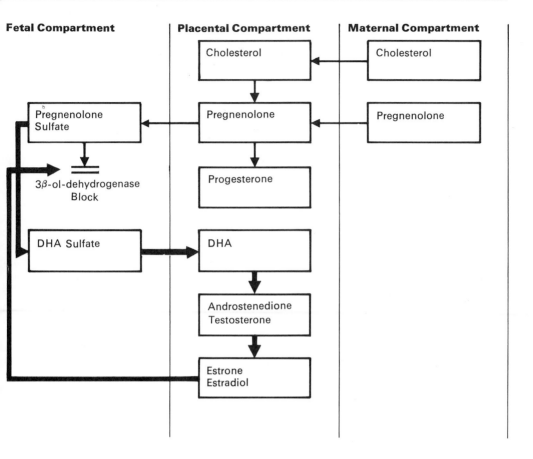

Fetal Compartment

Pregnenolone Sulfate

3β-ol-dehydrogenase Block

DHA Sulfate

Placental Compartment

Cholesterol

Pregnenolone

Progesterone

DHA

Androstenedione
Testosterone

Estrone
Estradiol

Maternal Compartment

Cholesterol

Pregnenolone

excreted. Only approximately 8–10% of the maternal blood estriol is unconjugated (or free).

The Fetal Adrenal Gland

The fetal adrenal cortex is differentiated by 7 weeks into a thick inner fetal zone and thin outer definitive zone. Early in pregnancy adrenal growth and development are remarkable, and the gland achieves a size equal to or larger than that of the kidney by the end of the first trimester. After the first trimester the adrenal glands slowly decrease in size until a second spurt in growth beginning at about 34–35 weeks. The glands remain proportionately larger than the adult adrenal glands. After delivery, the fetal zone (about 80% of the bulk of the gland) rapidly degenerates to be replaced by the adult definitive zone of the adrenal cortex. Thus the specific steroidogenic characteristics of the fetus are associated with a specific morphologic component of the adrenal gland which is limited in function to the time period of fetal life.

The regulation of steroidogenesis within the fetal adrenal gland is not understood. Early in pregnancy, the adrenal gland may function without ACTH. After 20 weeks gestation fetal ACTH is required, although its presence may only serve a permissive role. The disappearance of

191

the fetal zone with delivery suggests that this zone depends upon some influence which is unique to intrauterine life. Human chorionic gonadotropin (HCG) may serve this purpose. It also has been suggested that fetal prolactin may play this role. (5) The principal mission of the fetal zone may be to provide dehydroepiandrosterone sulfate as the basic precursor for placental estrogen production. The lack of 3β-hydroxysteroid dehydrogenase-isomerase activity in the fetal adrenal gland is due to inhibition imposed by the high pregnancy levels of estrogen. (6) Therefore the effect of estrogen on the fetal adrenal gland is to direct steroidogenesis along the Δ5 pathway leading to the secretion of dehydroepiandrosterone sulfate. Placental estrogen may influence the fetal hypothalamic-pituitary axis to increase fetal prolactin levels, which in turn may increase fetal adrenal zone activity. Cortisol production by the fetal adrenal gland may be chiefly derived from the definitive zone, perhaps under the major control of ACTH.

Measurement of Estrogen In Pregnancy

Because pregnancy is characterized by a great increase in maternal estrogen levels, and estrogen production is dependent upon fetal and placental steroidogenic cooperation, the amount of estrogen present in the maternal blood or urine reflects both fetal and placental enzymatic capability and hence, well-being. Attention has been focused on estriol in the maternal urine because 90% of the estrogen excreted is estriol derived from fetal precursors. The end product to be assayed in the maternal urine is influenced by a multitude of factors. Availability of precursor from the fetal adrenal gland is a prime requisite as well as the ability of the placenta to carry out its conversion steps. Maternal metabolism of the product as well as the efficiency of maternal renal excretion of the product may modify the daily amount of estrogen in the urine. Blood flow to any of the key organs in the fetus, placenta, and mother becomes important. In addition, drugs or diseases may affect any level in the cascade of events leading up to assay of the product in the urine

The Urinary Method. Determination of estrogen in the urine is usually based on Kober's observation in 1931 that estrogens form colored or fluorescent compounds when heated with concentrated sulfuric acid. This sulfuric acid reaction is referred to as the Kober reaction. Modifications by Ittrich substantially increased the sensitivity of the reaction. Extraction of the sulfuric acid-induced color and fluorescent compounds into an organic solvent containing ρ-nitrophenol further reduced the large and variable blank readings. Later, Ittrich found that the use of tetrabromoethane provided optimal color and fluorescent intensity, and that less concentrated sulfuric acid could be utilized in the presence of hydroquinone. These modifications improved the sensitivity of the methods and made the procedure less complicated and time-consuming.

With these technical modifications and utilizing either a spectrophotometer or a fluorometer, total estrogen content of pregnancy urine can be determined at the approximate rate of 10 urines per 4 hours. The lack of specific chromatographic separation of estriol is not a serious deficiency in the method, since after the 20th week of gestation, 90% of the total estrogen in maternal urine is estriol. More recently, antisera have been developed which allow the rapid radioimmunoassay of unextracted, diluted urine. The methods are sensitive to approximately 1–2 mg of estrogen per 24 hours. In all methods, accuracy must be monitored by the addition of a radioactive estrogen conjugate to correct for procedural losses.

The output of creatinine in a 24-hour urine is relatively constant except in times of strenuous physical activity. To insure that a sample is truly a 24-hour collection a creatinine measurement should be performed on every urine received in the laboratory for estriol assay, and the creatinine result should be available to the obstetrician the same day. The average daily creatinine excretion in the last month of pregnancy is 1.35 ± 0.14 gm (SD). (7) Creatinine levels below 1.0 gm per 24 hours in the absence of significant renal pathology indicate an unreliable urine collection. In addition, the creatinine may be utilized to calculate an estrogen/creatinine ratio. A significant fall in estriol excretion should be accompanied by a comparable fall in the estriol/creatinine ratio.

The result of the estrogen assay should be available to the clinician within 12 hours following completion of the urine collection. In the case of diabetic pregnancy a delay longer than 12 hours may result in fetal loss.

Normal Values and Interpretation. The normal 24-hour total estrogen excretion in urine throughout pregnancy is illustrated as ± two standard deviations. Notice the wide standard deviation for a 24 hour value: ±30%. This deviation is largely due to maternal factors, such as the accuracy of the 24 hour collection, variations in fluid intake and renal dynamics, and the amount of bedrest. Because of this variation, there are two essential aspects to the use of this assay clinically. First, a single specimen is meaningless unless it is extremely low, in the range incompatible with fetal survival. Serial assessment is essential in order to determine sequential changes. Second, to be significant, there must be a decrease in estrogen excretion of approximately 60% of the preceding values. To be conservative, we routinely consider a decrease of 50% as clinically significant, and we have found this magnitude of change to be reliable.

Diurnal changes in estrogen during the last trimester of pregnancy reflect the contribution of precursors from the maternal adrenal gland. Since this contribution is minimal, diurnal changes are not significant, at most reflecting a 10% change from mean levels.

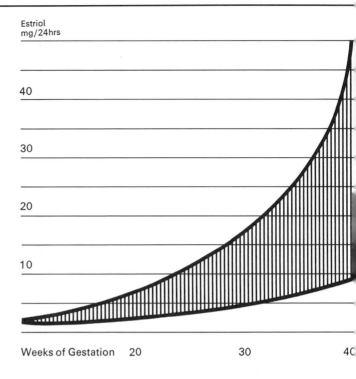

Estriol values in the last trimester correlate with the weight of the infant. This is directly related to the size of the fetal adrenal gland and its production of precursor. Excessive adrenal activity as in congenital adrenal hyperplasia is therefore associated with abnormally high urinary estrogen excretion. (8)

Problems. Drugs which affect the 24 hour urinary estrogen level include: methanimine mandelate (mandelamine), phenolphthalein, corticosteroids, and ampicillin. Mandelamine liberates formaldehyde during acid hydrolysis, destroying estrogen, and resulting in falsely low levels. The assay is reliable again two days after discontinuing the drug. Many laxatives contain phenolphthalein which inhibits hydrolysis of the estrogen conjugates. Because the use of a radioimmunoassay technique eliminate the need for hydrolysis, the problems encountered with mandelamine or phenolphthalein are eliminated. Corticosteroids administered to the mother cross the placenta poorly, and large amounts are required to suppress fetal adrenal production of estriol precursor. As a rule of thumb, the equivalent of 75 mg of cortisol daily is necessary to affect maternal estrogen excretion.

Ampicillin depresses maternal estriol excretion in pregnancy by interfering with its enterohepatic circulation. (9) The majority of the decrease is due to a decrease in estriol-2-glucuronide, which is of intestinal origin. Neomycin which is not absorbed has a similar effect on estriol excretion. Thus ampicillin inhibits the hydrolysis of the biliary estriol conjugates in the gut, preventing their reabsorption and reconjugation and leading to loss of estriol in the feces.

Bedrest is frequently accompanied by a transitory increase in estriol excretion. A variation such as this can be compensated for by calculating the estrogen/creatinine ratio. Estriol collections made while a patient is receiving oxytocin for the induction of labor may be invalid. Because of the antidiuretic action of oxytocin, a decrease in estriol and creatinine excretion, along with a decline in the urine output can occur. (10) Again calculation of the estrogen/creatinine ratio is helpful because a pathologic fall in the estriol excretion should be accompanied by a comparable fall in the estriol/creatinine ratio. Proteinuria and acetonuria have no effect on the assays.

New Approaches

Estriol/Creatinine Ratio. The major difficulty with the 24 hour urine method is the problem of collecting accurate specimens. The success of this biochemical surveillance depends upon patient motivation and reliability. Added to this human problem is the considerable variation seen from specimen to specimen, and the time lag for changes in estrogen production to be reflected in the maternal urine. An estriol/creatinine ratio performed on the first morning voided urine correlates well with 24 hour urine ratios. (11)

There are problems, however, with the estriol/creatinine ratio. Some individuals periodically excrete very high levels of creatinine per day making the ratio falsely low, while a low creatinine level with a low estriol will be clinically misleading because of a normal ratio. Furthermore, clearance of estriol and creatinine can vary independently. (12) Thus while an estriol/creatinine ratio performed on a single urine specimen generally correlates with the 24 hour urinary measurement of estriol, variations are of such significance that this method is not a reliable substitute for a 24 hour urinary estriol determination. (13)

Blood Estrogen Measurements. With the availability of radioimmunoassay techniques, rapid measurement of estrogen levels in the blood is now possible. The measurement of estriol in blood avoids the problems of urine collection, and the serum or plasma estrogen level does correlate with urinary estrogen excretion. However, there are difficulties of interpretation because of a wide range of variation in both unconjugated and total estrogen measurements.

No significant difference has been noted in the measure
ment of unconjugated estradiol between normal an
abnormal pregnancies. (14) Measurement of unconju
gated estriol also shows a wide spread of values. (14
Unconjugated estriol levels occasionally drop sharply an
abruptly without apparent cause. (2) In our opinion mor
reliable clinical information is obtained by the use of 2
hour urinary estrogen determinations along with the mea
surement of creatinine excretion.

Amniotic Fluid Estrogen Measurements. Amniotic flui
estriol is correlated with the fetal estrogen pattern rathe
than the maternal. Most of the estriol in the amnioti
fluid is present as 16-glucosiduronate or as 3-sulfate-16
glucosiduronate. A small amount exists as 3-sulfate. Ver
little unconjugated (free) estriol is present in the amnioti
fluid because free estriol is rapidly transferred across th
placenta and membranes. Estriol sulfate is low in concer
tration because the placental and fetal membranes hydro
lyze the sulfated conjugates, and the free estriol is the
passed out of the fluid.

Because the membranes and the placenta have no glucu
ronidase activity, the glucosiduronate conjugates are re
moved slowly from the fetus. The glucosiduronates there
fore predominate in the fetal urine and the amnioti
fluid. Because of the slow changes in glucosiduronate:
measurements of amniotic fluid estriol have wide varia
tions in both normal and abnormal pregnancies. A
important clinical use for amniotic fluid estrogen measure
ments has not emerged.

Estetrol. Estetrol (15α-hydroxy estriol) is formed from
fetal precursors, and is very dependent upon 15-hydrox
ylation activity in the fetal liver. The capacity for 15α
hydroxylation of estrogens increases during fetal life
reaching a maximum at term. This activity then decline
during infancy and is low, absent, or undetectable i
adults. (15)

In a series from Finland, urinary estetrol and estriol gav
the same information on the fetal state except in erythro
blastosis. (16) Estetrol was correlated with the cord bloo
hemoglobin concentration, while estriol showed no cor
relation. This may be due to the fact that 15α-hydroxyl
ation requires significant liver participation, and in eryth
roblastosis liver function is affected by the presence c
excess hematopoiesis.

Amniotic fluid estetrol assays do not seem to be c
predictive value, and thus are not useful. (17) The clinica
use of maternal blood and urine estetrol measurement
is of no advantage over the usual estriol assessment

Provocative Tests. In nonpregnant individuals circulating dehydroepiandrosterone sulfate (DS) is cleared via 19 carbon products such as 17-ketosteroids, and less than 0.2% is converted to estrogen. In late pregnancy, approximately 35% of maternal circulating DS is irreversibly converted to estradiol by placental aromatization, while 32% undergoes maternal 16α-hydroxylation. (18) Thus uteroplacental perfusion may be reflected by measuring DS clearance by placental aromatization to estradiol. The administration of DS followed by the measurement of blood estrogen levels may allow assessment and screening of high risk pregnancies. The response is variable, however, and apparently was of little clinical use in one study which utilized only estradiol measurements, (19), but was highly correlated with eventual fetal distress when both estradiol and estetrol were measured. (20) Utilizing the total metabolic clearance rate of DS, a decline in clearance has been demonstrated prior to the development of clinically evident toxemia of pregnancy. (21) Further development and testing of these techniques may lead to methods for revealing those patients destined to develop problems during their pregnancies.

A high risk population may be detected by routine screening of all pregnant patients with urinary estriol assays. In Australia, approximately 14% of pregnant women had a low estriol excretion at 30 or 36 weeks gestation, and this low estriol excretion was associated with a 5-fold increase in perinatal mortality, as well as an increased incidence of major fetal malformations and intrauterine growth retardation. (22) These associations are true whether glucose tolerance is normal or abnormal. However, there is a 6-fold increase in the incidence of small-for-dates babies when low estriol excretion is combined with hypoglycemia. (23) While hyperglycemia has been long recognized as a biochemical abnormality of pregnancy, the recent observation that perinatal mortality is increased with hypoglycemia as well as hyperglycemia, suggests that both measurement of estrogen excretion and glucose tolerance are effective screening procedures. Furthermore, in the hyperglycemic patient, the use of urinary estriol measurements is not just a screening method, but an essential part of management.

Diabetes Mellitus. The classic obstetric dilemma in diabetes has been when to deliver the patient. The risk of neonatal death when the infant is delivered before 38 weeks of gestation is significantly higher than in the normal population. On the other hand the risk of sudden intrauterine fetal loss rises when the pregnant diabetic is allowed to go to term.

What is it that makes the diabetic pregnancy unique in that fetal jeopardy is heralded by a drop in maternal estriol excretion? The answer to this question is not known. It is clinically recognized that the diabetic pregnancy is marked by the association between intrauterine fetal demise and a rapid decline in estriol excretion. Indeed, fetal death may follow a fall in the estriol excretion within 24 hours. Therefore monitoring the diabetic pregnancy with 24 hour urinary estriol measurements will detect those fetuses in jeopardy. The rapid change in estriol excretion suggests a sudden failure on the part of the fetal adrenal gland to provide precursors.

Despite many years use, the clinical value of estriol assays in the management of diabetic pregnancy is not without controversy. It is our contention, and well-documented by Goebelsmann, et al, (24) that success in avoiding fetal loss in diabetic pregnancies is dependent upon the frequency of estriol determinations. Goebelsmann, et al, (24) calculated (based on 60 diabetic patients) that the day-to-day variability in estriol excretion in diabetic pregnancies is 12.7%, and that falls in estriol excretion attributable to day-to-day variations do not exceed 35%. These authors have regarded a 40% fall as significant. In our experience a 50% decline has proved to be a reliable indicator.

In 14 of the 60 pregnancies monitored with daily estriol measurements by Goebelsmann, et al, (24), a significant (40%) fall in estriol was observed. Nine of the 14 would have been missed or detected later if estriol had been assayed only twice a week. Six of the 14 would have been missed if estriol had been assayed three times a week. Therefore, it is our practice to obtain daily 24 hour urine estrogen and creatinine measurements after the 35th week of gestation. Prior to the 35th week, urine is assayed twice a week from 28 to 32 weeks, and 3 times a week from 32 to 35 weeks.

Another explanation for the lack of confidence in urine estriol assays is the reliance on absolute numbers rather than percent decrease. For example, utilizing a figure of 12 mg as an indication of fetal jeopardy ignores the case where the 24 hour urinary estriol falls from 60 mg to 25 mg, and fetal death might be averted by rapid delivery. Establishment of a baseline with frequent measurements, and acting upon a 50% decrease produces better clinical results. In addition, we believe that a plateau in estriol excretion may be an indication of early fetal jeopardy.

During a diabetic pregnancy, a high estriol output is usually, but not always, associated with fetal macrosomia. Perhaps a large placenta even in the presence of a normal sized fetus may be responsible for an increase in estriol production. As in nondiabetic patients, substantial day-to-day variation occurs in both creatinine and estriol levels.

198

In the mild diabetic, it is our clinical practice to allow the patient to go into labor or to reach the point where she can easily be delivered by induction of labor unless there is a 50% fall in estriol as measured daily after the 35th week of pregnancy. In the more severe diabetic, estriol measurements are utilized to allow the patient to achieve that point in pregnancy when fetal pulmonic maturity is accomplished as measured by the L/S ratio. At that point a decision on delivery depends upon a variety of clinical factors, such as declining insulin requirement, fetal macrosomia, polyhydramnios and toxemia.

Other High Risk Pregnancies

Estriols and Hypertension. The use of serial estriol assays in patients with toxemia has a different orientation when compared to diabetic pregnancies. While in diabetic pregnancies urinary estriol is a means of detecting fetal distress and impending demise, in toxemia the obstetrician uses estriol measurements to assure himself that the fetus is growing and doing well, and that the pregnancy may be allowed to continue until fetal maturity has been attained. Because of rapid changes due to maternal renal function, and probably to utero-placental blood flow, sudden decreases of estriol in toxemia are not consistently associated with impending fetal demise. On the other hand, a rising, normal estriol excretion is very reassuring that the fetus is doing well.

Chronically low excretion of estriol during pregnancy is a grave prognostic sign for the fetus. Low estriol values during a pregnancy with hypertension are associated with elevated perinatal mortality, (25) and in a small series, we reported that chronically low estriol excretion in toxemic pregnancy was associated with a high incidence of neurologic defects. (26)

Our program for assessing fetal well-being in toxemia of pregnancy is as follows. This program only indicates considerations from the fetal point of view, and this information must be integrated with maternal considerations for proper decision-making. When a patient enters the category of high risk pregnancy because of hypertension, serial estriol measurements are obtained. After the 32nd week of gestation, estriol assays are performed three times per week. If the patient is hospitalized, daily estriol measurements are ordered. Normal rising values indicate that conservative management is justified from the fetal point of view. Chronically low estriol levels indicate fetal jeopardy, and delivery is indicated as soon as the L/S ratio predicts that the fetus has achieved pulmonic maturity. If the estriol level is falling, and maternal renal function is stable, intervention is justified if the L/S ratio is in the mature range. If the L/S ratio indicates immature pulmonic function, the clinical decision is difficult, and all other methods of assessment must be brought to bear (e.g. the oxytocin challenge test).

Erythroblastosis Fetalis. In pregnancies with erythroblastosis fetalis, the use of estriol assays has proven to be of no benefit. Normal estriol values do not predict the condition of the fetus, and in particular, there is no correlation with the fetal hemoglobin at birth.

Prolonged Gestation. Approximately 3.5% of all pregnancies continue past the 42nd week, but not all of these post-term pregnancies result in the birth of a postmature baby. Postmature infants have a 2 to 3-fold increase in perinatal mortality, a higher rate of intrapartum asphyxia, a 20% incidence of neonatal hypoglycemia, and a greater tendency to develop health problems in the first 3 years of life. Interruption of the pregnancy would be a simple matter if every patient undelivered after the 42nd week of gestation could be easily delivered by induction of labor. Unfortunately, this is often not the case, and some means of diagnosing the true postmature fetus is an important clinical issue.

In prolonged pregnancies assessment of estriol excretion may be rational, but it is usually not practical. One cannot predict which patients will carry their pregnancies to 42 weeks and beyond, therefore baseline serial assays are not available for comparison and proper judgment. The use of the oxytocin challenge test, combined with estriol and human placental lactogen (HPL) measurements, is the most practical approach to the management of a post-term pregnancy.

Intrauterine Growth Retardation. In general, it can be stated that the failure to demonstrate a rising estriol level is consistent with a failure of the fetus to grow normally. As such, the estriol assessment is an adjunct in the evaluation of suspected intrauterine growth retardation.

Child Development after Pregnancies Complicated by Low Estriol.

In the past few years, the question has arisen whether infants salvaged from complicated pregnancies would grow to be normal healthy children and adults. In the most complete study to date, Yssing (27) reported on the long term prognosis of surviving children from 158 diabetic pregnancies. The incidence of cerebral damaged children in the subnormal estriol group (51.5%) was significantly higher than in the normal group (22.4%). The incidence of children with major abnormalities in the subnormal estriol group (29.4%) was also significantly higher than in the normal group.

We studied the level of maternal estriol excretion and subsequent child development in 16 pregnancies complicated by pre-eclampsia. (26) Neurological abnormalities on follow-up examination were confined to children whose mothers had chronically low rather than precipitously dropping estriol levels. Chronically low urinary estriol excretion indicates intrauterine problems are present. Delivery into the environment of a modern neonatal intensive care unit may produce a healthier child than if the pregnancy is allowed to continue.

Placental Sulfatase Deficiency

A deficiency in placental sulfatase is usually discovered when patients go beyond term and are found to have extremely low estriol excretion and no evidence of fetal distress. Through 1976, less than 20 cases had been reported. (28, 29) All newborn children have been male, suggesting that the disorder is due to an X-linked recessive gene. The patients usually fail to go into labor and require delivery by cesarean section. The characteristic steroid findings are as follows: extremely low estriol and estetrol in the mother with extremely high amniotic fluid dehydroepiandrosterone sulfate (DS) and normal amniotic fluid dehydroepiandrosterone (DHA) and androstenedione. The normal DHA and androstenedione with a high DS rule out the adrenogenital syndrome. The small amount of estriol which is present in these patients probably arises from 16-hydroxylation of DS in the maternal liver, thus providing 16-hydroxylated DHA to the placenta for aromatization to estriol. The diagnosis may be confirmed by administration of nonradioactive DS into the amniotic fluid and demonstration of little change in maternal estriol excretion. (29) However, demonstration of a high level of DS in the amniotic fluid is probably adequate.

Protein Hormones of The Placenta

Human Chorionic Gonadotropin (HCG)

Human chorionic gonadotropin is a glycoprotein, a peptide framework to which carbohydrate sidechains are attached. Alterations in the carbohydrate components may alter biologic properties. For example, the half life of HCG is approximately 24 hours as compared to 2 hours for LH, a 10-fold difference which is due mainly to the greater sialic acid content of HCG. As with the other glycoproteins, FSH, LH, and TSH, HCG, consists of two non-covalently linked subunits, called alpha and beta. The alpha subunit in these glycoprotein hormones are virtually identical, consisting of 89 to 92 amino acids. Unique biological activity as well as specificity in radioimmunoassays must be attributed to the molecular differences in the beta subunits.

The 28 to 30 terminal amino acids of the beta-HCG on the carboxy terminal are unique and different from the sequence on LH. Despite this difference (which allows specific antisera to discriminate between HCG and LH in assays) HCG is biologically similar to LH. To this day, the only definitely known function for HCG is support of the corpus luteum, taking over for LH on about the 8th day after ovulation when beta-HCG can be first detected in maternal blood. Continued survival of the corpus luteum is totally dependent upon HCG, and in turn the survival of the pregnancy is dependent upon steroids from the corpus luteum until the 7th week of pregnancy. (1) From the 7th week to the 10th week, the corpus luteum is gradually replaced by the placenta, and by the 10th week, removal of the corpus luteum will not be followed by steroid withdrawal abortion.

It is very probable that HCG stimulates steroidogenesis in the early fetal testes, so that androgen production will ensue and masculine differentiation can be accomplished. It also appears that the function of the inner fetal zone of the adrenal cortex may depend upon HCG for steroidogenesis. The mechanism for control of placental steroidogenesis is unknown and it is not certain whether the presence of HCG is necessary.

HCG is secreted by the syncytiotrophoblast, reaching a maximum level of 500,000 to 1,000,000 IU/day at 10 weeks gestation (50–100 IU/ml in the blood). The old bioassay tests for pregnancy have been replaced with immunological agglutination tests for the presence of HCG in maternal urine. The tests are reliable with essentially no falsely positive reactions. Falsely negative results may occur prior to the 5th to 6th week of gestation because the sensitivity of the tests must be maintained at a level high enough to avoid cross-reactions with LH.

HCG levels close to term are higher in women bearing female fetuses. (30, 31) This is true of serum levels, placental content, urinary levels, and amniotic fluid concentrations. The mechanism and purpose of this difference are not known.

Human Chorionic Thyrotropin (HCT)

The human placenta contains two thyrotropic substances. One is called human chorionic thyrotropin (HCT), similar in size and action to pituitary TSH. The content in the normal placenta is very small. HCT differs from the other glycoproteins in that it does not appear to share the common alpha subunit. Antiserum generated to alpha HCG does not neutralize the biologic activities of HCT, but it does that of HCG and pituitary TSH. Rarely, patients with trophoblastic disease may have hyperthyroidism. Studies indicate that HCG has intrinsic thyrotropic activity, and thus represents the second placental thyrotropic substance. (32) On a molecular basis it is calculated that

HCG contains approximately 1/4000th of the thyrotropic activity of human TSH. (33) In conditions with very elevated HCG levels, the thyrotropic activity can be sufficient to produce hyperthyroidism.

Human Chorionic Adrenocortico-tropin Hormone (HCACTH)

There is evidence that the rise in free cortisol which takes place throughout pregnancy may be due to ACTH production by the placenta. (34) The placental content of ACTH is higher than can be accounted for by the contribution of sequestered blood. In addition, cortisol levels in pregnant women are resistant to dexamethasone suppression, suggesting that there is a component of maternal ACTH which does not originate in the maternal pituitary gland. One may speculate that placental ACTH raises maternal adrenal activity in order to provide the basic building blocks (cholesterol and pregnenolone) for placental steroidogenesis.

Human Placental Lactogen (HPL)

Human placental lactogen (HPL), also secreted by the syncytiotrophoblast, is a single chain polypeptide held together by two disulfide bonds. It is about 96% similar to human growth hormone (HGH), but has only 3% of HGH somatotropin activity. In addition, HPL has about 50% of the lactogenic activity of sheep prolactin. Its half life is short, about 30 minutes; hence its appeal as an index of placental problems. The level of HPL in the maternal circulation is correlated with fetal and placental weight, plateauing in the last 4 weeks of pregnancy. There is no circadian variation. Very high levels are found in association with multiple gestations; levels up to 40 μg/ml have been found with quadruplets and quintuplets. (35)

Physiologic Function. Experimentally, the maternal level of HPL can be altered by changing the circulating level of glucose. HPL is elevated with hypoglycemia and depressed with hyperglycemia. This information along with studies in fasted pregnant women have led to the following formulation for the physiologic function of HPL. (35–40)

The metabolic role of HPL is to mobilize lipids as free fatty acids. In the fed state, there is abundant glucose available, leading to increased insulin levels, lipogenesis, and glucose utilization. This is associated with decreased gluconeogenesis, and a decrease in the circulating free fatty acid levels, as the free fatty acids are utilized in the process of lipogenesis to deposit storage packets of triglycerides (see Chapter 13, Obesity).

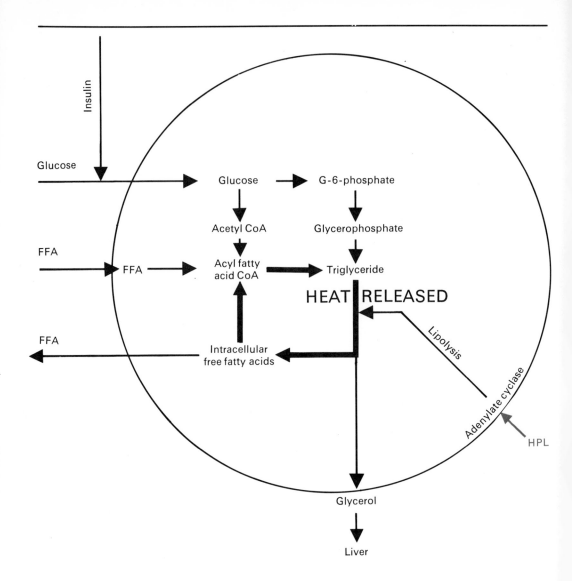

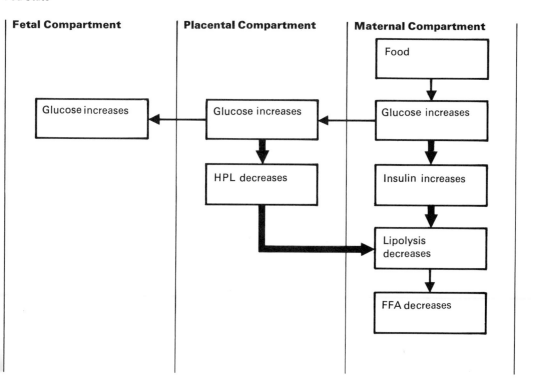

Pregnancy has been likened to a state of "accelerated starvation," (37) characterized by a relative hypoglycemia in the fasting state. This state is due to two major influences:

1. Glucose provides the major, although not the entire, fuel requirement for the fetus. A difference in gradient causes a constant transfer of glucose from the mother to the fetus.

2. Placental hormones, specifically estrogen and progesterone, and especially HPL, interfere with the action of maternal insulin. In the second half of pregnancy when HPL levels rise approximately 10-fold, HPL is a major force in the diabetogenic effects of pregnancy. The latter is characterized by increased levels of insulin associated with decreased cellular response.

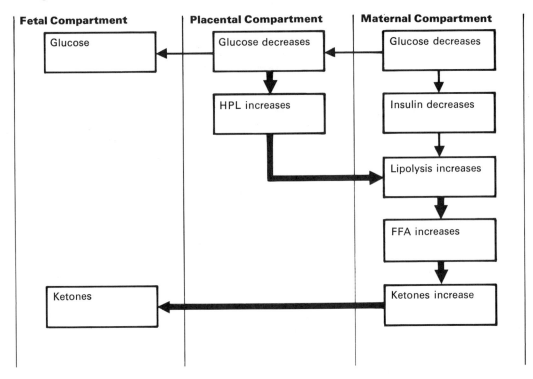

Fetal Compartment | **Placental Compartment** | **Maternal Compartment**

In the fasting state, as the supplies of glucose decrease, HPL levels rise, stimulating lipolysis leading to an increase in circulating free fatty acids in order to provide a different fuel for the mother so that glucose and amino acids can be conserved for the fetus. With sustained fasting, maternal fat is utilized for fuel to such an extent that maternal ketone levels rise. There is limited transport of free fatty acids across the placenta. Therefore, when glucose becomes scarce for the fetus, fetal tissues utilize the ketones which do cross the placenta. Thus, decreased glucose levels lead to decreased insulin and increased HPL, increasing lipolysis and ketone levels. HPL may also enhance the fetal uptake of ketones and amino acids. The mechanism for the insulin antagonism by HPL may be the HPL-stimulated increase in free fatty acid levels, which in turn directly interferes with insulin-directed entry of glucose into cells.

This mechanism can be viewed as an important means to provide fuel for the fetus between maternal meals. However, with a sustained state of inadequate glucose intake the subsequent ketosis may impair brain development and function. Pregnancy is not the time to severely restrict caloric intake.

HPL Clinical Uses. Blood levels of HPL are related to placental function. Assay of the maternal HPL levels during pregnancy appears to be of value in screening patients for potential fetal complications. In a series of 200 apparently normal pregnancies, 3 or more levels of HPL less than 4 μg/ml, when measured between 35 and 40 weeks of gestation, were associated with a 71% chance of fetal distress or neonatal asphyxia. (41) A single value of less than 4 μg/ml was associated with a 30% risk, while 2 values less than 4 μg/ml indicated a 50% risk. In a large Finnish study, a single subnormal HPL level during the third trimester of pregnancy was associated with a 49% risk of fetal distress. (42)

HPL is of little help in predicting fetal demise in diabetic pregnancies. However, it might be utilized as an indicator of poorly controlled diabetes in that an elevated level is an indication of macrosomia. In post-term pregnancies, an HPL level less than 4 μg/ml indicates a high chance of the postmaturity syndrome in the fetus. Most pregnancies complicated by intrauterine growth retardation will be associated with HPL levels below 4 μg/ml.

Spellacy has defined the area below 4 μg/ml after the 30th week of gestation as a fetal danger zone. (43) In particular, he has noted that in patients with hypertension, HPL values in the danger zone are associated with a significant risk of intrauterine demise. In a prospective randomized series, utilization of the HPL assay in clinical management of high risk patients was associated with a lowering of the fetal death rate from 14.2% to 2.6%. (44)

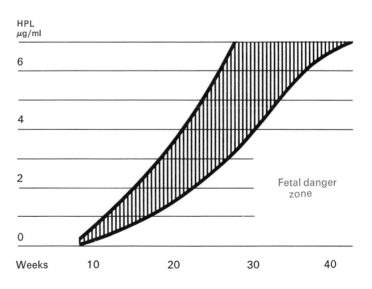

It appears useful to screen pregnant women by measuring the HPL level, ideally at 34, 36, and 38 weeks gestation. However, even a single measurement at 34–35 weeks is of value, with a repeat measurement if a low level is noted.

Previous suggestions that a low or declining level of HPL and a high level of HCG are characteristic of trophoblastic disease were not accurate. Because of the rapid clearance of HPL, aborting molar pregnancies are likely to have low levels of HPL, while the level of HCG is still high. However intact molar pregnancies may have elevated levels of both HPL and HCG. (55)

The Endocrinology of Parturition

Perhaps the best example of the interplay among fetus, placenta, and the mother is the initiation and maintenance of parturition. Human labor is the expression of a constellation of interrelated events, including fetal control, steroid hormone changes, prostaglandin production, the role of oxytocin, and myometrial cellular mechanisms. No single factor is the answer or key; rather parturition is the result of changes in all the compartments of pregnancy: fetal, placental, and maternal.

Drawing heavily on studies in a variety of mammals, we can construct the following overall hypothesis: The fetal pituitary secretes ACTH, oxytocin, and prolactin. The fetal oxytocin crosses the placenta readily and may contribute to the action of maternal oxytocin on the myometrium. By lowering membrane potential, oxytocin action increases propagation of spontaneous muscular activity by means of a calcium-dependent process. Prostaglandins may exert an oxytocic effect on uterine muscle by means of the same calcium transport mechanism. Increasing stimulation of the fetal adrenal by ACTH and perhaps prolactin raises the fetal cortisol level as well as precursors for estrogen production. The fetal cortisol may initiate uterine events and induce developmental effects such as surfactant production by the lung.

The uterine events, beginning about 35 to 36 weeks in human pregnancy, include a decrease in progesterone, which allows increased myometrial conduction and excitability, and a more rapid rise in estrogen, which enhances rhythmic contractions, increases vascularity and permeability, and increases responsiveness to oxytocin. Estrogen may stimulate prostaglandin production. Prostaglandins in turn stimulate estrogen production and may sustain the high levels of estrogen, in addition to contributing a major oxytocic effect. The increased uterine activity, along with activation of Ferguson's reflex (reflex release of oxytocin by cervical and vaginal distention), leads to enhanced uterine contractions. This occurs under the influence of oxytocin upon already estrogen-primed and progesterone-deprived myometrium. Oxytocin release may be minute and the response provoked is probably governed largely by the modifications in myometrial sensitivity noted above.

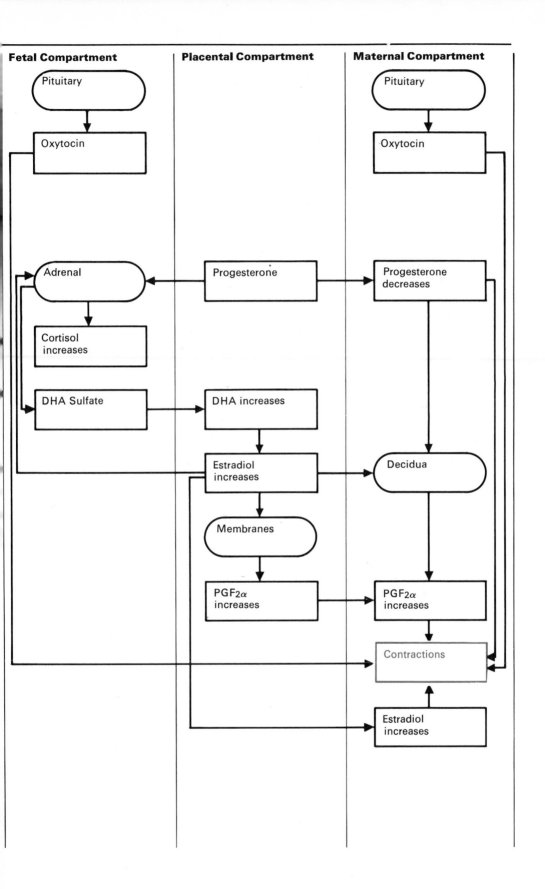

Fetal Compartment

Pituitary

Oxytocin

Adrenal

Cortisol
increases

DHA Sulfate

Placental Compartment

Progesterone

DHA increases

Estradiol
increases

Membranes

PGF$_{2\alpha}$
increases

Maternal Compartment

Pituitary

Oxytocin

Progesterone
decreases

Decidua

PGF$_{2\alpha}$
increases

Contractions

Estradiol
increases

There may be several sources for the prostaglandins. The uterus produces prostaglandins in both endometrial and myometrial tissues. Csapo has proposed that the myometrial content of prostaglandins is stretch-dependent. (46) Increasing uterine volume maintains stimulation of uterine prostaglandin synthesis and release, but the oxytocic effects of prostaglandin are held in check by progesterone. Even at a stable progesterone level the threshold may be overcome by a decrease in intranuclear progesterone translocation through binding changes, or an increase in prostaglandin production, or an increase in estrogen production. Although any one factor may remain stable, a critical change in the relationship among all the factors may trigger labor.

Another important source for prostaglandins, and perhaps a primary one, is the decidual tissue which utilizes arachidonic acid precursor released from storage in either the fetal membranes, the decidua, or both. Activation of the phospholipase enzyme may be a response to endocrine changes prior to parturition.

It is likely that endocrine changes in the utero-placental environment are the principal governing factors accounting for the eventual development of uterine contractions. Having the above overview in mind, let us now examine the individual parts of this formulation.

Fetal Control of Labor

The association between prolonged gestation and the anencephalic fetus in human pregnancy has long been recognized. Only in the past decade, however, has experimental work implicated the fetal pituitary-adrenal axis in normal parturition. This has largely been through the observations in sheep by Liggins and co-workers. (47)

Fetal adrenalectomy or hypophysectomy prolongs pregnancy, while infusion of ACTH or glucocorticoids into the sheep fetus stimulates premature labor. Implantation of chronic indwelling catheters into ewes and their lambs has allowed investigators to establish that the sequence of events begins about 10 days prior to labor with elevation of fetal cortisol, probably in response to fetal pituitary ACTH. (47)

Enzyme activity in the fetal adrenal gland increases very rapidly in the final few days of gestation. This is probably due to the effect of fetal ACTH, since its infusion into a lamb fetus induces labor even at premature dates. Furthermore, in sheep and human beings, there is little or no placental transfer of maternal ACTH into the fetal circulation. (47, 48)

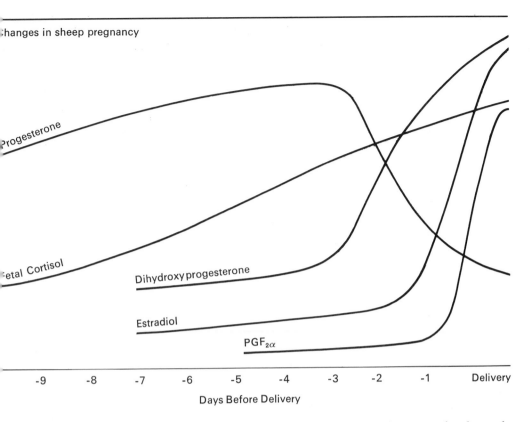

Progesterone

Fetal Cortisol

Dihydroxy progesterone

Estradiol

PGF$_{2\alpha}$

| -9 | -8 | -7 | -6 | -5 | -4 | -3 | -2 | -1 | Delivery |

Days Before Delivery

The activity of the fetal adrenal gland may not be dependent only upon fetal ACTH. Human chorionic gonadotropin (HCG) may also serve a role, especially in promoting steroidogenesis in the fetal zone. It has also been suggested that fetal prolactin plays a role, since there is a better correlation between growth of the fetal zone of the adrenal cortex with fetal prolactin levels than with fetal ACTH. (5) The precise stimulus and the control mechanism for the rise in cortisol secretion, however, remain to be determined.

Much of what is known in sheep also applies to human parturition. Murphy (49) has shown that cord blood cortisol concentrations are high in infants born vaginally or by cesarean section following spontaneous onset of labor. In contrast, cord blood cortisol levels are low in infants born without spontaneous labor, whether delivery is vaginal (induced labor) or by cesarean section (elective repeat section). If the rise in fetal cortisol were due to stress-induced maternal cortisol crossing the placenta, then the umbilical venous cortisol would be higher than the arterial level. However, the opposite is true: after spontaneous labor the umbilical arterial level is greater than the venous level. (50) It is unlikely that this A-V difference represents fetal response to the stress of labor, because levels are higher in spontaneous labor and induced labor after ruptured membranes when compared to levels with electively induced labor. Furthermore, as maternal cortisol crosses the placenta (which it does readily) it is largely metabolized to cortisone in the process. (51) This, in fact, may be the mechanism by which suppression of the fetal adrenal gland by maternal steroids is avoided. In contrast to the maternal liver, the fetal liver has a limited capacity for transforming the biologically inactive cortisone to the active cortisol.

Cortisol has also been shown to rise dramatically in amniotic fluid at term, (52, 53) correlating with maturation of the L/S ratio. (54) Neonatal plasma cortisol levels are lower in postmature neonates than they are in term neonates, (55) and labor has been initiated in post-term pregnancies with the instillation of cortisol into the amniotic fluid. (56) These studies strengthen the suggestion that a relationship exists between impaired pituitary adrenal function in the fetus and prolonged gestation in human pregnancy.

Increased glucocorticoid secretion by the fetal adrenal gland presumably starts a chain of events associated with labor. The sequence of changes in the sheep includes a decline in progesterone, a rise in estrogen, a rise in prostaglandin $F_{2\alpha}$ production, and the onset of uterine activity. At the same time, the increased fetal adrenal activity leads to important developmental accomplishments. These include increased pulmonary surfactant production and the accumulation of liver glycogen. Cortisol levels in cord serum are lower in infants who go on to develop respiratory distress. (57, 58)

Changes in Estrogen and Progesterone

Csapo has repeatedly emphasized the importance of the decline in progesterone concentrations associated with fetal growth and increase in uterine volume. (59) The over-all effect of increased uterine volume is to stimulate hypertrophy, excitability, and mechanical activity of the myometrium. Maintenance of myometrial activity, according to Csapo, is due to a balance between progesterone and prostaglandins. (46)

Much of the criticism of the concept of progesterone withdrawal has been based on the inability to demonstrate a clear-cut decline in peripheral blood levels of progesterone prior to human parturition. However, measurement of peripheral levels of progesterone may give only a gross hint of the dynamics of the situation. Metabolism, target tissue binding and utilization, and localized changes in uterine production are only a few of the many factors that complicate this consideration.

In this regard, a study of Turnbull and colleagues (60) has special value in that the steroids were measured serially in the same patients. Peripheral plasma levels of estradiol became elevated while progesterone decreased, beginning approximately 5 weeks prior to parturition. These changes began at the same time maturation of the L/S ratio occurs, and when cortisol levels increase.

Progesterone withdrawal is associated with a decrease in the resting potential of myometrium, i.e. an increased response to electric and oxytocic stimuli. Conduction of action potential through the muscle is increased and the myometrial excitability is increased. Estrogens enhance rhythmic contractions as well as increasing vascularity and permeability, and oxytocin response. Thus progesterone withdrawal and estrogen increase lead to an enhancement of conduction and excitation. It should be noted that patients with a placental sulfatase deficiency fail to produce significant amounts of estrogen and usually fail to go into labor. (28, 29)

How placental estrogen production is elevated and placental progesterone is decreased are not clear. Animal studies suggest that the effects are mediated via the placenta. In the sheep, progesterone metabolism is altered by glucocorticoids by the induction of a 17α-hydroxylase enzyme.

In *in vitro* studies of placental tissue, the rate of production of 17α, 20α-dihydroxypregn-4-en-3-one is increased by dexamethasone treatment. (61) This dihydroxyprogesterone compound has also been identified in fetal sheep placenta obtained after spontaneous labor. Thus direct synthesis of progesterone does not decline, but increased metabolism to a 17α-hydroxylated product results in less available progesterone. The 17α-hydroxylated compound also serves as a precursor for the rise in estrogen levels. Utero-ovarian venous levels of this compound rise at the time that progesterone levels decrease. (62) These findings indicate that the decline in progesterone and the rise in estrogen in the sheep are secondary to direct induction of a placental enzyme by a glucocorticoid.

Should endocrine events in human parturition bear any resemblance to those in the ewe, it might be expected that strategic hormonal administration would affect the labor process. Manipulation of the fetal pituitary-adrenal axis is a difficult, if not impossible, pursuit in human subjects. Administration of progestational drugs and estrogens, however, have produced general effects in keeping with the hypothesis of progesterone withdrawal and estrogen augmentation. Estrogen administration will be discussed later in this chapter in conjunction with prostaglandins.

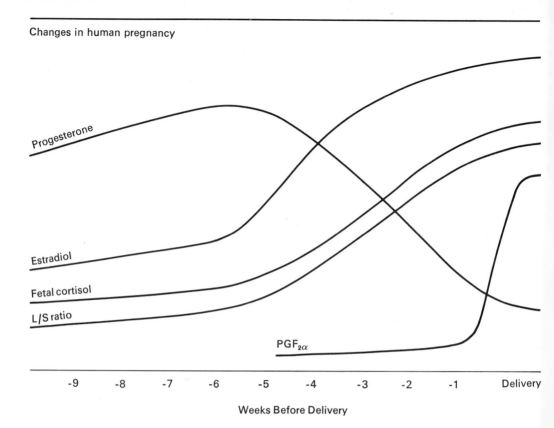

Progesterone

Estradiol

Fetal cortisol

L/S ratio

PGF$_{2\alpha}$

| -9 | -8 | -7 | -6 | -5 | -4 | -3 | -2 | -1 | Delivery |

Weeks Before Delivery

If progesterone withdrawal is a significant early event in human parturition, then administration of a progestational agent may delay premature delivery. It is widely recognized and accepted clinically that once labor has begun, the use of progestational agents, even when administered in very large doses, is ineffective. In a provocative report, Johnson and colleagues (63) presented compelling results in what appears to be the first carefully designed study utilizing a progestational agent prophylactically to prevent premature labor. Using a double-blind prospective approach, the administration of 17α-hydroxyprogesterone caproate significantly delayed delivery and reduced perinatal deaths in the treatment group.

The steroid events in human pregnancy appear to be similar to events in the ewe, with a very important difference: a more extended time scale. Steroid changes in the sheep occur over the course of several days, while in human pregnancy, the changes begin at approximately 34 to 36 weeks and occur over the last 5 weeks of pregnancy.

The respiratory distress syndrome consists of progressive atelectasis of the lungs of a newborn infant caused by an increase in surface tension. The pulmonary alveoli are lined with a surface-active phospholipid-protein complex called pulmonary surfactant. It is this surfactant which decreases surface tension, thereby facilitating lung expansion and preventing atelectasis. In full-term fetuses, surfactant is present at birth in sufficient amounts to permit adequate lung expansion and normal breathing. In premature fetuses, however, surfactant is present in lesser amounts, and when insufficient, postnatal lung expansion and ventilation are frequently impaired, presenting as the clinical syndrome of respiratory distress.

Phosphatidylcholine (lecithin) has been identified as a major lipid of the surfactant complex. (64) Beginning at 20 to 22 weeks of pregnancy, a less stable and less active lecithin, palmitoylmyristoyl lecithin is formed. Hence, a premature infant does not always develop respiratory distress syndrome; however, in addition to being less active, synthesis of this lecithin is more susceptible to stress and acidosis, making the premature infant more susceptible to respiratory distress. At about the 35th week of gestation, there is a sudden surge of dipalmitoyl lecithin, the major surfactant lecithin, which is stable and very active. Since the fetal lungs contribute to the formation of amniotic fluid and the sphingomyelin concentration of amniotic fluid changes relatively little throughout pregnancy, measurement of the lecithin/sphingomyelin (L/S) ratio indicates the change which occurs at approximately 34 to 36 weeks of pregnancy when the great increase in dipalmitoyl lecithin takes place.

Gluck, et al, were the first to demonstrate that the L/S ratio correlates with pulmonary maturity of the fetal lung. (64) In normal development sphingomyelin concentrations are greater than those of lecithin until about gestational week 26. Prior to 34 weeks, the L/S ratio is approximately 1:1. At 34 to 36 weeks, with a sudden increase in lecithin, the ratio rises acutely. In general, a ratio of 2.0 or greater indicates pulmonary maturity and that respiratory distress syndrome will not develop in the newborn. Respiratory distress syndrome associated with a ratio greater than 2.0 usually follows a difficult delivery with a low 5-minute Apgar score, suggesting that severe acidosis can inhibit surfactant production. A ratio in the transitional range (1.0 to 1.9) indicates that respiratory distress syndrome may develop but that the fetal lung has entered the period of lecithin production, and a repeat amniocentesis in 1 or 2 weeks usually reveals a mature L/S ratio. The rise from low to high ratios may actually occur within 3 to 4 days.

Abnormalities of pregnancy may affect the rate of maturation of the fetal lung, resulting either in an early mature L/S ratio or a delayed rise in the ratio. (65) Accelerated maturation of the ratio is associated with hypertension, advanced diabetes, hemoglobinopathies, heroin addiction, and poor maternal nutrition. Delayed maturation is seen with diabetes without hypertension, and Rh-sensitization.

Previously it was believed that delivery by cesarean section was associated with a greater incidence of respiratory distress syndrome when groups were corrected for gestational age. Since respiratory distress syndrome is related to the maturity of the fetal lung, and the L/S ratio is an index of pulmonary maturity, comparison of mode of delivery with the L/S ratio has allowed a more accurate appraisal of this problem. Gabert et al (66) and Donald, et al, (67) demonstrated that the maturity of the lungs as indicated by the L/S ratio determines the presence of respiratory distress syndrome regardless of the mode of delivery.

Since Liggins observed early labor and survival of premature lambs following the administration of cortisol to the fetus, the possibility of accelerating pulmonary maturity with corticosteroids has been investigated. Injection of corticosteroids directly into a fetus accelerates the appearance of surface activity and increases the viability of the fetuses in various animals. In a clinical trial for the prevention of respiratory distress syndrome, betamethasone was administered to patients in whom premature delivery was threatened and there was a significant decrease in the neonatal mortality rate in the group of infants treated with steroids more than 24 hours before delivery. (68) Administration of corticosteroids after delivery has no beneficial effect on respiratory distress. There is also an association between low thyroid activity and the respiratory distress syndrome, consistent with animal studies in which lung maturation is accelerated with thyroxine treatments. (69, 70) The mechanism for the steroid- and thyroxine-induced acceleration is thought to be due to induction of enzyme systems involving lecithin biosynthesis.

Prostaglandins

Prostaglandins are carboxylic acids that are formed enzymatically from polyunsaturated fatty acids. The nomenclature is at first rather confusing because letters, numbers, and Greek letter subscripts are combined. Once understood, the basic pattern allows one to appreciate the differences among the various prostaglandins. The 20-carbon structures contain a cyclopentane ring, numbered as in the basic molecule, prostanoic acid.

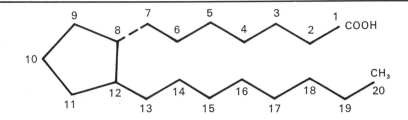

The character of the ring identifies four major groups, designated by the letters E, F, A, and B. Thus at the C-9 position, E prostaglandins contain a ketone group, and F prostaglandins a hydroxyl group. The A prostaglandins are derived from E prostaglandins by dehydration, whereas rearrangement of the ring in A prostaglandins gives rise to the B prostaglandins. In some animals, B prostaglandins are formed via the action of a PGA isomerase. The product of PGA isomerase is PGC with the double bond in the 11–12 position. PGB then arises as a result of the instability of PGC. PGC is not present in man.

The subscript number after each letter indicates the degree of unsaturation in the side chains. Thus subscript 2 indicates two double bonds, one at C-13,14, and a second at the C-5,6 position. The alpha notation in the F prostaglandins indicates that the hydroxyl group attached to carbon 9 is below the plane of the ring. PGF beta isomers have not been found in nature. All naturally occurring prostaglandins contain a hydroxyl group at C-15.

Interest in reproductive physiology focuses on the derivatives of arachidonic acid, PGE_2 and $PGF_{2\alpha}$. The precursors of the prostaglandins are released from phospholipids by phospholipase action. Only the free unesterified essential fatty acids can be utilized for synthesis to prostaglandins. Arachidonic acid and other essential free fatty acids are usually esterified in the 2 position of various glycerophospholipids or in cholesterol esters. Phospholipase A_2 catalyzes the hydrolysis of phospholipids releasing the fatty acids present in the 2 position, making them available for prostaglandin synthesis.

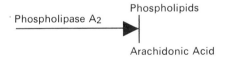

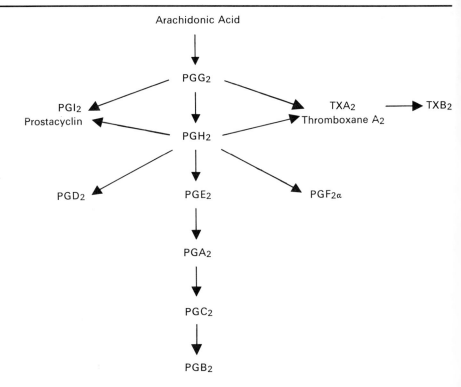

The rate limiting step in prostaglandin biosynthesis is the availability of the fatty acid precursor. Synthesis is accomplished by means of an enzyme complex, collectively referred to as prostaglandin synthetase. Well known anti-inflammatory agents, such as aspirin and indomethacin, inhibit the synthesis of prostaglandins by interfering with the action of the prostaglandin synthetase complex.

New compounds have now been isolated that are extremely short-lived, but that may be more potent than the prostaglandins. The prostaglandin endoperoxides PGG_2 and PGH_2, are precursors of the prostaglandins PGE_2 and $PGF_{2\alpha}$, but also of a new group of potent cellular regulatory agents, the thromboxanes and prostacyclin (prostaglandin I_2). The thromboxanes and the endoperoxide precursors may be the important agents in various physiologic functions. Thromboxane B_2 is the inactive metabolite of the active compound, TXA_2. Prostaglandin I_2 may serve to prevent the aggregation of platelets on normal, undamaged vascular walls while TXA_2 initiates platelet aggregation. It is still unknown which of these substances plays the key role in specific tissues, although in the kidney and the utero-placental unit, PGE_2 and $PGF_{2\alpha}$ appear to be the important substances. The availability of arachidonic acid remains as the initial essential step.

The initial step in the metabolism of prostaglandins is the oxidation of the hydroxyl group at the C-15 position. This important and rapid step is catalyzed by a specific enzyme, prostaglandin dehydrogenase, widely distributed in mammalian tissues, but especially rich in the lungs and in the placenta. Following conversion of the hydroxyl group to a ketone group, a reduction of the C-13,14 double bond usually follows. These metabolic changes at the C-15 position result in a reduction in biologic activity. Further metabolism results in 16-carbon dicarboxylic acids that are found in the urine.

Prostaglandin Regulation of Utero-Placental Blood Flow. Prostaglandins of the A and E families are potent vasodilators which decrease the peripheral resistance and systemic blood pressure by directly relaxing the smooth muscle of the arteriolar vessels. Because of the extremely rapid metabolism of E prostaglandins by the lungs, the activity of newly synthesized E prostaglandins appears to be limited to the immediate vicinity, within the synthesizing tissue itself. Thus E prostaglandins may act within a variety of organs as locally produced potent vasodilators to maintain basal blood flow, and as a determinant of the hemodynamic response to various acute and chronic stimuli. Such a role for E prostaglandins has been implicated within the kidney, the heart, the brain, and in regulating utero-placental blood flow. (71)

The approach to the study of prostaglandins as they might play a role in regulating utero-placental blood flow has utilized inhibition of prostaglandin biosynthesis and the demonstration of active prostaglandin production by the products of conception. The important observations in the monkey (72, 73), the dog (74), and the rabbit (75), are as follows:

1. Angiotensin-II increases uterine blood flow.

2. Angiotensin-II increases PGE production by the pregnant uterus.

3. Inhibition of prostaglandin synthesis lowers basal uterine blood flow, inhibits the blood flow and PGE respond to angiotensin-II, and raises the systemic maternal blood pressure.

These findings have suggested that E prostaglandin (in particular, PGE_2) plays a role in maintaining the resting utero-placental vasomotor tone, and the systemic maternal blood pressure. A change must take place in the vascular system along with the volume and flow changes during pregnancy. The plasma volume begins to increase about the 6th week of pregnancy and rapidly expands during the second trimester with only slight increases in the last trimester until term. In order to accomodate the increase in volume without a significant rise in the maternal blood pressure, there must be a decrease in the

219

peripheral vascular resistance. Maintenance of normal maternal blood pressure and also maintenance of utero-placental blood flow depend upon vasodilation, both in the systemic maternal circulation and locally within the utero-placental unit. Prostaglandin E_2 may serve this important function.

The clinical development of toxemia of pregnancy may represent defective prostaglandin production, loss of response to prostaglandins, or a combination of these events. The placental content of E prostaglandin has been found to be lower in placentas obtained from pregnancies associated with hypertension. (76, 77) The actual tissue source of the E prostaglandins is unknown. PGE synthesis has been demonstrated in the blood vessels themselves in response to angiotensin and bradykinin, and in our laboratory, to estrogen. Thus blood vessel production of prostaglandins in response to the endrocrine environment may be an important factor in influencing the exchange of substances between the fetal and maternal blood, as well as the maternal vasomotor response to pregnancy.

Prostaglandins and Parturition. Prostaglandin levels increase in association with labor. $PGF_{2\alpha}$ has been shown to increase significantly in amniotic fluid in labor as compared with levels in prelabor controls. (78, 79) PGE levels also increase in the amniotic fluid during labor, but there appears to be a greater association between contractions and $PGF_{2\alpha}$. (80) Arachidonic acid levels in the amniotic fluid also rise in labor, and arachidonate injected into the amniotic sac initiates parturition. (81) Measurement of the major urinary metabolite of F prostaglandins during pregnancy demonstrated a 2-fold to 5-fold increase compared with levels in nonpregnant women. (82)

These studies suggest that prostaglandins are associated with active labor. In the sheep, fetal cortisol levels increase during the last 8 to 10 days of gestation, followed by a decline in progesterone and a rise in estradiol. The last event to be observed is the appearance of $PGF_{2\alpha}$ in the uterine venous blood several hours before labor. A cause and effect relationship between the rise in estrogen and the appearance of the $PGF_{2\alpha}$ has been supported by the administration of estradiol (without cortisol) to the ewe and observation of increased production of $PGF_{2\alpha}$ in response. (47)

Estrogen administration to pregnant women at term does increase uterine activity and the sensitivity to oxytocin. However changes in PGF levels have not been detected. (83) The study of prostaglandin levels in physiologic events is handicapped by the rapid metabolism of these compounds. Prostaglandins of the E and F families are rapidly converted to the 13,14-dihydro-15-keto metabolites by lung, kidney, and placental tissues. Because of these considerations, attention must be directed to mea surements of the major metabolites. Indeed, there is a 10-fold to 30-fold increase during active labor in levels of the major metabolite of $PGF_{2\alpha}$, as measured by mass spectrometric-gas chromatographic methods. (84) This time consuming technique which requires large volumes of blood does not lend itself to establishing correlations among multiple substances in the same patient. Use of new radioimmunoassays for the prostaglandin metabolites will be required to establish these correlations.

Additional indirect evidence of a physiologic role for prostaglandins in labor comes from studies utilizing inhibitors of prostaglandin synthesis. In a retrospective study of labor in patients taking high doses of aspirin for various indications, a highly significant increase in the average length of gestation, incidence of postmaturity, and duration of spontaneous labor was demonstrated in the women taking aspirin. (85) Novy and colleagues (86) demonstrated that therapeutic doses of indomethacin given to rhesus monkeys in the last week of pregnancy prolong gestation and prevent the normal onset of parturition. In addition, indomethacin has been shown to be effective in stopping premature labor in human pregnancies. (87, 88)

The full effects of these agents on the fetus and newborn need to be determined prior to general clinical use. For example, in the presence of inhibited prostaglandin production, the fetal circulation may persist after delivery, especially in the presence of hypoxia, presenting as primary pulmonary hypertension due to elevated pulmonary vascular resistance. (89) This response is due to the fact that E prostaglandins maintain the ductus arteriosus in the open state in the fetus, while after birth, oxygen closes the ductus in a prostaglandin-mediated event. The vascular tone of the umbilical artery may be regulated in a similar fashion.

The site of prostaglandin production in parturition is thought to be the decidua, while the precursor fatty acid may be derived from storage pools in the fetal membranes or the decidua, or in both. Phospholipase A_2 has been demonstrated in both human chorioamnion and uterine decidua. (90, 91) Gustavii has suggested that progesterone withdrawal allows degeneration of decidual cells and release of lysosomal enzymes. (92) Schwarz and colleagues believe the major source of arachidonic acid is the fetal membranes. (93) The mechanism for initiating prostaglandin synthesis, presumably by activation of the enzyme phospholipase A_2, is unknown. It is possible that within the utero-placental unit, enzyme activation by cortisol is followed by estrogen and prostaglandin production. Both processes may have feedback effects upon the other in the cascade of events which results in uterine contractions.

The Role of Oxytocin

Until it was realized that a major difficulty existed in timing of sampling, oxytocin was detected in maternal blood during spontaneous human labor only sporadically or not at all. Brief spurts of secretion occur but may go undetected by infrequent or random sampling. With frequent sampling, an increase in the number of episodic oxytocin secretions may be noted during labor.

Chard has made the following conclusions in regard to oxytocin: (94) There is little evidence that increased maternal levels of oxytocin are responsible for initiating parturition, although a low fixed level may be an essential permissive factor. Once labor has begun, however, oxytocin levels do rise, especially during the second stage. Thus oxytocin may be important for developing the more intense uterine contractions. Extremely high concentrations of oxytocin can be measured in the cord blood at delivery. Therefore, release of oxytocin from the fetal pituitary during labor may play a part in uterine activity.

Myometrial Cellular Events

The final goal for the various endocrine permutations is contraction of the uterine smooth muscle cell. There is evidence to suggest that calcium flux is the basic intracellular expression of oxytocic action. Increased levels of intracellular free calcium ions are associated with increased muscle activity. With excitation of the smooth muscle, calcium moves across the cell membrane into the cell, and calcium is released from intracellular stores. The increased intracellular free calcium acts directly upon the regulatory proteins of the myofibril. The opposite situation also holds true: decreased intracellular free calcium relaxes muscle.

Prostaglandins and oxytocin may exert their effect through this calcium transport mechanism (95) Beta-receptor stimulating agents, used recently to inhibit premature labor, are known to increase calcium binding and to promote efflux of calcium from the myometrial cell. Thus calcium mediates the effects of agents which stimulate and relax the uterus.

The calcium ion utilized in this mechanism may originate from intracellular or extracellular sources. The sarcoplasma reticulum (the interfibrillar material of muscle tissue, i.e. the noncontracting tissue) serves as a site of intracellular calcium storage. Myometrium contains a microsomal protein fraction, largely derived from sarcoplasma reticulum, which binds calcium in the presence of ATP. Prostaglandins and oxytocin inhibit calcium binding in this subcellular fraction, thereby raising intracellular calcium levels and activating contractions.

References

1. **Csapo, AI, Pulkkinen, MO, and Wiest, WG,** Effects of Luteectomy and Progesterone Replacement in Early Pregnant Patients, Am J Obstet Gynec 115:759, 1973.

2. **Buster, JE, and Abraham, GE,** The Applications of Steroid Hormone Radioimmunoassays to Clinical Obstetrics, Obstet Gynec 46:489, 1975.

3. **Siiteri, PK, Febres, F, Chang, RJ, Clemens, LE, and Gondos, B,** Immunosuppressive Properties of Progesterone, Program, 58th Annual Meeting, The Endocrine Society, 1976, Abstract 247.

4. **Buster, JE, Sakakini, J, Jr., Killam, AP, and Scragg, WH,** Serum Unconjugated Estriol Levels in the Third Trimester and Their Relationship to Gestational Age, Am J Obstet Gynec 125:672, 1975.

5. **Winters, AJ, Colston, C, MacDonald, PC, and Porter, JC,** Fetal Plasma Prolactin Levels, J Clin Endocrinol Metab 41:626, 1975.

6. **Serra, GB, Perez-Palacios, G, and Jaffe, RB,** Enhancement of 3β-Hydroxysteroid Dehydrogenase-Isomerase in the Human Fetal Adrenal by Removal of the Soluble Cell Fraction, Biochim Biophys Acta 244:186, 1971.

7. **Wray, PM, and Russell, CS,** The Value of the Creatinine Estimation as a Gauge of the Completeness of the 24-Hour Specimen. J Obstet Gynaecol Br Emp 67:623, 1960.

8. **Cathro, DM, Betrand, J, and Coyle, MG,** Antenatal Diagnosis of Adrenocortical Hyperplasia, Lancet 1:732, 1969.

9. **Adlercreutz, H, Martin, F, Tikkanen, MJ, and Pulkkinen, M,** Effect of Ampicillin Administration on the Excretion of Twelve Estrogens in Pregnancy Urine, Acta Endocrinol 80:551, 1975.

10. **Jewelewicz, R, Bassett, M, and Levitz, M,** Estriol "Clearance" and Creatinine Clearance during Normal Spontaneous Labor and Labor Induced by Oxytocin Infusion, J Clin Endocrinol Metab 29:1539, 1969.

11. **Luther, ER, MacLeod, SC, and Langan, MJ,** The Value of Single Specimen Estriol/Creatinine Determinations during Pregnancy, Am J Obstet Gynec 116:9, 1973.

12. **Carrington, ER, Oesterling, MJ, and Adams, FM,** Renal Clearance of Estriol in Complicated Pregnancies, Am J Obstet Gynec 106:1131, 1970.

13. **Katagiri, H, Distler, W, Freeman, RK, and Goebelsmann, U,** Estriol in Pregnancy, IV. Normal Concentrations, Diurnal and/or Episodic Variations, and Day-to-Day Changes of Unconjugated and Total Estriol in Late Pregnancy Plasma, Am J Obstet Gynec 124:272, 1976.

14. **Lindberg, BS, Johansson, EDB, and Nilsson, BA,** Plasma Levels of Nonconjugated Estradiol-17β, and Estriol in High Risk Pregnancies, Acta Obstet Gynec, Gynec Scand, Suppl 32:37, 1974.

15. **Hagen, AA,** Formation of 15α-Hydroxyestriol from 4-^{14}C-17β-Estradiol and 6-7-^{3}H-Estriol by an Anencephalic, J Clin Endocrinol Metab 30:763, 1970.

16. **Heikkila, J, and Luukkainen, T,** Urinary Excretion of Estriol and 15α-Hydroxyestriol in Complicated Pregnancies, Am J Obstet Gynec 110:509, 1971.

17. **Sciarra, JJ, Tagatz, GE, Notation, AD, and Depp, R,** Estriol and Estetrol in Amniotic Fluid, Am J Obstet Gynec 118:626, 1974.

18. **Maden, JD, Siiteri, PK, MacDonald, PC, and Gant, NF,** The Pattern and Rates of Metabolism of Maternal Plasma Dehydroisoandrosterone Sulfate in Human Pregnancy, Am J Obstet Gynec 125:915, 1976.

19. **Korda, AR, Challis, JJ, Anderson, AB, and Turnbull, AC,** Assessment of Placental Function in Normal and Pathological Pregnancies by Estimation of Plasma Estradiol Levels after Injection of Dehydroepiandrosterone Sulphate, Brit J Obstet Gynec 82:656, 1975.

20. **Tulchinsky, D, Osathanondh, R, and Finn, A,** Dehydroepiandrosterone Sulfate Loading Test in the Diagnosis of Complicated Pregnancies, New Eng J Med 294:517, 1976.

21. **Gant, NF, Hutchinson, HT, Siiteri, PK, and MacDonald, PC,** Study of the Metabolic Clearance Rate of Dehydroisoandrosterone Sulfate in Pregnancy, Am J Obstet Gynec 111:555, 1971.

22. **Beischer, NA,** Low Estriol Excretion. Incidence, Significance and Treatment in an Obstetric Population, Med J Australia 2:379, 1975.

23. **Abell, DA, Beischer, NA, Papas, AJ, and Willis, MM,** The Association between Abnormal Glucose Tolerance (Hyperglycemia and Hypoglycemia) and Estriol Excretion in Pregnancy, Am J Obstet Gynec 124:388, 1976.

24. **Goebelsmann, U, Freeman, RK, Mestman, JH, Nakamura, RM, and Woodling, BA,** Estriol in Pregnancy II Daily Urinary Estriol Assays in the Management of the Pregnant Diabetic Woman, Am J Obstet Gynec 115:795 1973.

25. **MacLeod, SC, Mitton, DM, and Avery CR,** Relationship between Elevated Blood Pressure and Urinary Estriol during Pregnancy, Am J Obstet Gynec 109:375, 1971.

26. **Yogman, MW, Speroff, L, Huttenlocher, PR, and Kase, NG,** Child Development after Pregnancies Complicated by Low Urinary Estriol Excretion and Pre-Eclampsia, Am J Obstet Gynec 115:1069, 1972.

27. **Yssing, M,** Estriol Excretion in Pregnant Diabetics Related to Long-Term Prognosis of Surviving Children, Acta Endocrinol 75:Suppl 182:95, 1974.

28. **Osathanondh, R, Canick, J, Ryan, KJ, and Tulchinsky, D,** Placental Sulfatase Deficiency: A Case Study, J Clin Endocrinol Metab 43:208, 1976.

29. **Tabei, T, and Heinrichs, WL,** Diagnosis of Placental Sulfatase Deficiency, Am J Obstet Gynec 124:409, 1976.

30. **Wide, L, and Hobson, B,** Relationship between the Sex of the Foetus and the Amount of Human Chorionic Gonadotrophin in Placentae from the 10th to the 20th Week of Pregnancy, J Endocrinol 61:75, 1974.

31. **Boroditsky, RS, Reyes, FI, Winter, JSD, and Faiman, C,** Serum Human Chorionic Gonadotropin and Progesterone Patterns in the Last Trimester of Pregnancy: Relationship to Fetal Sex, Am J Obstet Gynec 121:238, 1975.

32. **Nisula, BC, Morgan, FJ, and Canfield, RE,** Evidence that Chorionic Gonadotropin has Intrinsic Thyrotropic Activity, Biochem Biophys Res Comm 59:86, 1974.

33. **Kenimer, JG, Hershman, JM, and Higgins, HP,** The Thyrotropin in Hydatidiform Moles is Human Chorionic Gonadotropin, J Clin Endocrinol Metab 40:482, 1975.

34. **Rees, LH, Buarke, CW, Chard, T, Evans, SW, and Letchworth, AT,** Possible Placental Origin of ACTH in Normal Human Pregnancy, Nature 254:620, 1975.

35. **Grumbach, MM, Kaplan, SL, and Vinik, A,** Chapter 2, HCS, in Berson, SA, and Yalow, RS, *Peptide Hormones,* Vol 2B, North-Holland Publishing Co., 1973, pp. 797–819.

36. **Spellacy, WN, Buhi, WC, Schram, JD, Birk, SA, and McCreary, SA,** Control of Human Chorionic Somatomammotropin Levels during Pregnancy, Obstet Gynec 37:567, 1971.

37. **Felig, P,** Maternal and Fetal Fluid Homeostasis in Human Pregnancy, Am J Clin Nutr 26:998, 1973.

38. **Felig, P, and Lynch, V,** Starvation in Human Pregnancy: Hypoglycemia, Hypoinsulinemia, and Hyperketonemia, Science 170:990, 1970.

39. **Kim, YJ, and Felig, P,** Plasma Chorionic Somatomammotropin Levels during Starvation in Mid-Pregnancy, Clin Endocrinol Metab 32:864, 1971.

40. **Felig, P, Kim, YJ, Lynch, V, and Hendler, R,** Amino Acid Metabolism during Starvation in Human Pregnancy, J Clin Invest 51:1195, 1972.

41. **Letchworth, AT, and Chard, T,** Placental Lactogen Levels as a Screening Test for Fetal Distress and Neonatal Asphyxia, Lancet 1:704, 1972.

42. **Ylikorkala, O,** Maternal Serum HPL Levels in Normal and Complicated Pregnancy as an Index of Placental Function, Acta Obstet Gynec Scand, Suppl 26, 1973.

43. **Spellacy, WN, Teoh, ES, and Buhi, WC,** Human Chorionic Somatomammotropin (HCS) Levels prior to Fetal Death in High-Risk Pregnancies, Obstet Gynec 35:685, 1970.

44. **Spellacy, WN, Buhi, WC, and Birk, SA,** The Effectiveness of Human Placental Lactogen Measurements as a Adjunct in Decreasing Perinatal Deaths, Am J Obstet Gynec 121:835, 1975.

45. **Dawood, MY, and Teoh, ES,** Serum Human Chorionic Somatomammotropin in Unaborted Hydatidiform Mole, Obstet Gynec 47:183, 1976.

46. **Csapo, AI,** The Prospects of the PGs in Postconceptual Therapy, Prostaglandins 3:245, 1973.

47. **Liggins, GC, Fairclaugh, RJ, Grieves, SA, Kendall, JZ, and Knox, BS,** The Mechanism of Initiation of Parturition in the Ewe, Recent Prog Horm Res 29:111, 1973.

48. **Allen, JP, Cook, DM, Kendall, JW, and McGilvray, B,** Maternal-Fetal ACTH Relationship in Man, J Clin Endocrinol Metab 37:230, 1973.

49. **Murphy, BEP,** Does the Human Fetal Adrenal Play Role in Parturition? Am J Obstet Gynec 115:521, 1973.

50. **Leong, MKH, and Murphy, BEP,** Cortisol Levels in Maternal Venous and Umbilical Cord Arterial and Venous Serum at Vaginal Delivery, Am J Obstet Gynec 124:471, 1976.

51. **Murphy, BEP, Clark, SJ, Donald, IR, Pinsky, M, and Vedady, D,** Conversion of Maternal Cortisol to Cortisone During Placental Transfer to the Human Fetus, Am J Obstet Gynec 118:538, 1974.

52. **Fench, M, and Tulchinsky, D,** Total Cortisol in Amniotic Fluid and Fetal Lung Maturation, New Eng J Med 292:133, 1975.

53. **Murphy, BEP, Patrick, J, and Denton, R,** Cortisol in Amniotic Fluid During Human Gestation, J Clin Endocrinol Metab 40:164, 1975.

54. **Tan, SY, Gewolb, IH, and Hobbins, JC,** Unconjugated Cortisol in Human Amniotic Fluid: Relationship to Lecithin/Sphingomyelin Ratio, J Clin Endocrinol Metab 43:412, 1976.

55. **Nwosw, VC, Wallach, E, Boggs, T, and Bongiovanni, A,** Possible Adrenocortical Insufficiency in Post-Mature Neonates, Am J Obstet Gynec 122:969, 1975.

56. **Nwosw, VC, Wallach, EE, and Bolognese, RJ,** Initiation of Labor with Intraamniotic Cortisol Instillation in Prolonged Human Pregnancy, Obstet Gynec 47:137, 1976.

57. **Murphy, BEP,** Cortisol and Cortisone Levels in the Cord Blood at Delivery of Infants with and without Respiratory Distress Syndrome, Am J Obstet Gynec 119:1111, 1974.

58. **Sybulski, S, and Maughan, GB,** Relationship between Cortisol Levels in Umbilical Cord Plasma and Development of the Respiratory Distress Syndrome in Premature Newborn Infants, Am J Obstet Gynec 125:239, 1976.

59. **Csapo, A,** The Four Direct Regulatory Factors of Myometrial Function, in Ciba Foundation Study Group No. 34 on Progesterone: Its Regulatory Effect on the Myometrium, ed. by Wolstenholme, GEW, and Knight, J, J and A Churchill, London, 1969.

60. **Turnbull, AC, Patten, PT, Flint, AP, Keirse, MJ, Jeremy, JY, and Anderson, AB,** Significant Fall in Progesterone and Rise in Estradiol Levels in Human Peripheral Plasma Before Onset of Labor, Lancet 1:101, 1974.

61. **Anderson, AB, Flint, AP, and Turnbull, AC,** Mechanism of Action of Glucocorticoids in Induction of Ovine Parturition: Effect on Placental Steroid Metabolism, J Endocrinol 66:61, 1975.

62. **Flint, AP, Goodson, JD, and Turnbull, AC,** Increased Levels of 17α, 20α, Dihydroxypregn-4-en-3-one in Utero-Ovarian Venous Plasma Near Parturition in Pregnant Sheep, J Endocrinol 65:41P, 1975.

63. **Johnson, JWC, Austin, KL, Jones, GS, Davis, GH, and King, TM,** Efficiency of 17α-Hydroxyprogesterone Caproate in the Prevention of Premature Labor, New Eng J Med 293:675, 1975.

64. **Gluck, L, Kulovich, MV, Borer, RC, Brenner, PH, Anderson, GG, and Spellacy, WN,** Diagnosis of Respiratory Distress Syndrome by Amniocentesis, Am J Obstet Gynec 109:440, 1971.

227

65. **Aubry, RH, Rourke, JE, Almanza, R, Cantor, RM, an**
Van Doren, JE, The Lecithin/Sphingomyelin Ratio in
High-Risk Obstetric Population, Obstet Gynec 47:2?
1976.

66. **Gabert, HA, Bryson, MJ, and Stenchever, MA,** Th
Effect of Cesarean Section on Respiratory Distress in th
Presence of a Mature Lecithin/Sphingomyelin Ratio, A?
J Obstet Gynec 116:366, 1973.

67. **Donald, IR, Freeman, RK, Goebelsmann, U, Cha?**
WH, and Nakamura, RM, Clinical Experience with th
Amniotic Fluid Lecithin/Sphingomyelin Ratio, Am J O?
stet Gynec 115:547, 1973.

68. **Liggins, GC, and Howie, RN,** A Controlled Trial ?
Antepartum Glucocorticoid Treatment for Preventio?
of the Respiratory Distress Syndrome in Premature I?
fants. Pediatrics 50:515, 1972.

69. **Cuestas, RA, Lindall, A, and Engel, RR,** Low Thyroi?
Hormone and Respiratory Distress Syndrome of th?
Newborn, New Eng J Med 295:297, 1976.

70. **Wu, B, Kikkawa, Y, Orzalesi, MM, Motoyama, EK?**
Kaibara, M, Zigas, CJ, and Cook, CD, Accelerate?
Maturation of Fetal Lungs by Thyroxin, Physiologis?
14:253, 1971.

71. **Speroff, L,** An Autoregulatory Role for Prostaglandin?
in Placental Hemodynamics: Their Possible Influence o?
Blood Pressure in Pregnancy, J Reprod Med 15:181
1975.

72. **Franklin, GO, Dowd, AJ, Caldwell, BV, and Speroff, L?**
The Effect of Angiotensin-II Intravenous Infusion o?
Plasma Renin Activity and Prostaglandins A, E, and ?
Levels in the Uterine Vein of the Pregnant Monkey?
Prostaglandins 6:271, 1974.

73. **Speroff, L, Haning, RV, Jr., Ewaschuk, EJ, Alberino?**
SL, and Kieliszek, FS, Uterine Artery Blood Flow Studie?
in the Pregnant Monkey, in Lindheimer, MD, Katz, A?
and Zuspan, FP (eds.) *Hypertension in Pregnancy*, Joh?
Wiley and Sons, NY, 1976, pp. 315–338.

74. **Terragno, NA, Terragno, DA, Pacholczyk, D, an?**
MacGiff, JC, Prostaglandins and the Regulation of Uter?
ine Blood Flow in Pregnancy, Nature 249:57, 1974.

75. **Venuto, RC, O'Dorisio, T, Stein, JH, and Ferris, TF?**
Uterine Prostaglandin E Secretion and Uterine Bloo?
Flow in the Pregnant Rabbit, J Clin Invest 55:193, 1975?

76. **Ryan, WL, Coronel, DM, and Johnson, RJ,** A Vasode?
pressor Substance of the Human Placenta, Am J Obste?
Gynec 105:1201, 1969.

77. **Demers, LM, and Gabbe, SG,** Placental Prostaglandin Levels in Pre-Eclampsia, Am J Obstet Gynec 126:137, 1976.

78. **Singh, EJ, and Zuspan, FP,** Content of Amniotic Fluid Prostaglandins in Normal, Diabetic and Drug-Abuse Human Pregnancy, Am J Obstet Gynec 118:358, 1974.

79. **Keirse, MI, Flint, AP, and Turnbull, AC,** Prostaglandins in Amniotic Fluid During Pregnancy and Labour, J Obstet Gynaec Br Commonw 81:131, 1974.

80. **Dray, F, and Frydman, R,** Primary Prostaglandins in Amniotic Fluid in Pregnancy and Spontaneous Labor, Am J Obstet Gynec 126:13, 1976.

81. **MacDonald, PC, Schultz, FM, Duenhoelter, JH, Gant, NF, Jimenex, JM, Pritchard, JA, Porter, JC, and Johnston, JH,** Initiation of Human Parturition; I, Mechanism of Action of Arachidonic Acid, Obstet Gynec 44: 629, 1974.

82. **Hamberg, M,** Quantitative Studies on Prostaglandin Synthesis in Man. III. Excretion of the Major Urinary Metabolites of Prostaglandins $F_{1\alpha}$ and $F_{2\alpha}$ during Pregnancy, Life Sci 14:247, 1974.

83. **Larsen, JW, Hanson, TM, Caldwell, BV, and Speroff, L,** The Effect of Estradiol Infusion on Uterine Activity and Peripheral Levels of Prostaglandin F and Progesterone, Am J Obstet Gynec 117:276, 1973.

84. **Green, K, Bygdeman, M, Toppozada, M, and Wiqvist, N,** The Role of $PGF_{2\alpha}$ in Human Parturition, Am J Obstet Gynec 120:25, 1974.

85. **Lewis, RB, and Schulman, JD,** Influence of Acetysalicylic Acid, an Inhibitor of Prostaglandin Synthesis, on the Duration of Human Gestation and Labour, Lancet 2:1159, 1973.

86. **Novy, MJ, Cook, MJ, and Manaugh, L,** Indomethacin Block of Normal Onset of Parturition in Primates, Am J Obstet Gynec 118:412, 1974.

87. **Zuckerman, HK, Reiss, V, and Rubinstein, I,** Inhibition of Human Premature Labor by Indomethacin, Obstet Gynec 44:787, 1974.

88. **Wiqvist, N, Lundstrom, V, and Green, K,** Premature Labor and Indomethacin, Prostaglandins 10:515, 1975.

89. **Manchester, D, Margolis HS, and Sheldon, RE,** Possible Association Between Maternal Indomethacin Therapy and Primary Pulmonary Hypertension of the Newborn, Am J Obstet Gynec 126:467, 1976.

90. **Schultz, FM, Schwarz, BE, MacDonald, PC, and Johnston, JM,** Initiation of Human Parturition; II. Identification of Phospholipase A_2 in Fetal Chorioamnion and Uterine Decidua, Am J Obstet Gynec 123:650, 1975.

91. **Kesson, B, and Gustavii, B,** Occurrence of Phospholipase A_1 and A_2 in Human Decidua, Prostaglandins 9:667, 1975.

92. **Gustavii, B,** Release of Lysosomal Acid Phosphatase into the Cytoplasm of Decidual Cells before the Onset of Labor in Human, Brit J Obstet Gynaec 82:177, 1975.

93. **Schwarz, BE, Schultz, FM, MacDonald, PC, and Johnston, JM,** Initiation of Human Parturition; III. Fetal Membrane Content of Prostaglandin E_2 and $F_{2\alpha}$ Precursor, Obstet Gynec 46:564, 1975.

94. **Chard, T,** The Posterior Pituitary and the Induction of Labor, *Endocrine Factors in Labour*, ed. by Klopper, A, and Gardner, J, Cambridge University Press, 1973, p. 61.

95. **Carsten, ME,** Prostaglandins and Oxytocin: Their Effects on Uterine Smooth Muscle, Prostaglandins 5:33, 1974.

11 Normal and Abnormal Sexual Development

Abnormalities of sexual differentiation are infrequently seen in an individual gynecologist's practice. However, there are few practitioners who have not been challenged at least once by a newborn with ambiguous genitalia or by a young woman with primary amenorrhea on a genetic basis. The categorization of the various syndromes in this area is confusing, and constant reference to multiple textbooks is essential for informed practice.

This chapter will present a catalogue of the major problems and our clinical approach to diagnosis. Normal sexual differentiation will be considered in order to provide a basis of understanding for the various types of abnormal development. This is followed by a section on the diagnosis and management of ambiguous genitalia. Some subjects are discussed in other chapters, but brief descriptions will be repeated here in order to present a complete picture. The text by Jones and Scott is recommended for greater detail, including descriptions of operative techniques used for the surgical repair of genital abnormalities.

Normal Sexual Differentiation

The gender identity (whether an individual identifies himself as a male or a female) is the end result of genetic, hormonal, and morphologic sex as influenced by the environment of the individual. It includes all behavior with any sexual connotation, such as body gestures and mannerisms, habits of speech, recreational preferences, and content of dreams. Sexual expression, both homosexual and heterosexual, can be regarded as the result of all influences on the individual, both prenatal and postnatal.

Prenatally, the sequence of events is as follows. First is the establishment of the genetic sex. Second, under the control of the genetic sex the gonads differentiate, determining the hormonal environment of the embryo, the differentiation of internal duct systems, and the formation of the external genitalia. Recently, it has become apparent that the embryonic brain is also sexually differentiated, probably via a control mechanism very similar to that which determines the sexual development of the external genitalia. The inductive influences of hormones on the central nervous system may have an effect on the patterns of hormone secretion and sexual behavior in the adult.

Gonadal Differentiation

The genital system arises in human embryos during the 5th and 6th weeks of pregnancy. The complete differentiation of normal gonads depends upon the arrival at the genital ridges of the dorsal mesentery of sufficient numbers of viable primordial germ cells. The germ cells arise extragonadally, and therefore must migrate into the sites of gonadal differentiation. If they fail to arrive, gonads do not develop. The germ cells are enveloped in the primitive gonad by cells which in the female are future granulosa cells, and in the male, Sertoli cells. At this stage the gonad is said to be bipotential; it may become either a testicle or an ovary. This period of sexual neutrality in human embryos is important in understanding the variety of sexual anomalies.

The primitive gonads consist of cortical and medullary areas. The medulla is a potential testis, while cortical development and degeneration of the medulla are required to make an ovary. Differentiation into a testicle depends upon the active influence of the Y chromosome. The Y chromosome induces medullary development and regression of the cortical zone in a process mediated by an antigen which appears to occur on the surface of all male cells. This antigen is known as Y-induced histocompatibility antigen, H-Y antigen for short. White blood cells can be tested for the presence of H-Y antigen, (H-Y assay), a reliable indicator for the presence of testicular tissue. In the absence of a Y chromosome, the cortical zone develops and contains the germ cells, while the medullary portion regresses with its remnant being the rete ovarii, a compressed nest of tubules and Leydig cells in the hilus of the ovary. The formation of the testicle precedes any other sexual development in time, and

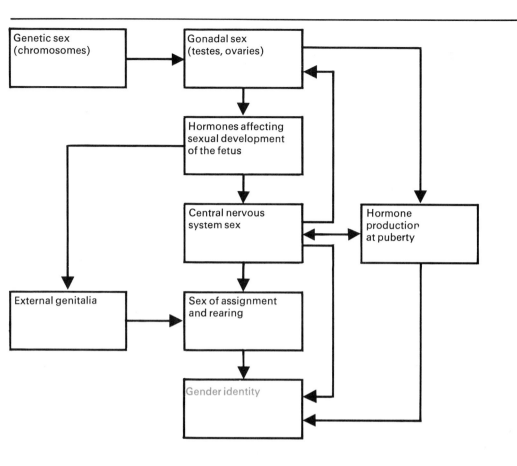

therefore the testes may control subsequent sexual development.

In an XX individual, without the active influence of a Y chromosome, the bipotential gonad develops into an ovary, about two weeks later than testicular development. In early fetal life, the female germ cells proliferate by mitosis, reaching a peak of 5–7 million at about 20 weeks of pregnancy. Degeneration (atresia) begins even earlier, and by birth approximately 1 million germ cells remain. These have become surrounded by a layer of follicular cells, forming primordial follicles with oocytes which have entered the first meiotic division. Meiosis is arrested in the prophase of the first meiotic division until reactivation of follicular growth which may not occur until years later.

Duct System Differentiation	The Wolffian and Müllerian ducts are discrete primordia which temporarily coexist in all embryos during the ambisexual period of development. One type of duct system persists normally and gives rise to special ducts and glands, whereas the other disappears during the 3rd fetal month, except for unimportant vestiges. The urogenital sinus and genital tubercle are neutral primordia which develop into either male or female structures depending upon whether the gonads develop into a testis or an ovary.

The elaboration of androgens by the medullary cells (forerunners of the Leydig cells) in the early testicle stimulates development of the Wolffian duct system into epididymis, vas deferens, and seminal vesicles. Another substance, yet unidentified (known as Müllerian Inhibiting Factor, MIF), is responsible for regression of the Müllerian duct system in the male. This influence from the fetal testis is unilateral. Duct system differentiation will proceed, therefore, according to the nature of the adjacent gonad.

In the absence of a Y chromosome, the lack of MIF allows the Müllerian duct system to develop into Fallopian tubes, uterus, and upper vagina, while in the absence of testosterone the Wolffian system regresses. Thus, in the presence of a normal ovary, or in the absence of any gonad, the Müllerian duct system will develop.

External Genitalia Differentiation	In the bipotential stage (8th fetal week), the external genitalia consist of a urogenital sinus, two lateral labioscrotal swellings, and a genital tubercle. Differentiation is under the active influence of androgen. In the presence of a Y chromosome and androgen production, the genital tubercle forms the penis, the labioscrotal folds fuse to form a scrotum, while the folds of the urogenital sinus form the urethra.

In the absence of a Y chromosome (in the presence of an ovary or in the absence of a gonad), the folds of the urogenital sinus remain open, forming the labia minora, the labioscrotal folds form the labia majora, and the genital tubercle forms the clitoris. The urogenital sinus differentiates into the vagina and the urethra; thus the lower vagina is formed as part of the external genitalia.

Exposure to androgens at this critical time period (about the 7th week of pregnancy) will masculinize a female, i.e. the phenotype will be masculinized regardless of the internal genitalia. An inadequate amount of androgens in a male will lead to incomplete masculinization.

234

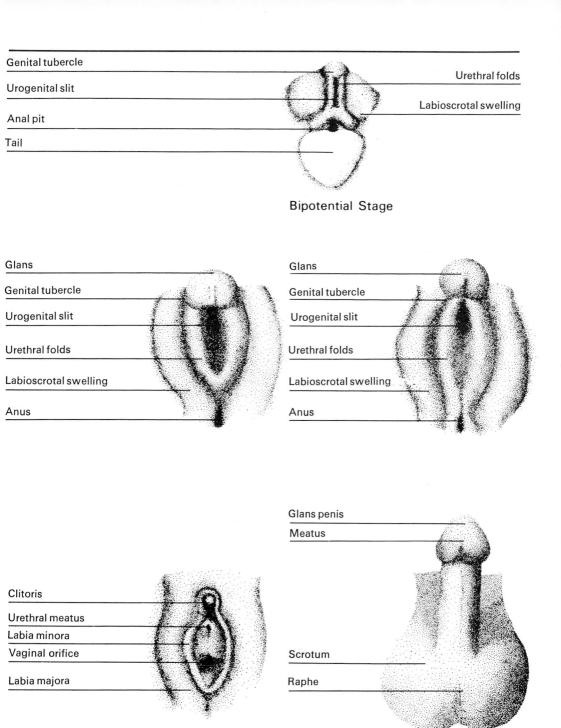

Genital tubercle

Urogenital slit

Anal pit

Tail

Urethral folds

Labioscrotal swelling

Bipotential Stage

Glans

Genital tubercle

Urogenital slit

Urethral folds

Labioscrotal swelling

Anus

Glans

Genital tubercle

Urogenital slit

Urethral folds

Labioscrotal swelling

Anus

Clitoris

Urethral meatus

Labia minora

Vaginal orifice

Labia majora

Glans penis

Meatus

Scrotum

Raphe

| Central Nervous System Differentiation | At the same time the presence or absence of androgens is playing a critical role in genitalia development, the neuroendocrine mechanism of the central nervous system is also being influenced. Androgens present in sufficient amounts during the appropriate critical stage of development may program the CNS to be masculine. Recent experimental and analytic evidence suggests that a behavioral effect may be traced to this early androgen influence. Inappropriate fetal hormonal programming may contribute, therefore, to the spectrum of psychosexual behavior seen in humans. |

Abnormal sexual Differentiation

Masculinized Females (Female Pseudo-hermaphrodites)

Masculinized females are female by genetic sex (XX) and possess ovaries, but the external genitalia are not those of a normal female. Of all infants with ambiguous genitalia, 40–50% have adrenal hyperplasia.

The Adrenogenital Syndrome. The adrenogenital syndrome in females is characterized by masculinized external genitalia, and diagnosed by demonstrating hyperfunction of the adrenal cortex with excessive androgen production, due either to tumor or hyperplasia. The syndrome may appear at birth or develop postnatally. If present at birth, it is invariably due to virilizing adrenal hyperplasia, while if first noted in an older child it is usually due to an adrenal tumor.

The presence of excessive androgens is manifested by varying degrees of fusion of the labioscrotal folds, clitoral enlargement, and anatomical changes of the urethra and vagina. Generally the urethra and vagina share a urogenital sinus formed by the fusion of labial folds. This sinus opens at the base of the clitoris which is usually enlarged. The degree of urogenital sinus deformity is related to the timing in prenatal development of the onset of masculinizing androgen effect. The size of the clitoris depends on the quantity of androgen. Cases of incorrect sex assignment in the female are due to the similarity between these external genitalia and hypospadias and bilateral cryptorchidism in a male infant.

If untreated, the female with adrenal hyperplasia will develop signs of progressive virilization. Pubic hair will appear by age 2–4, followed by axillary hair, then body hair and beard. Bone age is advanced by age 2, and because of early epiphyseal closure, height in childhood is achieved at the expense of shortened stature in adulthood. Progressive masculinization continues with the development of the male habitus, acne, deepened voice, and primary amenorrhea and infertility.

In addition to sexual changes, patients may present with metabolic disorders such as salt-wasting, hypertension, or rarely, hypoglycemia. An electrolyte imbalance of the salt-losing type is usually apparent within a few days of birth and occurs in approximately one-third of patients with virilizing adrenal hyperplasia. Beginning with a refusal to feed, failure to thrive, apathy, and vomiting, the infant goes on to an Addisonian-like crisis with hyponatremia, hyperkalemia, and acidosis. Rapid diagnosis and treatment are necessary to save these infants. Less frequent are cases with hypertension, which occurs in approximately 5% of patients with virilizing adrenal hyperplasia.

Virilizing adrenal hyperplasia is the result of an inherited abnormality of steroid biosynthesis which results in an inability to synthesize glucocorticoids. The hypothalamic-pituitary axis responds to the low level of cortisol by elevated ACTH secretion in an effort to achieve normal levels of cortisol production. This stimulation causes a hyperplastic adrenal cortex which produces androgens as well as corticoid precursors in abnormal quantities.

Therefore, one can see a well-compensated infant who has achieved normal cortisol levels, but at the expense of extensive masculinization.

Elevated levels of pregnanetriol excretion, the chief urinary metabolite of 17α-hydroxyprogesterone, suggest that an enzymatic defect of 21-hydroxylation is present, and it is this "simple" type that is the most common form of the syndrome. The hypertensive form is due to a deficiency of 11β-hydroxylase, leading to an accumulation of deoxycorticosterone, a salt-retaining mineralocorticoid. The salt-losing type is in all likelihood related to the severity of the enzyme block (probably a greater block in 21-hydroxylase with diminished ability to produce mineralocorticoids). In the 3β-dehydrogenase deficiency pregnanetriol will be absent and 17-ketosteroids will consist mainly of dehydroepiandrosterone (DHA). These infants are severely ill, and usually do not live. 17-Hydroxylase deficiencies are associated with similar blocks in the gonad, hence a failure of secondary sexual development is the problem, not abnormal genitalia at birth. Rarely, 20, 22 hydroxylation deficiency occurs with a total block in adrenal steroid production, and death occurs.

Genetic Aspects. The genetic defect in virilizing adrenal hyperplasia is an autosomal recessive gene. Within families the clinical picture is uniform, the type of syndrome (simple, salt-losing, hypertensive) is always the same in affected siblings. The ratio in offspring of unaffected parents is 1 affected to 3 nonaffected individuals. Treated patients have a 1:100 to 1:200 chance of producing an affected infant. Heterozygous carriers cannot be detected.

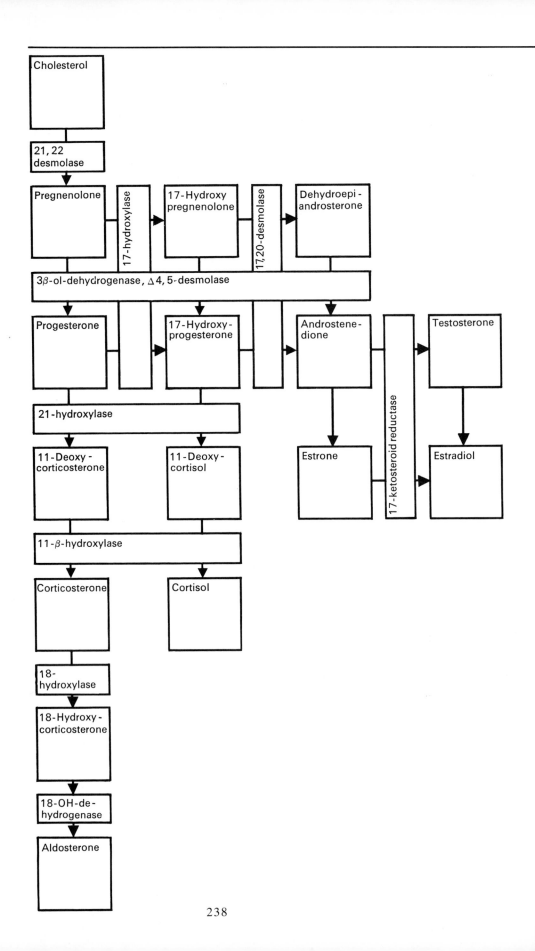

238

Diagnosis. Since the genetic sex is XX, the sex chromatin will be positive. The demonstration of a metabolic defect depends upon the study of urinary 17-ketosteroid excretion. The table shows the normal and abnormal values of 17-ketosteroids. Notice that in the first few days of life the excretion of 17-ketosteroids is normally slightly higher, however pregnanetriol excretion is not elevated.

Urinary 17-ketosteroid Excretion
mg per 24 hours

Age	Normal Values	Values in Virilizing Adrenal Hyperplasia
1–10 days	0.5–5.0	
2–3 weeks	0.5–1.0	2–6
1–6 months	0.5	1–10
7–12 months	0.5	3–10
1–5 years	1.0	4–30
6–9 years	2.0	11–40
10–15 years	7±3	16–50
over 15 years	10±3	21–80

Further study of the urine will reveal abnormal levels of pregnanetriol with 21 and 11β-hydroxylase blocks, elevated levels of tetrahydro-S and deoxycorticosterone (DOC) in the hypertensive type (11β-hydroxylase block), and elevated levels of DHA in the 3β-dehydrogenase defect. Total excretion of 17-ketosteroids may not be impressively elevated with the 3β-dehydrogenase block.

In recent years, radioimmunoassays of blood progesterone and 17-hydroxyprogesterone have proved useful in the diagnosis and management of congenital adrenal hyperplasia. With the 21 and 11β-hydroxylase blocks, the 17-hydroxyprogesterone level may be 50 to 400-fold above normal and progesterone may be 2 to 50 times normal (normal for both is less than 1 ng/ml). (1) In the first few days of life when urinary 17-ketosteroids are normally elevated, measuring these steroids in the blood may afford a more accurate diagnosis. The blood level of dehydroepiandrosterone sulfate (DS) correlates well with adrenal activity and may eventually replace the use of 17-ketosteroid measurements. (2)

Treatment. Treatment of virilizing adrenal hyperplasia is to supply the deficient hormone, cortisol. This decreases ACTH secretion and lowers production of androgenic precursors. Dosage is adjusted by maintaining the 17-ketosteroid excretion in the normal range. Single random blood samples for progesterone and 17-hydroxyprogesterone are not adequate to judge good control. (1) The additional use of a salt-retaining steroid is usually necessary in the salt-losing type, although it may eventually be discontinued. With major stress, however, the salt-retaining steroid may be needed again. Minor stresses will cause brief elevations of 17-ketosteroids, but usually do not require readjustment of dosage.

The surgical treatment of the anatomical abnormalities (see Jones and Scott) should be carried out in the first few years of life, when the patient is still too young to remember the procedure and too young to have developed psychological problems centered about the abnormal external genitalia. If clitoridectomy is necessary, it is important to know that women who undergo total clitoral amputations have no subsequent impairment of erotic responsiveness or capacity for orgasm.

With replacement therapy of the cortisol deficiency, normal reproduction is possible. Many cases come to cesarean section because normal anatomy of the perineum may be obscured by scar tissue from earlier plastic surgery; therefore greater blood loss and the risk of a hematoma with a vaginal delivery are significant factors. A masculine pelvis is not expected since the adult form and size of the inlet of the pelvis are assumed largely during the growth spurt in puberty. However, a small pelvis might be anticipated if the bone age is up to age 13–14 when treatment is initiated.

The maintenance steroid dose usually does not need to be changed during pregnancy. Urinary 17-ketosteroids do not alter appreciably during pregnancy, and may be used for monitoring the patient. The dosage of steroids used in the treatment of this syndrome is replacing the approximate amount normally produced, and therefore is a physiologic dose. At these low doses, teratogenic effects would be unlikely, and none have been noted.

The need for additional steroids during the stress of labor and delivery is obvious, and is usually met by the administration of cortisone acetate intramuscularly and cortisol intravenously. Wound healing and infection have not been problems. Aside from the liability associated with genetic transmission of this syndrome, the children born to patients with adrenal hyperplasia have been normal. The newborn should be closely observed for adrenal insufficiency due to steroid crossover and suppression of the fetal adrenal *in utero*.

Masculinization Due to Elevated Androgens in Maternal Circulation. Masculinization of the female fetus, while in most cases due to fetal virilizing adrenal hyperplasia, may be produced by an androgen-secreting maternal tumor, or may be due to the intake of exogenous androgenic substances. When not caused by an error in the metabolism of the fetal adrenal gland, virilization is not progressive, urinary 17-ketosteroids are not elevated, and no hormonal therapy is needed. Subsequent development will be normal. Therefore, surgical correction of abnormalities in the external genitalia is the only indicated treatment.

The occurrence of an androgen-secreting tumor in a mother during pregnancy is rarely seen. On the other hand, the iatrogenic cause of masculinization is a well-known story. The majority of these cases resulted from antenatal maternal treatment of threatened or recurrent abortion with various progestin compounds. In view of the lack of evidence for positive accomplishment with such therapy, the use of progestin compounds in pregnancy is contraindicated.

Incompletely
Masculinized
Males
(Male Pseudo-
hermaphrodites)

Incompletely masculinized males are male by genetic sex (XY) and possess testicles, but the external genitalia are not normally male. Male pseudohermaphrodites may arise in one of three ways:

1. An insensitivity to androgen,

2. Abnormal androgen synthesis,

3. Absent or defective Müllerian Inhibiting Factor.

Syndromes of Androgen Insensitivity.
Complete Androgen Insensitivity—Testicular Feminization. The phenotype of this condition (also discussed in Chapter 5) is female because there is a congenital insensitivity to androgens, transmitted by means of a maternal X-linked recessive gene responsible for the androgen intracellular receptor. (3) Therefore, androgen induction of Wolffian duct development does not occur. However, MIF activity is present, and the individual does not have Müllerian development (a natural experiment which indicates the presence of a Müllerian Inhibiting Factor). The vagina is short (derived from the urogenital sinus only) and ends blindly. The uterus and tubes are absent. There is no problem of sex assignment as there is no trace of androgen activity.

The "complete" form indicates that there is no androgen response, therefore, normal external female development occurs, and these infants should be reared as females. The gonads may be present in the inguinal canals, and children with inguinal hernias and/or inguinal masses should be suspected of testicular feminization. Because

241

of the lack of androgen response there is no virilization at puberty. In contrast to dysgenetic gonads with a Y chromosome, the occurrence of gonadal tumors is relatively late. (4, 5) Therefore gonadectomy should be performed at approximately age 16 to 18, to allow endogenous hormonal changes and a smooth transition through puberty.

Future apparent sisters of affected individuals have a 1 in 3 chance of being XY; female offspring of a normal sister of an affected individual have a 1 in 6 chance of being XY.

Incomplete Androgen Insensitivity. All incomplete forms may be divided into two categories: Type 1, due to an X-linked recessive trait; and Type 2, due to an autosomal recessive trait. (6, 7)

Type 1

This is a spectrum of disorders known as the incomplete form of testicular feminization. The clinical presentation ranges from almost complete failure of virilization to essentially complete masculinization. (6) Toward the feminine end of the spectrum is the Lubs syndrome, while toward the masculine end is the Reifenstein syndrome. The various syndromes represent variable manifestations of the same mutant gene. This single gene inheritance is compatible with the evidence that the single biochemical abnormality lies in the degree of function of the androgen receptor. (3)

Sex assignment may be a problem where there is a partial response to androgen and ambiguous genitalia occur. If sex assignment is female, early gonadectomy is necessary to avoid virilization and neoplasia. In the Reifenstein syndrome, the phallus is usually large enough to allow male sex assignment at birth, but there is a severe perineal hypospadias. After puberty, hypogonadism is evident and feminization occurs with gynecomastia. The minimal testicular androgen deficit early in life becomes more severe, and these men are infertile. The karyotype is normal male distinguishing this syndrome from other feminizing syndromes at puberty, e.g. Klinefelter's. Androgen therapy is necessary and effective.

Type 2

This form of familial incomplete male pseudohermaphroditism is due to an autosomal recessive trait and is characterized by severe hypospadias and underdevelopment of the vagina. (7) This condition has been known as pseudovaginal perineoscrotal hypospadias (PPH). It differs from incomplete androgen insensitivity (Type 1) because at puberty, masculinization occurs with normal testicular endocrine function, and there is no evidence of lack of response to androgens. At birth, however, appearance is similar to incomplete testicular feminization with hypospadias, varying failure of fusion of labioscrotal folds, and a urogenital opening or separate urethral and vaginal openings. The cleft in the scrotum appears to be a vagina, and these patients have been reared as girls with an enlarged clitoris. At birth, steroid excretion is normal, which rules out adrenal disorders. The karyotype is XY, and as with the other incompletely masculinized males, the sex of assignment is female if the phallus is inadequate. Gonadectomy is necessary if the infant is to be reared as a girl.

Recent study of this condition has revealed that the Wolffian duct virilizes in a normal male fashion, but the urogenital sinus and urogenital tubercle differentiate as female structures. (7) The failure is due to inadequate dihydrotestosterone formation in the urogenital sinus and urogenital tubercle at the time of virilization of the embryo. Seminal vesicles, ejaculatory ducts, epididymides, and vas deferentia are all present. The contrast between Type 1 and Type 2 incomplete male pseudohermaphrodites supports the contention that testosterone is the intracellular mediator for differentiation of the Wolffian duct, while dihydrotestosterone is the intracellular mediator necessary for virilization of the external genitalia, urethra, and prostate. Thus Type 2 or PPH is due to an autosomal recessive mutation responsible for a failure of DHT formation (absent 5α-reductase) in the urogenital sinus and tubercle at the time of sexual differentiation.

Abnormal Androgen Synthesis. Defects in testosterone synthesis can be at any one of the 5 required enzymatic reactions which lead from cholesterol to testosterone: 21, 22 desmolase; 3β-ol-dehydrogenase; 17α-hydroxylase, 17, 20 desmolase; and 17-ketosteroid reductase. These defects are inherited as autosomal recessive traits, and the phenotypes range from partial to complete male pseudohermaphroditism.

Patients with male pseudohermaphroditism who are considered variants of testicular feminization upon partial virilization at puberty may actually have a defect in androgen synthesis. The diagnosis is made by demonstrating elevated 17-ketosteroids, and elevated blood levels of androstenedione and estrogens, while the blood level of testosterone is low or low-normal. (8) When the enzyme involves a reaction which is active in the adrenal gland (all but the 17-ketosteroid reductase) the adrenal blocks are usually severe with adrenal failure and death in the newborn period.

The male pseudohermaphrodite due to deficient testicular 17-ketosteroid reductase activity has male internal genitalia and no Müllerian structures. However, masculinization is incomplete. These subjects may develop gynecomastia at puberty due to elevated estrogen levels arising from peripheral conversion of the increased androstenedione. Early gonadectomy is required to avoid virilization at puberty and testicular neoplasia.

243

Abnormal Müllerian Inhibiting Factor *Hernia Uterine Inguinale (Uterine Hernia Syndrome)*. Individuals with this syndrome appear to be normal males but relatively well-differentiated Müllerian duct structures are also found, usually as a uterus and tubes in an inguinal hernia sac. This is apparently an isolated failure of MIF and Müllerian regression, inherited as a recessive trait, either X-linked or autosomal. Fertility is usually preserved.

Bilateral Dysgenetic Testes (Swyer Syndrome). Affected individuals have an XY chromosomal component but normal female external and internal genitalia. There are streak gonads, and thus primary amenorrhea and lack of sexual development result. Virilization may occur on occasion due to androgen production in the gonads. These gonads have the potential for undergoing neoplastic change.

The pathogenesis of this condition in view of a normal XY sex chromosome complement must be early testicular degeneration which is usually total but may be incomplete. Therefore, usually androgen stimulation and Müllerian inhibition are both lost. Extragenital anomalies such as in Turner's syndrome are not found. The presence of a normal vagina, uterus, and tubes easily differentiates this syndrome from the variants of testicular feminization. However, Müllerian development may be rudimentary if testicular function was not lost early. The risk of gonadal neoplasm appears to be greater than in testicular feminization, therefore gonadectomy should be performed prior to puberty to avoid both neoplasia and unwanted virilization.

Anorchia. Affected individuals lack internal genitalia and may or may not have a vagina. Thus early testicular function must have occurred, enough to inhibit Müllerian development. Sex of assignment depends on the extent of external genitalia development. It is thought that the testicles degenerate and resorb, hence this syndrome is sometimes known as the vanishing testes syndrome.

True
Hermaphrodites

A true hermaphrodite possesses both ovarian and testicular tissue. Both types of tissue may be combined in one gonad, an ovotestis, or there may be an ovary on one side and a testicle on the other. The internal structures correspond to the adjacent gonad. The majority of cases have ambiguous external genitalia. Half are genetic females (XX), a few are males (XY), and the rest are mosaics with at least one cell line of XX.

244

Gonadal Dysgenesis	Gonadal dysgenesis due to the presence of only one X chromosome in all cell lines (X chromosome monosomy) is Turner's syndrome. The individual is 45,X or as written in the past, XO. In the absence of gonadal development, the individuals are phenotypic females. The well-known characteristics are short stature (48–58 inches), sexual infantilism, and streak gonads. The streak gonad is composed of fibrous tissue, containing no ova or follicular derivatives. Other congenital problems in this syndrome are: a webbed neck, coarctation of the aorta, a high arched palate, cubitus valgus, a broad shield-like chest with widely spaced nipples, a low hairline on the neck, short fourth metacarpal bones, and renal abnormalities. Usually the diagnosis is not made until puberty when amenorrhea and lack of sexual development become apparent. However, at birth, lymphedema of the extremities may indicate the condition. About 98% of conceptuses with only one X chromosome abort. The remaining 2% account for an incidence of 45,X in about 1 in 2,500 liveborn girls.

A large variety of mosaic patterns is seen with gonadal dysgenesis. From analysis of the various combinations, it is apparent that short stature is related to loss of the short arm of one X chromosome. Thus X, XXp-, and XXqi are all short. Xqi designates an isochromosome for the long arms, and Xp-, deletion of the short arm. The loss of the long arm of one of the X chromosomes (XXq-) is associated with amenorrhea and streak gonads, but the patients are not short and do not have the other malformations. Thus, loss of material from the short arms of the X chromosome leads to short stature and the other stigmata of Turner's syndrome. Streak gonads result if any part of an X chromosome is missing. This suggests that normal ovarian development requires two loci, one on the long arm and one on the short arm; loss of either results in gonadal failure.

Thyroid autoimmunity is common in Turner's syndrome, but Hashimoto's thyroiditis may be specific to the 46, XXqi cases.

Menstrual function and reproduction in a patient with Turner's phenotype must be due to a mosaic complement, such as a 46,XX line in addition to 45,X. Multiple X females (47,XXX) have normal development and reproductive function, although mental retardation may be more frequent. Secondary amenorrhea and/or eunuchoidism may be seen.

Mixed Gonadal Dysgenesis	In gonadal dysgenesis, the gonadal structures are streak gonads. In mixed gonadal dysgenesis, testicular tissue may be present on one side and a streak gonad on the other. Mosaicism is the likely underlying abnormality, even if it is not detected in the cell line studied. Regardless of apparent karyotype, the existence of the H-Y antigen

245

(e.g. on white blood cells) may be a clue to the presenc of hidden testicular tissue. Ambiguous genitalia are prc duced if testicular tissue is functional. In this instanc gonadectomy will be necessary if sex assignment is female Furthermore, gonadectomy is also necessary if sex assign ment is male to avoid neoplastic change, which ma occur prior to puberty.

Noonan's Syndrome

Both affected males and females have apparently norma chromosome complements and normal gonadal function The phenotypic appearance of the female is that of patient with Turner's syndrome: short stature, webbe neck, shield chest, and cardiac malformations. The car diac lesions, however, are different. Pulmonic stenosis i most frequent in Noonan's syndrome as opposed to aorti coarctation in Turner's. Apparently this syndrome result from a mutant gene or genes (9). In the past these patients have been referred to as male Turner's o Turner's with normal chromosomes.

Adrenal Hyperplasia with 17-Hydroxylase Deficiency

The clinical triad associated with 17-hydroxylase defi ciency is amenorrhea, hypertension, and hypokalemi alkalosis. Thus this enzyme defect occurs in the ovary a well as the adrenal. The patient is unable to mak estrogen, and secondary sexual characteristics do no develop. In addition, the patient will be infertile an require estrogen replacement. Deoxycorticosterone an corticosterone are produced in excess, since they do no require 17-hydroxylation, and this leads to hypertensio and hypokalemia. Treatment as with other adrenal en zyme deficiencies, is with replacement of cortisol.

Diagnosis of Ambiguous Genitalia

Ambiguous external genitalia in a newborn infant repre sents a major diagnostic challenge. The physician ma find himself in a pressure-filled situation because of th necessity for making such an influential decision as th sex of rearing. Diagnostic procedures, however, ma delay the decision, and it is well-recognized that a perio of delay is far better than later reversal of the se assignment. Parental education and guidance are essentia in this anxiety-ridden situation.

The most important point to be remembered when con fronted with a newborn infant with ambiguous genitali or an apparently male infant with bilateral cryptorchidism is that the prime diagnosis until ruled out is congenita adrenal hyperplasia. The reason is clear: adrenal hyper plasia is the only condition which is life-threatening. Sign of adrenal failure such as vomiting, diarrhea, dehydration and shock may develop rapidly.

246

The history of a previously affected relative may aid in the diagnosis of testicular feminization or any of its variants. Similarly, the history of a sibling with genital ambiguity or the history of a previous neonatal death in a sibling strongly suggest the possibility of adrenal hyperplasia. A history of maternal exposure to androgenic compounds may be difficult to elicit. The mother may be unaware of the nature of her medications and the obstetrician should be consulted.

Palpation of the genital and inguinal regions is the most important part of the physical examination. Careful examination of the phallus may differentiate between a clitoris and a penis. The penis has a midline ventral frenulum, while the clitoris has two folds which extend from the lateral aspects of the clitoris to the labia minora. The position of the urethral meatus may range from a mild hypospadias to an opening in the perineal area into a urogenital sinus.

Ovaries are rarely found in scrotal folds or in the inguinal regions. Therefore, palpable masses in these locations usually represent testicles. However, the testicles may be intra-abdominal. If testicles are not palpable, the infant should be considered to have virilizing adrenal hyperplasia until demonstrated otherwise. A uterus may be palpable on rectal examination, especially shortly after birth when the uterus is a little enlarged in response to maternal estrogen.

The buccal smear for the sex chromatin pattern along with serum electrolytes and urinary 17-ketosteroids should be ordered immediately in all newborns with ambiguous genitalia. The Lyon hypothesis states that in females one of the two normal X chromosomes is functionally inactive in all somatic cells. This inactivation occurs at an early embryonic age, is irreversible, and is random and independent. Thus the normal female is a mosaic made of two cell populations, one consisting of cells in which the X chromosome inherited from the mother is active, and the other in which the paternal X is active. During interphase the inactive X is detected as the nuclear chromatin or Barr body. In the normal female, the percentage of buccal smear cells which contain a sex chromatin mass should be greater than 20%. The sex chromatin percentage may be low in normal females until the 3rd day of life.

Because both masculinized females and incompletely masculinized males may result from enzyme blocks in the adrenal, urinary 17-ketosteroids are necesary regardless of the sex chromatin pattern. In 3β-dehydrogenase and 17-hydroxylase enzyme blocks, the urinary pregnanetriol will not be elevated. 21-Hydroxylase and 11-β-hydroxylase blocks will be associated with pregnanetriol excretion of 2 or more mg/24 hours (in some laboratories, up to 4 mg is normal). The 17-ketosteroids may not be impres-

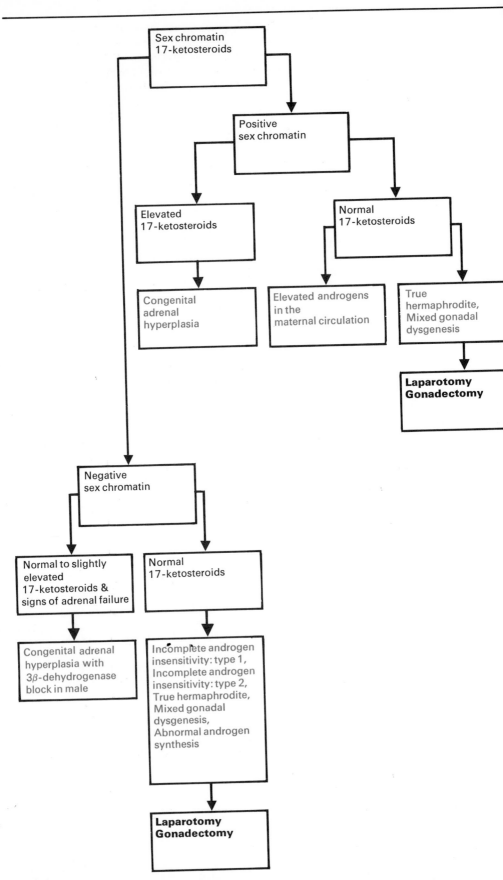

sively increased with a 3β-dehydrogenase block. *Clinical signs of adrenal failure indicate that the newborn has adrenal hyperplasia regardless of the urinary steroid excretion pattern.* If such an infant is hyperkalemic and hyponatremic, the diagnosis is certain.

Endoscopy and special x-ray studies are not necessary for assigning sex; however, the information gained will be helpful in delineating the exact structures and abnormalities present.

Although laparotomy is not necessary for assignment of sex, it may be the only way to arrive at a definitive diagnosis. Laparotomy is indicated in the following situations (Laparoscopic evaluation is inadequate because gonads may be small and hidden in the inguinal canal):

1. The sex chromatin-positive infant with ambiguous genitalia, normal 17-ketosteroid excretion, in apparent good health, and no history of maternal androgen exposure. This is either a true hermaphrodite or a variant of mixed gonadal dysgenesis and gonadectomy is indicated.

2. The sex chromatin-negative patient with ambiguous genitalia, without palpable gonads, and normal 17-ketosteroid excretion. The possibilities are incompletely masculinized males (variants of testicular feminization), a true hermaphrodite, mixed gonadal dysgenesis, and PPH. Sex of rearing will be female and gonadectomy is necessary to avoid virilization at puberty and the propensity to develop gonadal neoplasia.

    Chromosome analysis is not necessary for the assignment of sex, and indeed, requires too much time. For the purposes of documentation, a karyotype is indicated except in patients with adrenal hyperplasia.

In a newborn who presents a problem of correct sex assignment, it is better to delay than to reverse the sex assignment at a later date. Generally the decision can be made within a few days, at most a few weeks. In dealing with the parents, terms with unfortunate connotations, such as hermaphrodite, should be avoided. An easy way to explain ambiguous genital development to parents is to indicate that the genitals are unfinished, rather than abnormal from a sexual point of view. Chromosome discrepancies are probably best left unmentioned.

The future fertility in all masculinized females is unaffected. With proper treatment, reproduction is possible, since the internal genitalia and gonads are those of a normal female. Therefore, all masculinized females should be reared as females.

ssignment
Sex of
earing

The only other category of patients with ambiguous genitalia with reproductive capability consists of males with (1) isolated hypospadias; (2) the male with repaired isolated cryptorchidism; and (3) the male with the uterine hernia syndrome.

All other patients with ambiguous genitalia will be sterile. Except for salt-losing adrenal hyperplasia, the physician's prime concern is not with physical survival, but to enable the patient to grow into a psychologically normal, healthy, and well-adjusted adult. The sex of assignment depends upon only one judgement: whether the phallus can ultimately develop into a penis adequate for intercourse. The success of a penis is dependent upon erectile tissue, and the genitalia should not only be serviceable, but also erotically sensitive. Technically, the construction of female genitalia is easier, and therefore, the physician must be convinced that a functional penis is possible.

All decisions regarding sex of rearing and the overall treatment program should be made early in life. If a case has been neglected, sex reassignments must be made according to the gender identity in which a child has developed. Reassignment of sex can probably be safely made up to age 18 months.

It is recommended that older individuals requesting sexual changes be referred to research-oriented clinical programs established in univerity medical centers.

References

1. **Lippe, BM, LaFranchi, SH, Lavin, N, Parlow, A, Coyotupa, J, and Kaplan, SA,** Serum 17α-hydroxyprogesterone, Progesterone, Estradiol, and Testosterone in the Diagnosis and Management of Congenital Adrenal Hyperplasia, J Pediatrics 85:782, 1974.

2. **Korth-Schutz, S, Levine, LS, and New, MI,** Dehydroepiandrosterone Sulfate (DS) Levels, A Rapid Test for Abnormal Adrenal Androgen Secretion, J Clin Endocrinol Metab 42:1005, 1976.

3. **Meyer, WJ, Migeon, BR, and Migeon, CJ,** Locus on Human X Chromosome for Dihydrotestosterone Receptor and Androgen Insensitivity, Proc Nat Acad Sci 72:1469, 1975.

4. **Manuel, M, Katayama, KP, and Jones, HW, Jr.,** The Age of Occurrence of Gonadal Tumors in Intersex Patients With a Y Chromosome, Am J Obstet Gynec 124:293, 1976.

5. **Morris, J, McL,** Gonadal Anomalies and Dysgenesis in Behrman, SJ, and Kistner, RW, eds, *Progress in Infertility*, Little Brown and Co., Boston, 1975, pp. 265–279.

6. **Wilson, JD, Harrod, MJ, Goldstein, JL, Hemsell, DL, and MacDonald, PC,** Familial Incomplete Male Pseudohermaphroditism, Type 1, New Eng J Med 290:1097, 1974.

7. **Walsh, PC, Madden, JD, Harrod, MJ, Goldstein, JL, MacDonald, PC, and Wilson, JD,** Familial Incomplete Male Pseudohermaphroditism, Type 2, New Eng J Med 291:944, 1974.

8. **Givens, JR, Wiser, WL, Summitt, RI, Kerber, IJ, Anderson, RN, Pittaway, DE, and Fish, SA,** Familial Male Pseudohermaphroditism Without Gynecomastia Due to Deficient Testicular 17-Ketosteroid Reductase Activity, New Eng J Med 291:938, 1974.

9. **Summit, RL,** Turner's Syndrome and Noonan's Syndrome, J Pediat 74:155, 1969.

Especially recommended

Jones, HW, Jr., and Scott, WW, *Hermaphroditism, Genital Anomalies, and Related Endocrine Disorders*, Williams and Wilkins, Baltimore, 1971.

2 Abnormal Puberty and Growth Problems

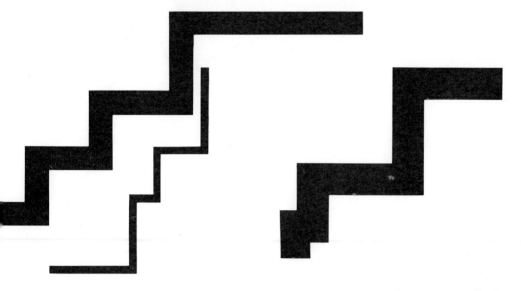

The mechanism of puberty, as outlined in Chapter 2, Neuroendocrinology, is presumably a changing sensitivity of the hypothalamic centers to gonadal steroids. This results in a gradual increasing level of gonadotropin and steroid production until adult levels are reached. *The purpose of this chapter is to discuss abnormalities of this process which produce accelerated or retarded sexual maturation, and to consider problems of growth which might be presented to a gynecologist.*

The first sign of puberty is generally an acceleration of growth followed by the appearance of the breast bud; pubic hair generally appears after breast development, although the sequence may be reversed. Axillary hair appears about 2 years after the beginning of pubic hair growth; however, in a few children axillary hair may be the first to appear. Menarche is a late event, occurring after the peak of the height spurt has been passed.

The growth of pubic and axillary hair is due to an increased production of adrenal androgens at puberty. Thus, this phase of puberty is often referred to as adrenarche or pubarche. Premature pubarche by itself is occasionally seen, i.e. pubic and axillary hair without any other sign of sexual development. Premature thelarche (breast development) without any other signs of puberty is very rare, but does occur, and it may be due to prolactin secretion, since gonadotropins and estrogens are not elevated.

Height Gain in Centimeters

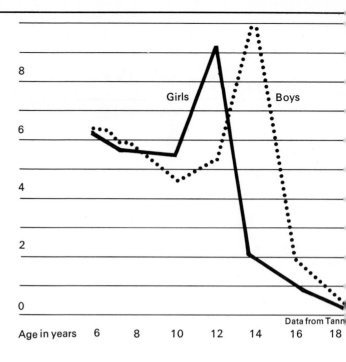

8

6

4

2

0

Age in years   6   8   10   12   14   16   18

Girls   Boys

Data from Tann

The adolescent growth spurt of the typical girl occurs years earlier than that of the boy, but it is less marked For one year or more at adolescence the rate of growth approximately doubles. In the year of peak growth, a girl will grow between 6 and 11 cm. The average middle class British girl reaches her peak of growth at 12 ± 0.9 year (1)

The relationship between menarche and the growth spurt is a relatively fixed sequence, i.e., menarche occurs after the peak growth in height has passed. A good rule of thumb is that the average growth in height after menarche is about 2.5 inches. (2)

The normal range of menarche is from 9.1 to 17.7 years in the United States with a mean of 12.8 years. (3 Because of the extreme variability in onset, there is no particular age or size at which an individual should be expected to experience menarche. Early cycles are usually anovulatory, and therefore, irregular and occasionally heavy. This anovulation usually lasts 12–18 months after menarche. There is a fairly good correlation between the times of menarche of mothers and daughters, and between sisters. (1)

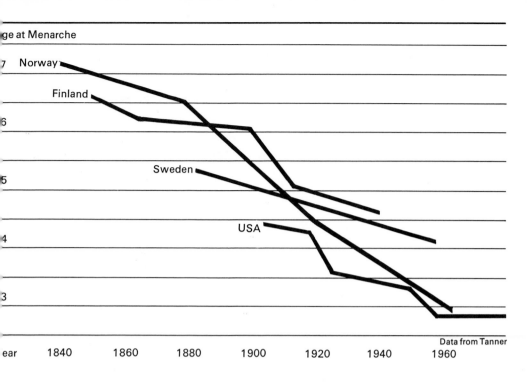

Data from Tanner

In general it can be said that environmental factors are important in the onset of puberty. Children have been maturing progressively earlier in most of the world in the last century, and improved living standards and nutrition in the mother antenatally and in children postnatally have played a significant role in producing taller, heavier children with earlier maturation. Studies of identical twins and non-identical twins show that the age at menarche is chiefly controlled by genetic factors when the environment is optimum. In affluent cultures, the trend toward lowering of the menarcheal age and puberty has now been halted. (3)

Precocious Puberty

Pubertal changes before the age of nine are best regarded as precocious. Increased growth is often the first change in precocious puberty. This is usually followed by breast development and growth of pubic hair. On occasion, simultaneous pubarche, thelarche, and linear growth may occur. Menarche, however, may be the very first sign.

Classically, precocious puberty has been divided into true sexual precocity in which the hormones are secreted by maturing gonads, and precocious pseudopuberty in which maturing normal gonads are *not* the source of the sex steroids. These classifications are of little practical use since the physician is obligated to rule out a serious disease process in the face of precocious development, and the above classification can only be made after full evaluation.

255

Sexual development does *not* require ovulatory capabilit. Evaluation of a patient's possible fertility, for exampl with basal body temperatures or progesterone assays, an unnecessary procedure. More importantly, true sexu precocity with potential fertility and adult levels of gonad otropins does not rule out the possibility of a seriou disease process (e.g. a CNS tumor). While it is true th the most common form of sexual precocity in females idiopathic or constitutional precocity (true sexual precoc ity), this must be a diagnosis by exclusion with prolonge follow-up in an effort to detect slowly developing lesion of the brain, ovary, or adrenal gland.

Diagnosis of Precocious Puberty

A classification of sexual precocity is presented in th table to provide a guide to the possible conditions an their relative incidence encountered in a large series c cases. (4) The cause of precocious development may b immediately suggested by the history and physical exam nation. A familial occurrence renders unlikely a variet of causes, mainly tumors.

Particular attention should be given to the followin possibilities: drug ingestion, cerebral problems such cranial trauma or encephalitis, retarded growth wit symptoms of hypothyroidism, and a pelvic or abdomin mass. A left hand-wrist film (for use with Atlases) shoul be obtained for bone age. Determination of thyroid func tion is indicated, and the urinary excretion of 17-ketc steroids should be measured. An electroencephalograr and brain scan are probably indicated in patients wit premature precocious puberty, even in the face of a no mal overall evaluation, including normal routine sku x-rays. Other procedures should be dictated by the find ings. Virilization, of course, demands a full adrenal eva uation, while further neuroradiologic procedures shoul probably be reserved for patients with demonstrabl intracranial problems.

Precocious Development Due to Stimulation of Gonadotropin Secretion

The signs of constitutional sexual precocity are due t premature maturation of the hypothalamic-pituitary-ova ian axis, resulting in production of gonadotropins and se steroids. This diagnosis should be made only by exclusio and deserves long-term follow-up, as cerebral abno malities may not become apparent until adulthood Despite the precocious sexual development, thes children fortunately resemble children of their ow chronologic age in other parameters. Adult fertility an time of menopause are not affected.

A number of cerebral problems can cause precociou development including abnormal skull development du to rickets. The various tumors include: craniophary gioma, optic glioma, astrocytoma, and suprasellar terat mas—all usually near the hypothalamus. Pineal tumor

Classification of Sexual Precocity	Total numbers of cases of three series		Approximate numbers described in literature	
	Girls	Boys	Girls	Boys
True sexual precocity:				
Cerebral	19	14		
Pineal gland			0	50
Hamartoma			8	22
Neurofibromatosis				6
Cryptogenic, constitutional or idiopathic	114	18		
Hypothyroid sexual precocity			9	2
Polyostotic fibrous dysplasia	5	1		
Gonadotropin-producing tumors:				
Chorionepithelioma			8	3
Hepatoma		1		5
Presacral tumor				3
Precocious pseudopuberty:				
Ovarian tumors (excluding chorionepithelioma)	3		80	
Scrotal tumors		3		30
Congenital virilizing adrenal hyperplasia in boy		31		
Adrenal adenoma	2	2		
Adrenal carcinoma	1	2		
Incomplete sexual precocity:				
Premature adrenarche or pubarche	12	5		
Premature Thelarche	11			
Total	167	77		

for unknown reasons, are associated with precocious puberty only in boys. Nontumorous causes include en cephalitis, meningitis, hydrocephalus, and von Recklinghausen's disease. An injury to the skull may stimulate sexual development. The mechanism is unknown and latent period of 1–2 months is usually seen. A hamartoma is a hyperplastic malformation at the base of the hypothalamus which usually produces precocity in the first few years of life.

Albright's syndrome (polyostotic fibrous dysplasia) consists of multiple disseminated cystic bone lesions which easily fracture, *café au lait* skin areas of various sizes and shapes, and sexual precocity. Premature menarche may be the first sign of the syndrome. The etiology is unknown. Skeletal abnormalities may become evident following the onset of puberty. The combination of multiple bone fractures, *café au lait* patches, and premature development should lead to the diagnosis.

Sexual precocity occurs in a small number of children with long-standing hypothyroidism. While reported cases have been severe and therefore clinically obvious, laboratory evaluation of thyroid function is probably indicated in all cases of sexual precocity.

Precocious
Development
Due to
Availability
of Sex Steroids

Only 1–2% of girls with precocious puberty have an ovarian tumor. The tumor is usually an estrogen-producing neoplasm or cyst. To emphasize again the rarity of this condition, only 5% of granulosa cell tumors and 1% of theca cell tumors occur before puberty. (5) Teratomas, dysgerminomas, and choriocarcinomas may produce gonadotropin which, by its high local concentration, stimulates ovarian hormone production. The production of gonadotropin may be so great that a pregnancy test will be positive. Palpation of a pelvic or abdominal mass demands surgical exploration.

A feminizing adrenal tumor is very rare, and is associated with increased excretion of 17-ketosteroids.

Drug ingestion should be suspected when there is dark pigmentation of the nipples and breast areola, an effect of certain synthetic estrogens such as stilbestrol.

Special Cases of
Precocious
Development

Special cases of precocious development include the isolated appearance of one sexual characteristic: premature adrenarche or pubarche (pubic hair) or premature thelarche (breast development). Sparse hair growth on the vulva does not represent precocious pubarche. Little known about these conditions other than that they are associated with an increased incidence of central nervous system abnormalities, such as mental deficiency. The usual effort should be made to exclude a serious disease process. If the bone age is advanced, treatment is indicated.

Treatment of precocious development when no cause can be found, or when a cause cannot be removed, is limited to the use of a potent progestational agent to inhibit gonadotropin production. The agent of choice is medroxy-progesterone acetate in depot form (Depo-Provera) given in large doses, 400 mg intramuscularly every 3 months.

Pubic hair will not disappear, but further menstruation, breast development, and growth may be inhibited. It is important to inhibit growth until the chronologic age can catch up with the bone age, otherwise the prematurely tall child will be a short adult due to accelerated bone growth and early epiphyseal closure. The response to progestin therapy is not uniformly good. However, it is impossible to determine which child will respond favorably, therefore all children should be treated. The psychologic management of the sexually precocious child is a serious matter deserving of time and attention, and one must be careful to consider the family dynamics and parental attitudes.

Even if the only achievement is inhibition of menses, this is useful. Precocious menses can be a psychologic and a social problem, both of which are easily avoided with the use of progestin therapy. Treatment should be continued until the chronologic age matches the bone age or until age 12. Hand-wrist films should be obtained every 6 months until epiphyseal closure is demonstrated. Breakthrough bleeding can be stopped by the use of an estrogen (e.g. conjugated estrogens 2.5 mg or ethinyl estradiol 20 μg daily for 10 days). Reoccurence of bleeding is unusual.

Delayed Puberty

Since there is such a wide variation in normal development, it is difficult to define the patient with abnormally delayed sexual maturation. Only 1% of all girls will not have had menarche by the age of 18, and complete absence of breast budding by the age of 13 is probably abnormal. However, whenever a patient or parents are concerned enough to seek a physician's advice, some evaluation is indicated.

Delayed puberty is a rare condition in girls, and a genetic problem or hypothalamic-pituitary disorder must be suspected.

Chronic systemic disease or malnutrition must be excluded along with primary CNS-pituitary and ovarian failure. *The latter problems will be detected if the patient is managed according to the program outlined in the chapter on amenorrhea.* A malnourished individual may complete adolescence with fused epiphyses, without achieving a full height potential. This situation is possible because the bone age effects of the sex steroids may be expressed while the suboptimal state of nutrition will inhibit full growth-promoting activity.

Growth Problems in Normal Adolescents

Perhaps the worst thing about an adolescent grow[t] problem is that it makes the individual "different." It [is] probably true that more than anyone else the adolesce[nt] does not like to be different. Therefore, excessive [or] insufficient growth is not a problem to be dismiss[ed] lightly, and psychologic support and reassurance are k[ey] features in the management of such problems. A willing ness to listen to problems, together with an adult-to-adu[lt] attitude, will place the adolescent-physician relationsh[ip] at the proper level of mutual respect.

The basic and essential laboratory procedure is a le[ft] hand-wrist x-ray for bone age. The Bayley-Pinneau Tabl[es] (6) predict future adult height, utilizing the bone age a[nd] present height. To use the tables, one needs a measur[e] ment of height, the patient's age, and an x-ray of the l[eft] hand and wrist for bone age. All of the hand epiphys[es] and those of the distal end of the arm are used [to] determine the skeletal age. The Bayley-Pinneau Tabl[es] begin on page 264.

To estimate a patient's adult height, use the tables [as] follows: Go down the left hand column to the patien[t's] present height, follow this horizontal row to the colum[n] under the bone age which is given by 6-month interva[ls] across the top. The number at the intersection represen[ts] the predicted adult height. If figures do not fall at the [1] inch or 6-month intervals used on the tables, the predict[ed] height can be easily extrapolated.

It is important to use the table suitable for the rate [of] maturing. If the bone age is within 1 year of the chron[ol] ogic age, use the table for average girls; if the bone age [is] accelerated 1 year or more, use the table for accelerat[ed] girls; if the bone age is retarded 1 year or more, use t[he] table for retarded girls.

The tables are for use with bone age films of the ha[nd] and wrist only in conjunction with the Greulich-P[yle] atlas. (7) Use with bone age determined by any oth[er] method is less accurate.

Short Stature

Thorough medical history and physical examination w[ill] eliminate the usual disorders associated with short statur[e:] malnutrition, chronic urinary tract disease, chronic infe[c] tious disease, hypothyroidism, mental illness, panhypo[pi] tuitarism, and gonadal dysgenesis. In the history, t[he] heights and weights of parents, siblings, and relativ[es] should be obtained along with timing of growth in t[he] family, dietary history, daily activities, and sleep habi[ts.] Normal history and examination in an individual with [a] bone age only 1 year behind the chronologic age sugge[sts] a constitutional pattern which does not require treatmen[t.]

Generally, endocrine disease is an uncommon basis for impairment of growth. Congenital hypothyroidism is the most frequent problem of this type, followed by hypopituitarism, hypothyroidism with onset during childhood, and excess cortisol.

It is unlikely that a patient with congenital hypothyroidism will present undiagnosed and untreated to a gynecologist. However, juvenile hypothyroidism must be suspected in an adolescent with obesity and short stature and a normal early childhood development. Similarly, an adolescent with hypopituitarism due to a slow growing pituitary tumor may present with a failure to develop secondary sexual characteristics and a failure to grow. Cortisol excess may be due to Cushing's disease (rare in childhood) or to therapy with corticosteroids. Excess endogenous or exogenous corticosteroids suppress skeletal maturation and growth. Moderate overdosage of cortisol, when treating children with adrenal hyperplasia, for example, may suppress growth.

Treatment of Short Stature. If the physician concludes that an adolescent suffers from a delay of normal growth and no disease process is present, support and observation are indicated. If the bone age is more than 1 year below the chronologic age, but the family history reveals a consistent pattern of retarded but eventual normal growth, reassurance is essential. It is helpful to point out the x-ray, indicating that the individual has 1 year or more of unused potential in which to catch up with her friends.

When continued failure to grow is evident in the absence of disease, hormone treatment can be considered. Presently the use of growth hormone is restricted by short supplies, and is limited to use in growth hormone-deficient dwarfs. Fortunately, it is rare to see a female adolescent with this problem. More commonly it is an adolescent boy who is sensitive to reduced growth, and in whom the use of testosterone may be indicated. In cases of gonadal failure estrogen may be used in a female to stimulate epiphyseal growth, bringing the bone age to match the chronologic age. Conjugated estrogen can be given in a dose of 10 mg daily from the 1st through the 24th of each month, and medroxyprogesterone acetate (Provera), 10 mg, is added on the 20th through the 24th to ensure consistent and predictable menstrual bleeding. Patients should be observed at 6 month intervals to document the pattern of growth and development. Hormone treatment may be discontinued when the bone age matches the chronological age.

all Stature

This is rarely a problem in boys (basketball provides a ready outlet), but girls who are the daughters of very tall parents may come to the gynecologist for help. A predicted height greater than 6 feet probably deserves treatment. The Bayley-Pinneau tables are accurate in predicting the height of tall girls. (8)

If a family history for tallness is not elicited, an earnest search for a problem is indicated, although little more than a thorough history, examination, and routine laboratory tests are necessary. A hand-wrist x-ray for bone age is also necessary. The degree of development of secondary sexual characteristics is important, since the more mature a girl is, the less effective treatment is in influencing her eventual height.

Treatment of Tall Stature. It is difficult to make a decision for treatment, and parental participation in the decision is essential. In a case where some success can be achieved, the patient is relatively young and may find it hard to know what to think about the future problem.

Since the adolescent growth spurt precedes menarche, treatment must begin before menarche in order to be optimally successful. This would be as early as 8 or 9 years, and certainly before the age of 12. However, treatment begun after menarche may still achieve up to an inch of growth reduction. (9) Once begun, treatment must continue until epiphyses are fused. If treatment is stopped earlier, further growth will occur. The parents and patient must be informed of possible problems with menorrhagia, breast symptoms, water retention, etc.

We recommend the use of conjugated estrogens rather than diethylstilbestrol. The latter causes pigmentation of the nipples and this effect can be easily avoided. In addition, diethylstilbestrol is associated with a significant incidence of nausea. Conjugated estrogen may be given in a dose of 10 mg daily from the 1st through the 24th of each month, and medroxyprogesterone acetate (Provera), 10 mg, is added on the 20th through the 24th to ensure consistent and predictable menstrual bleeding. Hand-wrist films should be taken every 6 months until epiphyseal closure is demonstrated.

References

1. **Tanner, JM,** *Growth at Adolescence,* 2nd edition, Blackwell Scientific Publications, Oxford, 1962.

2. **Fried, RI, and Smith, EE,** Postmenarcheal Growth Patterns, J Pediatr 61:562, 1962.

3. **Zacharias, L, Rand, WM, and Wurtman, RJ,** A Prospective Study of Sexual Development and Growth in American Girls: The Statistics of Menarche, Obstet Gynec Survey 31:325, 1976.

4. **van der Werff ten Bosch, JJ,** Isosexual Precocity, in Gardner, LI, ed., *Endocrine and Genetic Diseases of Childhood,* W.B. Saunders, Philadelphia, 1969.

5. **Pedowitz, P, Felmus, LB, and Mackles, A,** Precocious Pseudopuberty Due to Ovarian Tumors, Obstet Gynec Surv 10:633, 1955.

6. **Bayley, N, and Pinneau, SR,** Tables for Predicting Adult Height from Skeletal Age: Revised for Use with the Greulich-Pyle Hand Standards, J Pediatr 40:423, 1952.

7. **Greulich, WW, and Pyle, SL,** *Radiographic Atlas of Skeletal Development of the Hand and Wrist,* Stanford University Press, Stanford, California, 1950.

8. **Schoen, EJ, Solomon, IL, Warner, D, and Wingerd, J,** Estrogen Treatment of Tall Girls, Am J Dis Child 125:71, 1973.

9. **Norman, H, Wettenhall, B, Cahill, C, and Roche, AF,** Tall Girls: A Survey of 15 Years of Management and Treatment, Adolesc Med 86:602, 1975.

**Bayley-Pinneau Table
for Average Girls**
(J. Pediat. 40:423, 1952)

To predict height, find vertical column corresponding to skeletal age and horizontal row for the present height. The number at the intersection is the predicted height in inches. If figures do not fall at the whole inch or 6-month intervals, the predicted height must be extrapolated.

Skeletal age	6/0	6/6	7/0	7/6	8/0	8/6	9/0	9/6	10/0	10/6	11/0	11/6	12/0
Height 37	51.4												
in inches 38	52.8	51.5											
39	54.2	52.8	51.5										
40	55.6	54.2	52.8	51.8									
41	56.9	55.6	54.2	53.1	51.9								
42	58.3	56.9	55.5	54.4	53.2	51.9							
43	59.7	58.3	56.8	55.7	54.4	53.1	52.0						
44	61.1	59.6	58.1	57.0	55.7	54.3	53.2	52.1	51.0				
45	62.5	61.0	59.4	58.3	57.0	55.6	54.4	53.3	52.2				
46	63.9	62.3	60.8	59.6	58.2	56.8	55.6	54.5	53.4	52.0			
47	65.8	63.7	62.1	60.9	59.5	58.0	56.8	55.7	54.5	53.2	51.9	51.4	51.0
48	66.7	65.0	63.4	62.2	60.8	59.3	58.0	56.9	55.7	54.3	53.0	52.5	52.1
49	68.1	66.4	64.7	63.5	62.0	60.5	59.3	58.1	56.8	55.4	54.1	53.6	53.1
50	69.4	67.8	66.1	64.8	63.3	61.7	60.5	59.2	58.0	56.6	55.2	54.7	54.2
51	70.8	69.1	67.4	66.1	64.6	63.0	61.7	60.4	59.2	57.7	56.3	55.8	55.3
52	72.2	70.5	68.7	67.4	65.8	64.2	62.9	61.6	60.3	58.8	57.4	56.9	56.4
53	73.6	71.8	70.0	68.7	67.1	65.4	64.1	62.8	61.5	60.0	58.5	58.0	57.5
54		73.2	71.3	69.9	68.4	66.7	65.3	64.0	62.6	61.1	59.6	59.1	58.6
55		74.5	72.7	71.2	69.6	67.9	66.5	65.2	63.8	62.2	60.7	60.2	59.7
56			74.0	72.5	70.9	69.1	67.7	66.4	65.0	63.3	61.8	61.3	60.7
57				73.8	72.2	70.4	68.9	67.5	66.1	64.5	62.9	62.4	61.8
58					73.4	71.6	70.1	68.7	67.3	65.6	64.0	63.5	62.9
59					74.7	72.8	71.3	69.9	68.4	66.7	65.1	64.6	64.0
60						74.1	72.6	71.1	69.6	67.9	66.2	65.6	65.1
61							73.8	72.3	70.8	69.0	67.3	66.7	66.2
62								73.5	71.9	70.1	68.4	67.8	67.2
63								74.6	73.1	71.3	69.5	68.9	68.3
64									74.2	72.4	70.6	70.0	69.4
65										73.5	71.7	71.1	70.5
66										74.7	72.9	72.2	71.6
67											74.0	73.3	72.7
68												74.4	73.8
69													74.8
70													
71													
72													
73													
74													

12/6	13/0	13/6	14/0	14/6	15/0	15/6	16/0	16/6	17/0	17/6	18/0	
												37
												38
												39
												40
												41
												42
												43
												44
												45
												46
												47
51.0												48
52.1	51.1											49
53.1	52.2	51.3	51.0									50
54.2	53.2	52.4	52.0	51.7	51.5	51.4	51.2	51.2	51.1	51.0	51.0	51
55.3	54.3	53.4	53.1	52.7	52.5	52.4	52.2	52.2	52.1	52.0	52.0	52
56.3	55.3	54.4	54.1	53.8	53.5	53.4	53.2	53.2	53.1	53.0	53.0	53
57.4	56.4	55.4	55.1	54.8	54.5	54.4	54.2	54.2	54.1	54.0	54.0	54
58.4	57.4	56.5	56.1	55.8	55.6	55.4	55.2	55.2	55.1	55.0	55.0	55
59.5	58.5	57.5	57.1	56.8	56.6	56.4	56.2	56.2	56.1	56.0	56.0	56
60.6	59.5	58.5	58.2	57.8	57.6	57.4	57.2	57.2	57.1	57.0	57.0	57
61.6	60.5	59.5	59.2	58.8	58.6	58.4	58.2	58.2	58.1	58.0	58.0	58
62.7	61.6	60.6	60.2	59.8	59.6	59.4	59.2	59.2	59.1	59.0	59.0	59
63.8	62.6	61.6	61.2	60.9	60.6	60.4	60.2	60.2	60.1	60.0	60.0	60
64.8	63.7	62.6	62.2	61.9	61.6	61.4	61.2	61.2	61.1	61.0	61.0	61
65.9	64.7	63.7	63.3	62.9	62.6	62.4	62.2	62.2	62.1	62.0	62.0	62
67.0	65.8	64.7	64.3	63.9	63.6	63.4	63.3	63.2	63.1	63.0	63.0	63
68.0	66.8	65.7	65.3	64.9	64.6	64.4	64.3	64.2	64.1	64.0	64.0	64
69.1	67.8	66.7	66.3	65.9	65.7	65.5	65.3	65.2	65.1	65.0	65.0	65
70.1	68.9	67.8	67.3	66.9	66.7	66.5	66.3	66.2	66.1	66.0	66.0	66
71.2	69.9	68.8	68.4	68.0	67.7	67.5	67.3	67.2	67.1	67.0	67.0	67
72.3	71.0	69.8	69.4	69.0	68.7	68.5	68.3	68.2	68.1	68.0	68.0	68
73.3	72.0	70.8	70.4	70.0	69.7	69.5	69.3	69.2	69.1	69.0	69.0	69
74.4	73.1	71.9	71.4	71.0	70.7	70.5	70.3	70.2	70.1	70.0	70.0	70
	74.1	72.9	72.4	72.0	71.7	71.5	71.3	71.2	71.1	71.0	71.0	71
		73.9	73.5	73.0	72.7	72.5	72.3	72.2	72.1	72.0	72.0	72
		74.9	74.5	74.0	73.7	73.5	73.3	73.2	73.1	73.0	73.0	73
				74.7	74.5	74.3	74.2	74.1	74.0	74.0		74

**Bayley-Pinneau Table
for Accelerated Girls**

To predict height, find vertical column corresponding to skeletal age and horizontal row for the present height. The number at the intersection is the predicted height in inches. If figures do not fall at the whole inch or 6-month intervals, the predicted height must be extrapolated.

Skeletal age		7/0	7/6	8/0	8/6	9/0	9/6	10/0	10/6	11/0	11/6	12/0
Height in inches	37	52.0										
	38	53.4	51.9									
	39	54.8	53.3	52.0								
	40	56.2	54.6	53.3	51.9							
	41	57.6	56.0	54.7	53.2	51.9						
	42	59.0	57.4	56.0	54.5	53.2	51.9					
	43	60.4	58.7	57.3	55.8	54.4	53.2	51.9				
	44	61.8	60.1	58.7	57.1	55.7	54.4	53.1	51.4			
	45	63.2	61.5	60.0	58.4	57.0	55.6	54.3	52.6	54.0		
	46	64.6	62.8	61.3	59.7	58.2	56.9	55.6	53.7	52.1	51.6	51.1
	47	66.0	64.2	62.7	61.0	59.5	58.1	56.8	54.9	53.2	52.7	52.2
	48	67.4	65.6	64.0	62.3	60.8	59.3	58.0	56.1	54.4	53.9	53.3
	49	68.8	66.9	65.3	63.6	62.0	60.6	59.2	57.2	55.5	55.0	54.4
	50	70.2	68.3	66.7	64.9	63.3	61.8	60.4	58.4	56.6	56.1	55.5
	51	71.6	69.7	68.0	66.1	64.6	63.0	61.6	59.6	57.8	57.2	56.6
	52	73.0	71.0	69.3	67.4	65.8	64.3	62.8	60.7	58.9	58.4	57.7
	53	74.4	72.4	70.7	68.7	67.1	65.5	64.0	61.9	60.0	59.5	58.8
	54		73.8	72.0	70.0	68.4	66.7	65.2	63.1	61.2	60.6	59.9
	55			73.3	71.3	69.6	68.0	66.4	64.3	62.3	61.7	61.0
	56			74.7	72.6	70.9	69.2	67.6	65.4	63.4	62.8	62.2
	57				73.9	72.2	70.5	68.8	66.6	64.6	64.0	63.3
	58					73.4	71.7	70.0	67.8	65.7	65.1	64.4
	59					74.7	72.9	71.3	68.9	66.8	66.2	65.5
	60						74.2	72.5	70.1	68.0	67.3	66.6
	61							73.7	71.3	69.1	68.5	67.7
	62							74.9	72.4	70.2	69.6	68.8
	63								73.6	71.3	70.7	69.9
	64								74.8	72.5	71.8	71.0
	65									73.6	72.9	72.1
	66									74.7	74.1	73.3
	67											74.4
	68											
	69											
	70											
	71											
	72											
	73											
	74											

12/6	13/0	13/6	14/0	14/6	15/0	15/6	16/0	16/6	17/0	17/6	
											37
											38
											39
											40
											41
											42
											43
											44
											45
											46
											47
51.9											48
53.0	51.9	50.9									49
54.1	52.9	51.9	51.4	51.0							50
55.2	54.0	53.0	52.5	52.0	51.7	51.5	51.4	51.3	51.1	51.0	51
56.3	55.0	54.0	53.5	53.1	52.7	52.5	52.4	52.3	52.1	52.0	52
57.4	56.1	55.0	54.5	54.1	53.8	53.5	53.4	53.3	53.1	53.0	53
58.4	57.1	56.1	55.6	55.1	54.8	54.5	54.4	54.3	54.1	54.0	54
59.5	58.2	57.1	56.6	56.1	55.8	55.5	55.4	55.3	55.1	55.0	55
60.6	59.3	58.2	57.6	57.1	56.8	56.5	56.4	56.3	56.1	56.0	56
61.7	60.3	59.2	58.6	58.2	57.8	57.6	57.4	57.3	57.1	57.0	57
62.8	61.4	60.2	59.7	59.2	58.8	58.6	58.4	58.3	58.1	58.0	58
63.9	62.4	61.3	60.7	60.2	59.8	59.6	59.4	59.3	59.1	59.0	59
64.9	63.5	62.3	61.7	61.2	60.9	60.6	60.4	60.3	60.1	60.0	60
66.0	64.6	63.3	62.8	62.2	61.9	61.6	61.4	61.3	61.1	61.0	61
67.1	65.6	64.4	63.8	63.3	62.9	62.6	62.4	62.3	62.1	62.0	62
68.2	66.7	65.4	64.8	64.3	63.9	63.6	63.4	63.3	63.1	63.0	63
69.3	67.7	66.5	65.8	65.3	64.9	64.6	64.4	64.3	64.1	64.0	64
70.3	68.8	67.5	66.9	66.3	65.9	65.7	65.5	65.3	65.1	65.0	65
71.4	69.8	68.5	67.9	67.3	66.9	66.7	66.5	66.3	66.1	66.0	66
72.5	70.9	69.6	68.9	68.4	68.0	67.7	67.5	67.3	67.1	67.0	67
73.6	72.0	70.6	70.0	69.4	69.0	68.7	68.5	68.3	68.1	68.0	68
74.7	73.0	71.7	71.0	70.4	70.0	69.7	69.5	69.3	69.1	69.0	69
	74.1	72.7	72.0	71.4	71.0	70.7	70.5	70.3	70.1	70.0	70
		73.7	73.0	72.4	72.0	71.7	71.5	71.4	71.1	71.0	71
		74.8	74.1	73.5	73.0	72.7	72.5	72.4	72.1	72.0	72
				74.5	74.0	73.7	73.5	73.4	73.1	73.0	73
						74.4	74.5	74.4	74.1	74.0	74

**Bayley-Pinneau Table
for Retarded Girls**

To predict height, find vertical column corresponding to skeletal age and horizontal row for the present height. The number at the intersection is the predicted height in inches. If figures do not fall at the whole inch or 6-month intervals, the predicted height must be extrapolated.

Skeletal age		6/0	6/6	7/0	7/6	8/0	8/6	9/0	9/6	10/0	10/6	11/0	11/6
Height in inches	38	51.8											
	39	53.2	51.9										
	40	54.6	53.3	51.9									
	41	55.9	54.6	53.2	52.0								
	42	57.3	55.9	54.5	53.3	52.2	51.0						
	43	58.7	57.3	55.8	54.6	53.5	52.2	51.1					
	44	60.0	58.6	57.1	55.8	54.7	53.5	52.3	51.3				
	45	61.4	59.9	58.4	57.1	56.0	54.7	53.5	52.4	51.5			
	46	62.8	61.3	59.7	58.4	57.2	55.9	54.7	53.6	52.6	51.3		
	47	64.1	62.6	61.0	59.6	58.5	57.1	55.9	54.8	53.8	52.5	51.2	
	48	65.5	63.9	62.3	60.9	59.7	58.3	57.1	55.9	54.9	63.6	52.3	51.8
	49	66.9	65.2	63.6	62.2	60.9	59.5	58.3	57.1	56.1	54.7	53.4	52.9
	50	68.2	66.6	64.9	63.5	62.2	60.8	59.5	58.3	57.2	55.8	54.5	54.0
	51	69.6	67.9	66.2	64.7	63.4	62.0	60.6	59.4	58.4	56.9	55.6	55.1
	52	70.9	69.2	67.5	66.0	64.7	63.2	61.8	60.6	59.5	58.0	56.6	56.2
	53	72.3	70.6	68.8	67.3	65.9	64.4	63.0	61.8	60.6	59.2	57.7	57.2
	54	73.7	71.9	70.1	68.5	67.2	65.6	64.2	62.9	61.8	60.3	58.8	58.3
	55		73.2	71.4	69.8	68.4	66.8	65.4	64.1	62.9	61.4	59.9	59.4
	56		74.6	72.7	71.1	69.7	68.0	66.6	65.3	64.1	62.5	61.0	60.5
	57			74.0	72.3	70.9	69.3	67.8	66.4	65.2	63.6	62.1	61.6
	58				73.6	72.1	70.5	69.0	67.6	66.4	64.7	63.2	62.6
	59				74.9	73.4	71.7	70.2	68.8	67.5	65.8	64.3	63.7
	60					74.6	72.9	71.3	69.9	68.7	67.0	65.4	64.8
	61						74.1	72.5	71.1	69.8	68.1	66.4	65.9
	62							73.7	72.3	70.9	69.2	67.5	67.0
	63							74.7	73.4	72.1	70.3	68.6	68.0
	64								74.6	73.2	71.4	69.7	69.1
	65									74.4	72.5	70.8	70.2
	66										73.7	71.9	71.3
	67										74.8	73.0	72.4
	68											74.1	73.4
	69												74.5
	70												
	71												
	72												
	73												
	74												

12/0	12/6	13/0	13/6	14/0	14/6	15/0	15/6	16/0	16/6	17/0	
											40
											41
											42
											43
											44
											45
											46
											47
51.5											48
52.6	51.6										49
53.6	52.7	51.9	51.2								50
54.7	53.7	52.9	52.2	51.9	51.6	51.3	51.2	51.1	51.1	51.0	51
55.8	54.8	53.9	53.2	52.9	52.6	52.3	52.2	52.1	52.1	52.0	52
56.9	55.8	55.0	54.2	53.9	53.6	53.3	53.2	53.1	53.1	53.0	53
57.9	56.9	56.0	55.3	54.9	54.6	54.3	54.2	54.1	54.1	54.0	54
59.0	58.0	57.1	56.3	56.0	55.6	55.3	55.2	55.1	55.1	55.0	55
60.1	59.0	58.1	57.3	57.0	56.6	56.3	56.2	56.1	56.1	56.0	56
61.2	60.1	59.1	58.3	58.0	57.6	57.3	57.2	57.1	57.1	57.0	57
62.2	61.1	60.2	59.4	59.0	58.6	58.3	58.2	58.1	58.1	58.0	58
63.3	62.2	61.2	60.4	60.0	59.7	59.4	59.2	59.1	59.1	59.0	59
64.4	63.2	62.2	61.4	61.0	60.7	60.4	60.2	60.1	60.1	60.0	60
65.5	64.3	63.3	62.4	62.1	61.7	61.4	61.2	61.1	61.1	61.0	61
66.5	65.3	64.3	63.5	63.1	62.7	62.4	62.2	62.1	62.1	62.0	62
67.6	66.4	65.3	64.5	64.1	63.7	63.4	63.3	63.1	63.1	63.0	63
68.7	67.4	66.4	65.5	65.1	64.7	64.4	64.3	64.1	64.1	64.0	64
69.7	68.5	67.4	66.5	66.1	65.7	65.4	65.3	65.1	65.1	65.0	65
70.8	69.5	68.5	67.6	67.1	66.7	66.4	66.3	66.1	66.1	66.0	66
71.9	70.6	69.5	68.6	68.2	67.7	67.4	67.3	67.1	67.1	67.0	67
73.0	71.7	70.5	69.6	69.2	68.8	68.4	68.3	68.1	68.1	68.0	68
74.0	72.7	71.6	70.6	70.2	69.8	69.4	69.3	69.1	69.1	69.0	69
	73.8	72.6	71.6	71.2	70.8	70.4	70.3	70.1	70.1	70.0	70
	74.8	73.6	72.7	72.2	71.8	71.4	71.3	71.1	71.1	71.0	71
		74.7	73.7	73.3	72.8	72.4	72.3	72.1	72.1	72.0	72
			74.7	74.3	73.8	73.4	73.3	73.1	73.1	73.0	73
					74.8	74.4	74.3	74.1	74.1	74.0	74

13 Obesity

One of the least rewarding experiences in clinical medicine is treating obesity. Because from 25% to 45% of American adults over 30 years old are more than 20% overweight, the unrewarding fight against obesity is all too common, not only with our patients but also with ourselves.

The lack of success is not due to an unawareness of the implications of obesity; there is a clear-cut relationship between mortality and weight. The death rate from diabetes mellitus, for example, is approximately 4 times higher among obese diabetics than among those who control their weight. Also higher among obese individuals is the incidence of gallbladder disease, cardiovascular disease, renal disease, and cirrhosis of the liver. The death rate from appendicitis is double, presumably from anesthetic and surgical complications. Even the rate of accidents is higher, perhaps because fat people are awkward or because their view of the ground or floor is obstructed. When the personal and social problems encountered by obese persons are also considered, it is no wonder that a physician without a weight problem cannot comprehend why fat individuals remain overweight.

The frequency with which a practitioner encounters the obese patient whose weight does not decrease despite a sworn adherence to a limited-calorie diet makes one question if there is something physiologically different about this patient. Is the problem due to lack of discipline and cheating on a diet, or does it also involve a pathophysiologic factor? Is the physiology of obese people unusual, or are they simply gluttons?

As a basis for a more understanding approach to obesity this chapter reviews the physiology of adipose tissue, discusses differences between normal and obese people, and comments on treatment.

**Physiology of
Adipose Tissue**

A person is obese when the amount of adipose tissue is sufficiently high (30% or more over the ideal weight) to detrimentally alter biochemical and physiologic functions and to shorten life expectancy. The ideal weight for any adult is believed to correspond to his or her ideal weight from age 20 to 30. The following formulas give ideal weight in pounds:

Man: 120 + [4 X (height in inches minus 60)]

Woman: 100 + [4 X (height in inches minus 60)]

Adipose tissue serves 3 general functions:

1. It is a storehouse of energy.

2. Fat serves as a cushion from trauma.

3. Adipose tissue plays a role in the regulation of body heat.

Each cell of adipose tissue may be regarded as a package of triglyceride, the most concentrated form of stored energy. There are 8 calories per gram of triglyceride as opposed to one calorie per gram of glycogen. The total store of tissue and fluid carbohydrate in adults (about 300 calories) is inadequate to meet between-meal demands. The storage of energy in fat tissue allows us to do other things beside eating.

The mechanism for mobilizing energy from fat involves various enzymes and neurohormonal agents. Following ingestion of fat and its breakdown by gastric and pancreatic lipases, absorption of long-chain triglycerides and free fatty acids takes place in the small bowel. Chylomicrons (microscopic particles of fat) transferred through lymph channels into the systemic venous circulation are normally removed by hepatic parenchymal cells where a new lipoprotein is released into the circulation. When this lipoprotein is exposed to adipose tissue, lipolysis takes place through the action of lipoprotein lipase, an enzyme derived from the fat cells themselves. The fatty acids that are released then enter the fat cells where they are re-esterified with glycerophosphate into triglycerides.

272

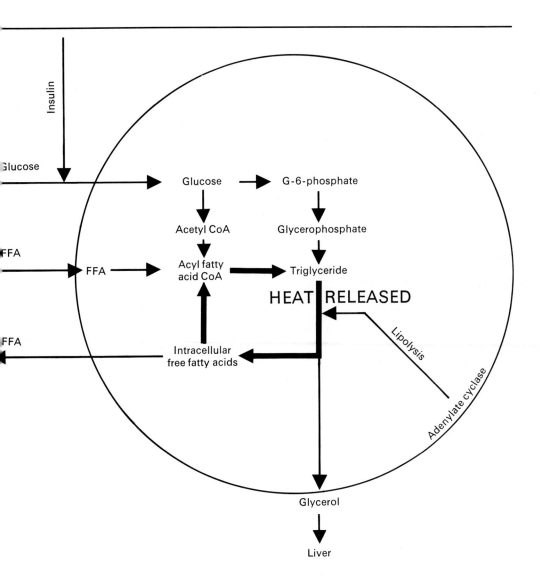

Glucose serves three important functions:

1. Glucose supplies carbon atoms in the form of acetyl CoA.

2. Glucose provides hydrogen for reductive steps.

3. Glucose is the main source of glycerophosphate.

    The production and availability of glycerophosphate (required for re-esterification of fatty acids and their storage as triglycerides) are considered rate-limiting in lipogenesis, and this process depends on the presence of glucose.

After esterification, subsequent lipolysis results in the release of fatty acids and glycerol. In the cycle of lipolysis and re-esterification, energy is freed as heat. A low variable level of lipolysis takes place continuously; its basic function may be to provide body heat.

The chief metabolic products produced from fat are the circulating free fatty acids. Their availability is controlled by adipose tissue cells. When carbohydrate is in short supply, a flood of free fatty acids can be released. The free fatty acids in the peripheral circulation are almost wholly derived from endogenous triglyceride that undergoes rapid hydrolysis to yield free fatty acid and glycerol. The glycerol is returned to the liver for resynthesis of glycogen.

Free fatty acid release from adipose tissue is stimulated by physical exercise, fasting, exposure to cold, nervous tension, and anxiety. The release of fatty acids by lipolysis varies from one anatomic site to another. Omental, mesenteric, and subcutaneous fat are more labile and easily mobilized than fat from other sources. Areas from which energy is not easily mobilized are retrobulbar and perirenal fat where the tissue serves a structural function. Adipose tissue lipase is sensitive to stimulation by both epinephrine and norepinephrine. Other hormones that activate lipase are ACTH, TSH, growth hormone, T-4, T-3, cortisol, glucagon, as well as vasopressin and HPL.

Lipase enzyme activity is inhibited by insulin, which appears to be alone as the major physiologic antagonist to the array of stimulating agents. When both glucose and insulin are abundant, transport of glucose into fat cells is high, and glycerophosphate production increases to esterify fatty acids.

The carbohydrate and fat composition of the fuel supply is constantly changing, depending upon stresses and demands. Since the central nervous system and some other tissues can utilize only glucose for energy, a homeostatic mechanism for conserving carbohydrate is essential. When glucose is abundant and easily available, it is utilized in adipose tissue for producing glycerophosphate to immobilize fatty acids as triglycerides. The circulating level of free fatty acids in muscle will, therefore, be low, and glucose will be used by all of the tissues.

When carbohydrate is scarce, the amount of glucose reaching the fat cells declines and glycerophosphate production is reduced. The fat cell releases fatty acids, and their circulating levels rise to a point where glycolysis is inhibited. Thus carbohydrate is spared in those tissues capable of using lipid substrates. If the rise of fatty acids is great enough, the liver is flooded with acetyl CoA. This is converted into ketone bodies, and clinical ketosis results.

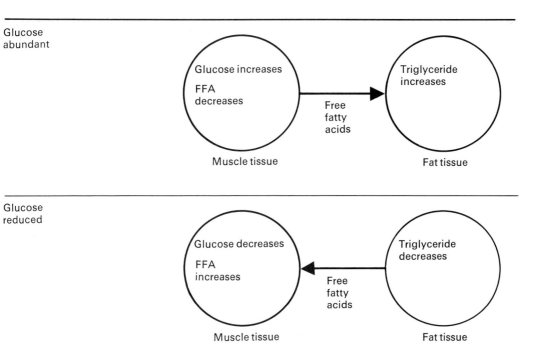

Glucose
abundant

Glucose increases

FFA
decreases

Free
fatty
acids

Triglyceride
increases

Muscle tissue

Fat tissue

Glucose
reduced

Glucose decreases

FFA
increases

Free
fatty
acids

Triglyceride
decreases

Muscle tissue

Fat tissue

In the simplest terms, when a person eats, glucose is available, insulin is secreted, and fat is stored. In starvation, the glucose level falls, insulin secretion decreases, and fat is mobilized.

If only single large meals are consumed, the body learns to convert carbohydrate to fat very quickly. Epidemiologic studies on school children demonstrate a positive correlation between fewer meals and a greater tendency toward obesity. (1) The person who does not eat all day and then stocks up at night is perhaps doing the worst possible thing.

Clinical Obesity

Obesity and the Brain

The hypothalamic location of the appetite center was established in 1940 by the demonstration that bilateral lesions of the ventromedial nucleus produce experimental obesity in rats. Such lesions lead to hyperphagia and decreased physical activity. Interestingly, this pattern is similar to that seen in human beings — the pressure to eat is reinforced by the desire to be physically inactive. The ventromedial nucleus was thought to represent an integrating center for appetite and hunger information. Destruction of the ventromedial nucleus was believed to result in a loss of satiety signals, leading to hyperphagia.

Recent studies, however, suggest that overeating and obesity are not due to ventromedial nucleus damage but rather to destruction of the nearby ventral noradrenergic bundle. (2) Hypothalamic noradrenergic terminals are derived from long fibers ascending from hindbrain cell bodies. Lesions of the ventromedial nucleus produced by radio frequency currents fail to cause obesity. These lesions lead to overeating and obesity only when they extend beyond the ventromedial nucleus. Selective destruction of the ventral noradrenergic bundle results in hyperphagia. The lesions that produce hyperphagia also reduce the potency of amphetamine as an appetite suppressant. This noradrenergic bundle may function as a satiety system and be the site of amphetamine action.

There may be two kinds of obesity: obesity stemming from a CNS regulatory defect, or obesity due to a metabolic problem occurring despite a normal central mechanism.

Psychologic Factors (3)

Obese and lean people respond differently to their environments. Obese people appear to regulate their desire for food through external signals. Lean people, on the other hand, regulate their intake by endogenous signals of hunger and satiety.

Fear does not inhibit gastrointestinal activity and dull the appetite in obese persons as it does in others. Fat people eat because it is mealtime, and food looks, smells, and tastes good. They also eat because other people are eating, but not necessarily because they themselves are hungry.

Obese people are also less physically active than are people of normal weight. The obese person will drive a car around the block repeatedly until a parking space is available, rather than walk a few blocks. Time-lapse photography studies show that obese people when in a swimming pool spend most of their time floating; lean people move around actively. (4) An obese baby is more willing than is a normal baby to take formula after it has been sweetened, but will take less formula, even though it is sweetened, if the work of eating is increased by a nipple with a smaller hole.

There may be two classes of obesity: One class may include those individuals who clearly eat too much. The other class would be composed of individuals who eat relatively normal diets but who are extremely inactive.

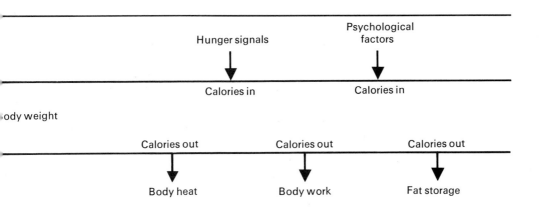

| | Hunger signals | Psychological factors |
| | Calories in | Calories in |

Body weight

| Calories out | Calories out | Calories out |
| Body heat | Body work | Fat storage |

Fat Cells

Fat cells develop from connective tissue early in fetal life. An important question is whether new fat cells are produced by metaplasia in the adult, or whether an individual achieves a total complement during a certain period of life. In other words, is excess fat stored by increasing the size of the fat cell, or by increasing the number of cells? The possibility arises that there is an increase in the total number of fat cells, which just wait to be packed full of storage fat. Furthermore the total number of fat cells may depend upon an infant's nutritional state during the neonatal period, and perhaps in utero as well.

Studies of fat obtained at surgery indicate that the mean fat cell volume is increased threefold in obese people, but an increase in the number of fat cells is seen only in the grossly obese. (5) When patients diet, the fat cells decrease in size but not in number. Thus hypercellular obesity may be a more difficult problem to overcome, since an individual may be saddled with a permanent increase in fat mass.

Some researchers think that at some period in a person's life, a fixed number of fat cells is obtained. Adolescence, infancy, and intrauterine life seem particularly critical. (6, 7) This premise is not solidly established, since there is no certain way to identify an empty fat cell, and potential fat cells cannot be recognized. Nevertheless, a hyperplastic type of obesity (more fat cells) may be associated with childhood and have a poor prognosis; a hypertrophic type (enlarged fat cells) that is responsive to dieting may occur in adults.

Endocrine Changes

The most important endocrine change in obesity is elevation of the basal blood insulin levels. Insulin response to either carbohydrates or amino acids is also increased. Because glucose levels are normal, it is apparent that a state of insulin resistance or antagonism exists. This is associated with triglyceride and free fatty acid levels approximately 20% higher than those in normal people.

277

With an increase in adipose tissue, fatty acid levels rise. This, in turn, may interfere with insulin action, causing increased insulin production. On the other hand, the distended cell may become resistant to insulin, and insulin levels increase to overcome this resistance. The latter explanation seems unlikely since fat cells have been shown to demonstrate normal binding and affinity between insulin and the membrane receptors.

Other endocrine changes associated with obesity include decreased growth hormone secretion, and increased cortisol production and metabolic clearance rates (thus plasma and urinary cortisol are relatively normal). The fasting level of growth hormone is decreased as well as the response to insulin, arginine, starvation, and sleep. There is evidence of decreased pancreatic alpha cell function in obese nondiabetic people. (8) Glucagon secreted by the alpha cells acutely raises blood glucose levels by stimulating hepatic glycogenolysis and the production of new glucose from amino acids in the liver. Glucagon also activates lipolysis in the fat cell and stimulates insulin secretion. The basal levels of glucagon are equal in obese and nonobese patients, but the glucagon response to alanine is reduced by 50% in the obese group.

Obese people are relatively unable to excrete both salt and water, especially while dieting. During dieting this seems to be mediated by increased output of aldosterone and vasopressin. Since water produced from fat outweighs the fat, people on diets often show little initial weight loss. The use of a diuretic may encourage a patient to persist with dieting.

The basic question is whether metabolic changes observed in obesity represent adaptive reponses to a markedly enlarged fat organ, or whether they are representative of a metabolic or hormonal defect. It appears that the former is true. These changes are secondary responses; they are totally reversible with weight loss. Four year follow-up in a group of patients who did not regain their weight after dieting revealed persistently normal insulin and glucose responses; patients who regained their weight showed further deterioration in these metabolic factors. (9)

Experimental
Obesity

In a Vermont study, 28 male volunteers in the state prison underwent induced weight gain to about 20% above their basal weights. (10) Subjective changes were noted that correlate with the behavior of obese patients. The volunteers experienced increased appetite late in the day and decreased desire for physical activity. Once the weight gain was achieved, these normal people required about twice as many calories to maintain their obesity as did spontaneously obese people; there was no difficulty in returning to normal weight. These results suggest that there is something different about obese people.

With the gain in weight, the subjects showed an increase in fasting plasma insulin levels, decreased glucose tolerance, and decreased responses of adipose tissue to insulin stimulation of lipolysis. There was no increase in adipose cell number. These metabolic changes reverted to normal when the gained weight was lost. Hence, the hyperinsulinemia of obesity does not seem to be an etiologic, primary response, but rather a secondary change.

Management of Obesity

The two radical methods for treating obesity are starvation in the hospital, and the intestinal bypass operation. Both involve many potential problems and are reserved for extreme situations. For most patients, after a routine evaluation to rule out pathology such as diabetes mellitus and hypothyroidism, the physician is left with the frustrating task of prescribing a diet. Careful studies (performed in hospitalized subjects on metabolic wards) have indicated that the carbohydrate and fat composition of the diet has no effect on the rate of weight loss. (3) Since protein contains just as many calories as carbohydrate (per gram) a high protein diet (replacing carbohydrate) offers no advantage. Restriction of calories remains the important principle.

Despite various fads and dietbooks, the best diet continues to be the following: A limitation of calories to between 900 and 1200 calories per day, the actual amount depending on what the individual patient will accept and pursue. The carbohydrate content should be at least 150 grams per day, and the protein content should be 1.0 gram per Kg per day.

The discouraging aspect is that to lose a pound of fat, the equivalent to a 3,500 calorie intake must be expended. Dieting has to be slow and steady to be effective. As an index of the general lack of success with diets, a summary of ten studies (approximately 1200 patients) revealed that only 30% lose 20 pounds or more; only 4% lose 40 pounds or more. (5) Thus it is obvious why gimmicks abound in this area of patient management.

Many studies have demonstrated that amphetamines effectively lead to a weight loss over an approximately two-week period. (3) However, this is followed by a return to the initial weight after discontinuing the drug, or a failure to lose further weight in most patients even if the drug is continued. Controlled studies have not demonstrated the effectiveness of thyroid preparations. Similarly, the usefulness of human chorionic gonadotropin (HCG) has not been substantiated in double-blind studies. (11, 12) It is clear that these adjunctive measures are not successful unless the patient is also motivated either to limit caloric intake or to increase the exercise level, in what will be a lifelong battle.

Most frustrating is the problem of some patients wh limit caloric intake, yet do not lose weight. In fact, as th weight of certain patients increase, the number of calorie required to remain in equilibrium decreases, probab due to a combination of reduced activity and a change i metabolism. The Vermont study demonstrated that th normal person with induced obesity requires 2700 calorie to remain in equilibrium; spontaneously obese patien require only about 1300 calories. (10) The physicia must be careful to avoid a condemning or punitive att tude, and understand that it is possible to significantl restrict caloric intake and not lose weight.

Patients appear doomed to frustration and despair unles the physician can motivate them to increase physici activity. In all individuals dieting is more effective whe combined with physical exercise, but this is especiall true in chronically obese patients. In other words, the lif style of an obese person must be changed to overcom the desire to be inactive (walk instead of riding). Only b significantly increasing caloric expenditure will the inpu output equilibrium be disturbed.

The obese person feels trapped. Obesity leads to charac teristic behavioral manifestations, including passive pei sonality, frequent periods of depression, decreased sel respect, and a sense of being hopelessly overwhelmed b problems. But just as the endocrine and metaboli changes seem to be secondary to obesity, many of th psychosocial attributes surrounding obesity may also b secondary. (13)

Motivation to change and emotional support during th the change are important. They can be provided b friends, relatives, physicians, or self-help organizations If the vicious circle of failed diets, resignation to fate guilt, and shame can be broken, a more effective, happie person will emerge.

1. **Fabry, P, Hejda, S, and Cerny, K,** Effect of Meal Frequency in School Children. Changes in Weight-height Proportion and Skinfold Thickness, Am J Clin Nutr 18:358, 1966.

2. **Gold, RM,** Hypothalamic Obesity: The Myth of the Ventromedial Nucleus, Science 182:488, 1973.

3. **Gordon, ES,** Metabolic Aspects of Obesity, Adv Metab Disord 4:229, 1970.

4. **Mayer, J,** Inactivity as a Major Factor in Adolescent Obesity, Ann NY Acad Sci 131:502, 1965.

5. **Bray, GA, Davidson, MB, and Drenick, EJ,** Obesity: A Serious Symptom, Ann Int Med 77:787, 1972.

6. **Ravelli, G, Stein, ZA, and Susser, MW,** Obesity in Young Men After Famine Exposure in Utero and Early Infancy, New Eng J Med 295:349, 1976.

7. **Charney, E, Goodman, HC, McBride, M, Lyon, B, and Pratt, R,** Childhood Antecedents of Adult Obesity, New Eng J Med 295:6, 1976.

8. **Wise, JK, Hendler, R, and Felig, P,** Obesity: Evidence of Decreased Secretion of Glucagon, Science 178:513, 1972.

9. **Hewing, R, Liebermeister, H, Daweke, H, Gries, FA, and Gruneklee, D,** Weight Regain After Low Calories Diet: Long Term Pattern of Blood Sugar, Serum Lipids, Ketone Bodies, and Serum Insulin Levels, Diabetologia 9:197, 1973.

10. **Sims, EAH, Danforth, E, Jr., Horton, ES, Bray, GA, Glennon, JA, and Salans, LB,** Endocrine and Metabolic Effects of Experimental Obesity in Man, Rec Prog Hor Res 29:457, 1973.

11. **Young, RL, and Woltjen, MJ,** Use of Human Chorionic Gonadotropin in Weight Reduction Program, 58th Annual Meeting, The Endocrine Society, 1976, Abstract No. 441.

12. **Stein, MR, Julis, RE, Peck, C, Hinshaw, W, Swaicki, J, and Deller, JJ, Jr.,** A Detailed Double-blind Study of Human Chorionic Gonadotropin in Weight Reduction Program, 58th Annual Meeting, The Endocrine Society, 1976, Abstract No. 444.

13. **Solow, C, Silberfarb, PM, and Swift, K,** Psychosocial Effects of Intestinal Bypass Surgery for Severe Obesity, New Eng J Med 290:300, 1974.

14

Steroid Contraception

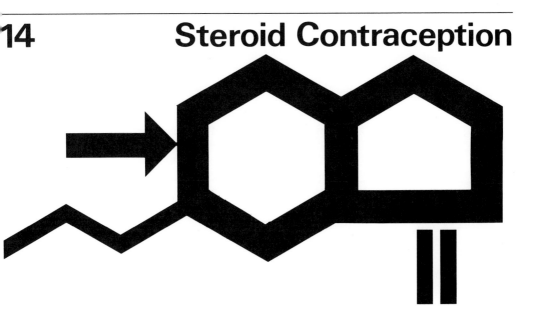

The clinical trials with steroids for contraception started with combination pills in 1958 and sequentials in 1962. There are now more than 50 million women throughout the world using steroids for contraception, and evaluation of coincidental medical problems and side effects continues to be a pressing issue.

Contraceptive steroids are not natural hormones and should not be so considered, i.e. a woman on the pill is not the same as a pregnant woman in more ways than the obvious one, nor can the effects be equated with phases of the menstrual cycle. Contraceptive steroids induce a pharmacologic state, not a physiologic one. Furthermore, the contraceptive drugs differ in their biochemical and metabolic effects, and thus far the contraceptive actions have not been separated from the metabolic effects.

The consistent effect of the pills is to challenge the physiologic reserve. The challenge to the physician is to identify the patient with less than ample reserve. *This chapter will survey those physiologic mechanisms under stress in the patient taking oral contraception, and review our methods for patient management.* Since an understanding of the basic chemical components of the pill is essential, a good starting point is a brief pharmacologic survey.

Pharmacology of Steroid Contraception

The Estrogen Component

The major obstacle to the use of steroids for contraception was inactivity of the compounds when given orally. A major breakthrough occurred in 1938 when it was discovered that the addition of an ethinyl group at the 17 position made estradiol orally active. Ethinyl estradiol is, therefore, a very potent oral estrogen and is one of the two forms of estrogen in every oral contraceptive. The other estrogen is the 3 methyl ether of ethinyl estradiol, mestranol.

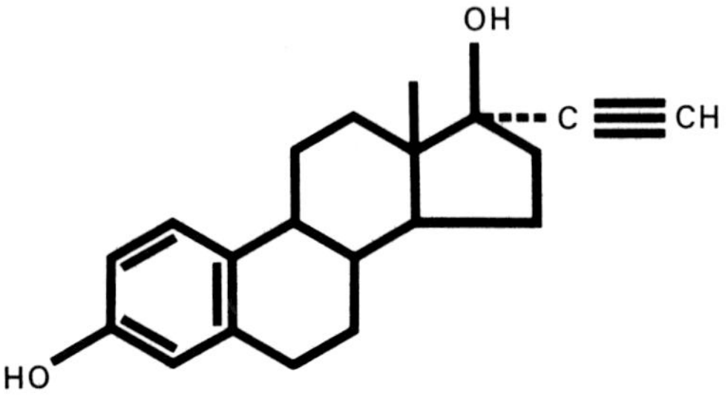

Ethinyl estradiol

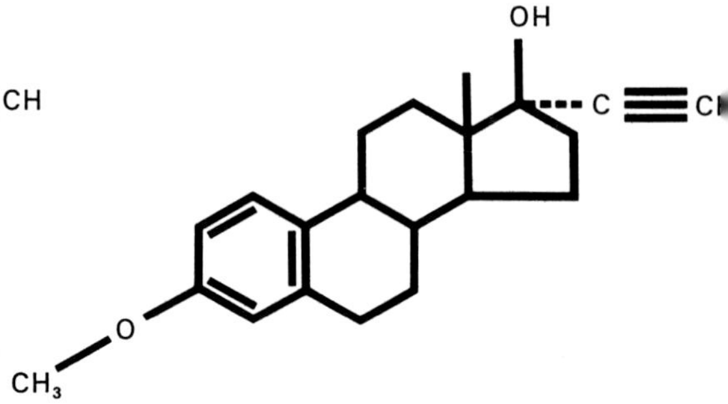

Mestranol

Mestranol and ethinyl estradiol are different from natural estradiol and must be regarded as pharmacologic drugs. A variety of animal studies have suggested that mestranol is weaker than ethinyl estradiol, presumably because mestranol must first be converted to ethinyl estradiol in the body. However in the human body, differences in potency between ethinyl estradiol and mestranol do not appear to be significant, certainly not as great as indicated by laboratory assays in rodents. (1, 2, 3)

The discovery of ethinyl substitution and oral potency led to the preparation of ethisterone, an orally active derivative of testosterone. In 1954, it was found that removal of the 19 carbon from ethisterone did not destroy the oral activity, but most importantly, it changed the major hormonal effect from that of an androgen to that of a progestational agent. Accordingly, these progestational derivatives of testosterone were designated as 19 nortestosterones (denoting the missing 19 carbon). The androgenic properties of these compounds, however, were not totally eliminated, and minimal anabolic and androgenic potential remains within the structure. Clinical effects, however, are rare, especially in the new low dose pills.

The "impurity" of the 19 nortestosterones, i.e. androgenic as well as progestational effects, is complicated further by the fact that they are metabolized within the body to estrogenic compounds. This conversion to estrogens varies in degree among the various steroids and probably between individuals. The clinician should be aware that the progestational agent in the combination pills contributes to the total estrogenic effect in the body, and the impact of this factor varies. However this effect has not been measured in human studies.

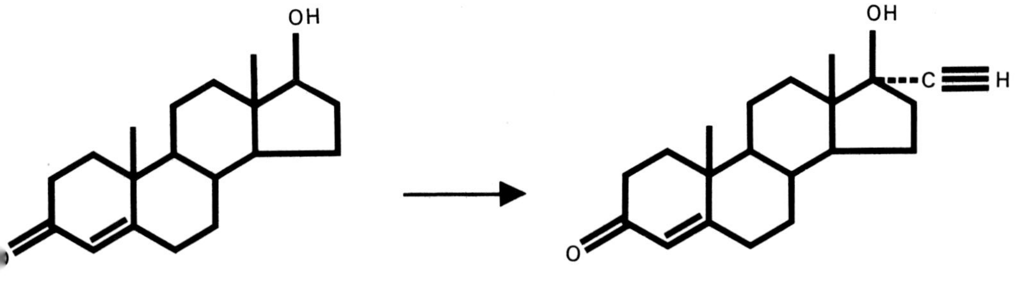

Testosterone

Ethisterone

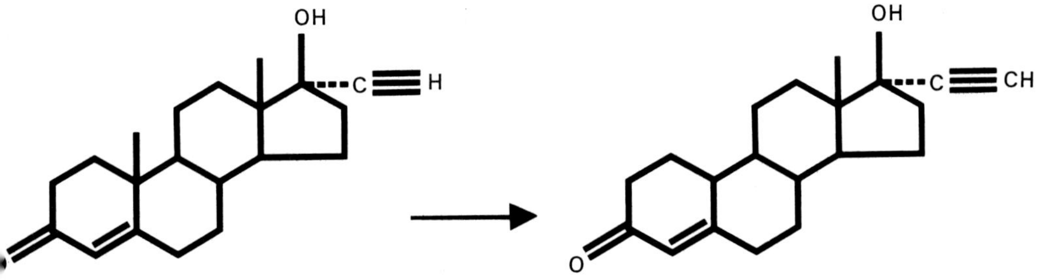

Ethisterone

Norethindrone

Norethindrone is the prototype of this family of compounds.

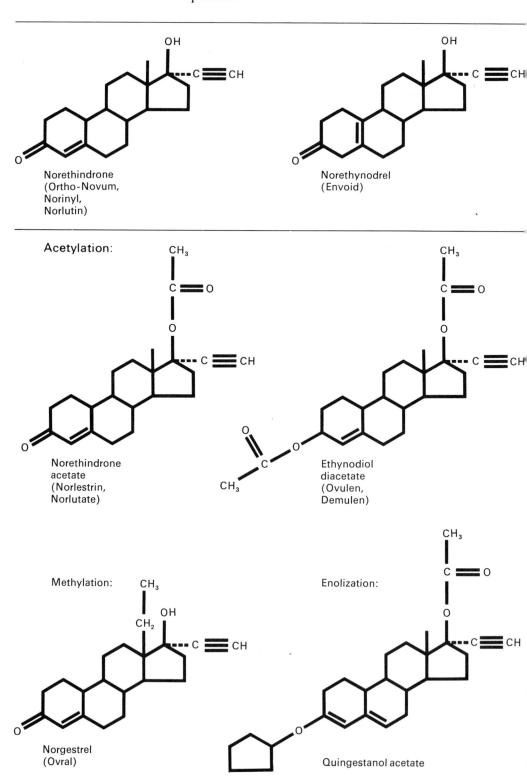

Norethindrone
(Ortho-Novum,
Norinyl,
Norlutin)

Norethynodrel
(Envoid)

Acetylation:

Norethindrone
acetate
(Norlestrin,
Norlutate)

Ethynodiol
diacetate
(Ovulen,
Demulen)

Methylation:

Norgestrel
(Ovral)

Enolization:

Quingestanol acetate

A second group of progestins became available for use when it was discovered that acetylation of the 17α-hydroxyl group of 17-hydroxyprogesterone produced oral activity. Acetylation at the 17 position gives oral potency, but hydroxylation at the 6 position is necessary to give sufficient progestational strength for human use, probably by inhibiting metabolism.

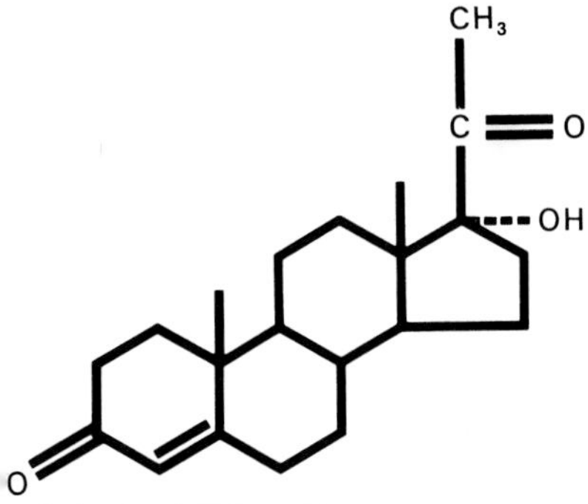

17α-Hydroxyprogesterone

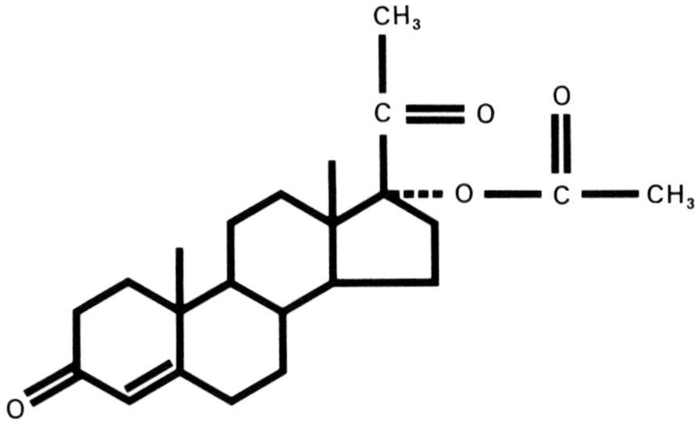

17-Acetoxy progesterone

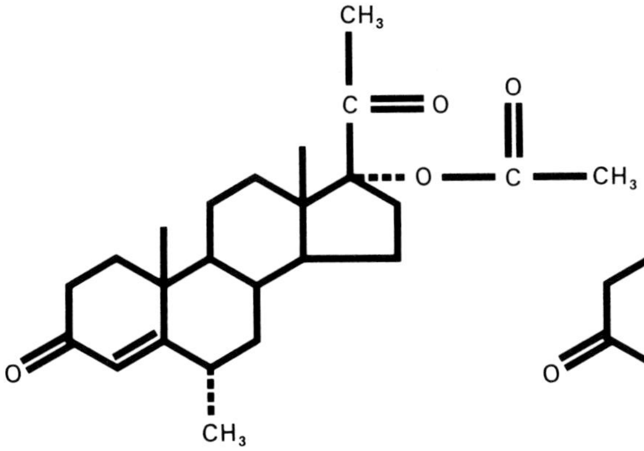

Medroxyprogesterone acetate
(Provera)

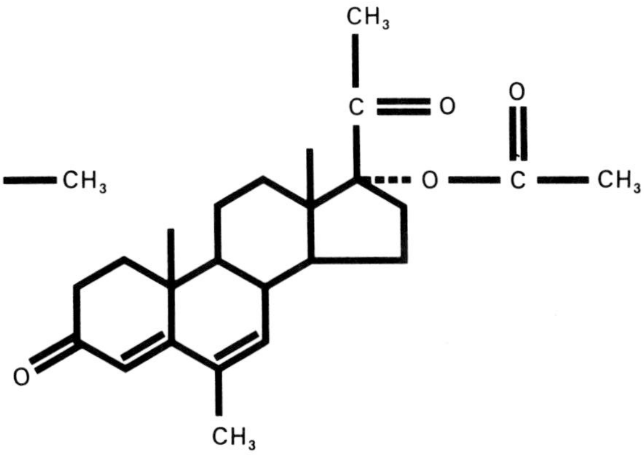

Megestrol acetate

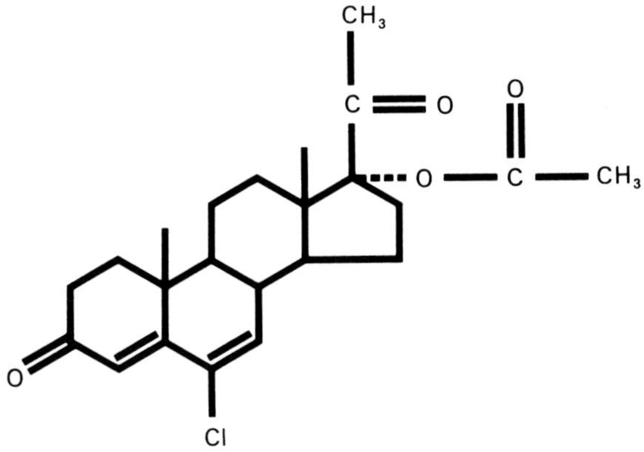

Chlormadinone acetate

| Mechanism of Action | The combination pill prevents ovulation by inhibition of gonadotropin secretion, exerting its principal effect on hypothalamic centers. The progestational agent in the pill suppresses LH secretion by a negative feedback action on the hypothalamus. The estrogenic agent suppresses FSH secretion in a similar fashion. The estrogen in the pill serves two other important purposes: It provides stability to the endometrium so that irregular shedding and unwanted break-through bleeding can be avoided and the presence of estrogen is required to potentiate the negative feedback action of the progestational agents. The latter function of estrogen has allowed reduction of the progestational dose in the pill. A certain pharmacologic level of estrogen is necessary to maintain the potency of the combination pill. The mechanism for this action may be the fact that the concentration of intracellular progestin receptors is increased by estrogen. |

Since the effect of a progestational agent will always take precedence over estrogen (unless the dose of estrogen is increased many, many fold), the endometrium, cervical mucus, and perhaps tubal function reflect progestational stimulation. The progestin in the combination pill produces an endometrium which is not receptive to ovum implantation, a decidualized bed with exhausted and atrophied glands. The cervical mucus becomes thick and impervious to sperm transport. It is possible that further contraceptive effects are obtained by progestational influences on egg movement within the Fallopian tube.

Weighing against the remarkable effectiveness of oral contraception is the growing concern to both patient and physician with the major metabolic effects.

Failure Rates Per Year:

Oral Contraceptives	0.1%
IUD	2.0
Condoms and Diaphragms	15.0
Rhythm	25.0
Nothing	80.0

Metabolic Effects

| Oncogenic Potential | A major concern about the impact of the pill on human health is whether steroid contraception causes cancer. The major concern in this area has been directed toward the uterus (corpus and cervix) and the breast. It must be acknowledged that the duration of use of steroids has not been long enough to permit absolute statements on this critical issue. Nevertheless, reasonably secure judgments can be made on the basis of a large body of experimental work. |

Estrogen not only supports normal endometrium, but prolonged unopposed estrogen is associated with a progression of histologic change from hyperplasia to adenomatous hyperplasia to atypia. The chemotherapeutic use of progestational agents for endometrial neoplasia would suggest that periodic progestin may prevent or hinder these estrogen-induced changes. As currently constituted the combined progestin and estrogen pill has a protective effect and there have been no abnormal endometrial changes associated with this form of oral contraception. Adverse experience with endometrial neoplasia on sequential therapy points out the delicate balance of hormones required to sustain the protective effects. Too much estrogen or too little progestin would not confer the safety seen with current formulations.

No causal relationship has been established between oral contraceptives and pathologic changes of the uterine cervix. (4) A definitive long-term prospective study, however, has not yet been accomplished. Certainly steroid contraceptives do not mask abnormal cervical changes, and the necessity for prescription renewals should improve screening for cervical disease.

There does not seem to be a major concern in regard to uterine cancer; however, there continues to be worry over the effects of estrogen on breast tissue.

Estrogens have not produced breast tumors in hamsters, guinea pigs, goats, cows, dogs, or monkeys. This includes long-term administration, high dosage, and long follow-up. The induction of breast and genital tumors is limited to rats and mice, and to specific strains of rats and mice.

In December, 1974, an important monograph was published. (5) This document was the first report of an ongoing prospective study involving 46,000 women, carried out by the Royal College of General Practitioners in England. In this study there was no evidence of an association of breast cancer with pill usage in the 5 year period (1968–1974) of the report. This has also been a consistent finding in retrospective studies. (6, 7) Worth noting is an apparent protective effect toward benign disease of the breast associated with the progestin component of the pill, an effect which becomes apparent after 2 years of continuous usage. (5) Retrospective studies have also found a lower incidence of benign breast tumors in pill users. (6) However one retrospective study has indicated that women with already established benign breast disease may have an increased incidence of breast cancer with long-term use of the pill. (8)

A lingering concern is the possibility that the latent period between stimulus and neoplasia may be 10–20 years or more. Information bearing on this area can be found in surveys looking for changes in the incidence and mortality rates of breast cancer. There has been no increase in breast or genital cancer since 1930 in women over the age of 50, and the data by Feinleib and Garrison from the Connecticut Registry show no increase in mortality. (8, 9) However a long-term epidemiologic study is necessary to absolutely rule out an oncogenic potential for estrogen.

In women with breast cancer, hormonal treatment should, of course, be avoided. There is no evidence to suggest that women with a family history of breast cancer will increase their possibility of developing this disease by using oral contraceptives.

Thromboembolic Disease

There has been a striking rise in idiopathic thromboembolism in the Western world since 1958, but it has occured in both sexes, making an evaluation of this problem in pill users very difficult.

In the most recent retrospective study, The Boston Collaborative Drug Surveillance Program found an 11-fold increase in the relative risk for thromboembolism among pill users. (6) The estimated actual incidence among pill users was estimated to be 60 per 100,000 users per year (1:1700). Of significance is the fact that an increase in relative risk was not discovered among postmenopausal women using estrogen replacement therapy. (7) This is circumstantial evidence that the dose of estrogen is an important factor, since the dose of estrogen used in replacement therapy is not intended to be pharmacologic, but merely replacement for waning endogenous production.

In the English prospective study, the risk of deep thrombosis of the leg was 5.7 times that of controls, and the risk of superficial thrombosis in the leg was 1.5 times higher than the controls. (5)

The difference between a retrospective study and a prospective study should be emphasized. In a retrospective study, the percent of women using the pill is analyzed in patients who already have thromboembolism. In a prospective study, the percent of women who develop thromboembolism is compared between a group on the pill and a control group. The significance of the English study is that for the first time, a long term ongoing prospective study has provided risk estimates which support the previous retrospective reports.

Certain statistical information in the English report may be of the utmost importance. In December, 1969, The British Committee on the Safety of Drugs issued a recommendation that only the lowest estrogen dose brands should be used. Hence data from the early part of the prospective study was derived from brands containing more than 50 μg of estrogen, while data after 1969 largely reflected usage of brands containing 50 μg of estrogen. Thus the dose effect of estrogen could be studied.

The attributable risk of deep thrombosis was 81 per 100,000 pill users per year with the 50 μg dose. This incidence of 1:1200 compares remarkably with that estimated in retrospective studies. The attributable risk of deep thrombosis with estrogen doses greater than 50 μg was 112 per 100,000 per year. Therefore the attributable risk decreased by 28 percent upon using a lower estrogen dose.

Although previous retrospective studies had suggested that risk was lower for users of lower estrogen doses, these data are the first solid evidence that reducing the estrogen dose can significantly affect the incidence of what is probably the most serious side effect of the pill. Currently there is no information as to the incidence of thromboembolism with the new lower dose pills (20, 30, and 35 μg ethinyl estradiol). However it seems logical to assume that the lower the dose of estrogen the lower the risk of thrombosis.

The data from the English prospective study, along with the consistency among the retrospective studies appear to be very convincing. Especially significant to the clinician is the demonstrated relationship to estrogen. The implications go beyond contraceptive use of estrogens. A number of studies of women treated with estrogen during the puerperum to suppress lactation have shown an increased incidence of venous thrombosis. In addition, birth control pills should be discontinued at least one month prior to surgery and not resumed until full recovery is achieved. The risk of postoperative thromboembolism is estimated to be 3 to 4 fold higher in pill users. (10)

Neurovascular Accidents

Clinical reports are consistent with an association between the use of oral contraceptives and cerebrovascular disease in otherwise healthy young women. (11) Most impressive is the occurrence of lesions in the vertebrobasilar posterior cerebral arterial system, a rare site of thrombosis in younger persons. In comparing strokes in user and nonuser groups, about 25% of the strokes in the user group were in the vertebrobasilar area and essentially none occurred in this area in the nonuser group.

The information on stroke is derived from a large collaborative retrospective study in the United States. (12, 13) Since stroke in young women is a relatively rare phenomenon, significant data are yet to be generated in a prospective study. According to the retrospective studies, pill use increases the risk of thrombotic stroke 3-fold, and that of hemorrhagic stroke, 2-fold. No correlation was found with the various progestin doses. Stroke patients were found to be using both high estrogen pills and the 50 μg estrogen dose.

No significant potentiation of hypertension among pill users was noted. On the other hand, smoking and migraine headaches had variable effects on thrombotic and hemorrhagic stroke. Heavy smoking by pill users was associated with an increased risk of hemorrhagic stroke (1.2 to 7.6), while thrombotic stroke was not influenced. Migraine headache was not associated with a change in the incidence of hemorrhagic stroke, but the risk of thrombotic stroke was apparently increased from 2.0 to 5.9. However the data on migraine were inconclusive because of inconsistencies in the control groups.

Because of the seriousness of this potential complication, the onset of visual symptoms, or severe headaches should be regarded as warning signs. Rather than immediately discontinuing the pill, however, the physician and patient should consider switching to another brand within the same low dose range. Often this relieves the symptoms.

Myocardial Infarction

Two retrospective studies in England have suggested that the pill increases the risk of myocardial infarction. (14, 15) In a group of women admitted to hospitals with nonfatal myocardial infarction, the risk in pill users 30 to 39 years of age was increased 2.7 times, while the relative risk in women 40 to 44 was 5.7. A similar study analyzing women who did not survive myocardial infarction revealed relative risks of 2.8 for women 30 to 39 and 4.8 for women 40 to 44. The attributable mortality was approximately 3.5 deaths per 100,000 users yearly in women 40 to 44. Also, consideration of other risk factors (hypertension, cigarette smoking, obesity, diabetes) indicated that oral contraceptives acted synergistically, rather than additively. These data have indicated that the risk of circulatory diseases is increased with increasing age and is even higher when associated with other risk factors.

Adrenal Gland

For some time it has been known that estrogen increases cortisol-binding globulin, transcortin. It had been thought that the increase in plasma cortisol while on the pill was due to increased binding by the globulin and not an increase in free active cortisol. Now it is apparent that free and active cortisol levels are also elevated. (16) In addition, progesterone and related compounds may displace cortisol from transcortin, and thus contribute to the elevation of unbound cortisol. Estrogen decreases the ability of the liver to metabolize cortisol, and this also may contribute to elevated levels. The effects of these elevated levels over prolonged periods of time are unknown.

The adrenal gland responds to ACTH normally, therefore, there is no suppression of the adrenal gland itself. Initial studies showed that the response to metyrapone (a 11β-hydroxylase blocker) was abnormal, suggesting that the pituitary was suppressed. It has now been shown that estrogen accelerates the conjugation of metyrapone by the liver, and therefore the drug has less effect, explaining the subnormal responses initially reported. (17) The pituitary-adrenal reaction to stress is normal in women on oral contraceptive pills.

Thyroid

As with transcortin, estrogen increases thyroxine-binding globulin, and prior to the new methods of calculating the free thyroxine levels, evaluation of thyroid function was a problem. Estimation of the free thyroxine level utilizes the measurement of thyroid binding globulin levels, the total thyroxine level, and the percentage of thyroxine saturation of the binding globulin. The free thyroxine level is an accurate assessment of a patient's thyroid state. Birth control pills affect the total thyroxine level in the blood as well as the amount of binding globulin, but the free thyroxine level is unchanged.

Carbohydrate Metabolism

There is an impaired oral glucose tolerance test in 15–40% of women on the pill, and in these women plasma levels of insulin as well as the blood sugar are elevated. Generally the effect of the pill is to produce an increase in peripheral resistance to insulin action. Most women can meet this change by increasing insulin secretion, and there is no change in the glucose tolerance test. Individuals who cannot respond with an appropriate increase in insulin may have an abnormal glucose tolerance.

Carbohydrate metabolism is affected by both the progestin and estrogen components of the pill. (18) Compounds with a positive charge at the 5 carbon (3-keto structures and estrogens) have insulinogenic and insulin antagonistic effects. Not all progestins, however, are diabetogenic. 6-Dehydro derivatives (unsaturation of the B ring at the 6 carbon) such as chlormadinone and megestrol actually may improve glucose tolerance because they increase insulin response but have no antagonistic effects. The derangement of carbohydrate metabolism may also be affected by estrogen influences on lipid metabolism, hepatic enzymes, and elevation of free cortisol.

The clinical significance of the elevated blood sugar remains uncertain. The elevation of glucose while taking the pill may be a functional change which is not deleterious and is completely reversible.

In the English prospective study (5), there was no evidence that the altered carbohydrate metabolism increased the likelihood of developing clinical diabetes or its complications. In clinical practice it may, at times, be necessary to prescribe oral contraception for the overt diabetic. Although one would expect the insulin requirement to increase, close follow-up is indicated, for the effect is neither consistent nor predictable.

Lipid Metabolism	There are three major groups of lipoproteins: cholesterol, phospholipids, and triglycerides. Progestins have no apparent effect on these lipids, while plasma triglycerides and phospholipids are elevated by estrogen. (19) Cholesterol levels are essentially unchanged. These effects can be produced in subjects on fat-free diets, indicating that estrogen increases synthesis in the liver or impairs removal into adipose tissue.

Lipogenesis in the liver requires the presence of insulin, and the removal of triglycerides from plasma involves the action of an enzyme, lipoprotein lipase, located in or near adipose tissue capillaries. The effect of estrogen may be two-fold: (1) to increase insulin levels and thus lipogenesis; and (2) to inhibit lipase activity. Heparin causes release of the lipase enzyme into the circulation, and estrogen blocks this action of heparin.

Still unanswered is the question of the clinical significance of these changes. Elevated serum lipid and lipoprotein levels are associated with the development of clinical manifestations of atherosclerosis. In women with strong family histories of coronary disease, it would seem wise to obtain a plasma triglyceride level periodically. Those who have high serum lipid levels probably should not be on the pill.

Liver

The liver is affected in more ways and with more regularity and intensity by gonadal steroids than any other extragenital organ. Estrogen influences the synthesis of hepatic DNA and RNA, hepatic cell enzymes, serum enzymes formed in the liver, and plasma proteins. Estrogenic hormones also affect hepatic lipid and lipoprotein formation, the intermediary metabolism of carbohydrates, and intracellular enzyme activity. The active transport of biliary components is impaired by a large number of estrogens as well as some progestins. The mechanism is unclear, but cholestatic jaundice and pruritus are occasional complications of the pill, and are similar to the recurrent jaundice of pregnancy, i.e. benign and reversible. BSP retention is abnormal in approximately 20% of patients and alkaline phosphatase is increased in 2%, but SGOT elevation, if persistent, is not due to the pill.

The only absolute contraindication to pill use is acute or chronic cholestatic hepatic disease. Cirrhosis and previous hepatitis do not seem to be aggravated. In these days, with the increasing incidence of hepatitis, it is important to know that once recovered from the acute phase of the disease, a patient may take oral contraceptive pills.

As of 1976, a registry of liver adenomas in women on the pill had collected a total of 71 cases. (20) Statistically it was noted that the apparent risk increased after 5 years of pill usage. The adenomas may be solitary or there may be multiple nodules. Since the tumors are not malignant, the significance of this problem lies in the hemorrhagic consequences of tumor growth (8 deaths in 71 cases).

The most common presentation is acute right upper quadrant or epigastric pain. However the tumors may be asymptomatic or present suddenly with hematoperitoneum. There is some evidence that the tumors may regress when the pill is stopped. In addition to the adenomatous change, there is a vascular component, termed peliosis hepatis, characterized by dilated blood spaces without endothelial linings. Peliosis may occur in the absence of adenomatous changes.

No reliable screening test or procedure is currently available, and routine blood tests are normal. Computerized axial tomography (CAT scanning) may be the best means of diagnosis. Angiography and ultrasonography are not reliable. Palpation of the liver should be part of the 6 month evaluation.

An association between the pill and gallbladder disease was first noted in the Boston Collaborative Drug Surveillance Program. (6) The relative risk in pill users was 2.0 with an annual estimated incidence of 158 per 100,000 per year. A similar increase in risk was noted with the use of replacement estrogen therapy in postmenopausal women.

The English prospective study verified the retrospective data, finding a 2-fold increase in risk of gallstones and cholecystitis. (5) The incidence of gallstones rose after the first 2 years of use, and plateaued after 4–5 years at a rate twice that of the control group. The mechanism for this problem appears to be induced alterations in the composition of gallbladder bile, specifically a rise in cholesterol saturation which is presumably an estrogen effect. (21)

The first mention of hypertension and oral contraceptive pills was a brief paragraph in 1962 in the Canadian Medical Association Journal by Brownrigg, reporting a patient who had the onset of hypertension while being treated for endometriosis. (22) The first well-documented cases are in what is already a classic paper by Laragh, et al, in 1967. (23)

The mechanism is thought to involve the renin-angiotensin system. (24, 25) The most consistent finding is a marked increase in plasma angiotensinogen, up to 8 times normal values. In the majority of women, excessive vasoconstriction may be prevented by a compensatory decrease in plasma renin concentration. It is also possible that excessive volume due to sodium retention plays the predominant role in the mechanism of pill-induced hypertension.

If hypertension develops, the renin-angiotensin changes may take 3–6 months to disappear after stopping the pill. This is an estrogen effect and can be produced in normal males by ethinyl estradiol. The problem is to identify the susceptible patient, and at this time there is no way to do so. A history of pre-eclampsia does not appear to be an added risk factor, nor is pill-induced hypertension known to predispose a woman to develop pre-eclampsia.

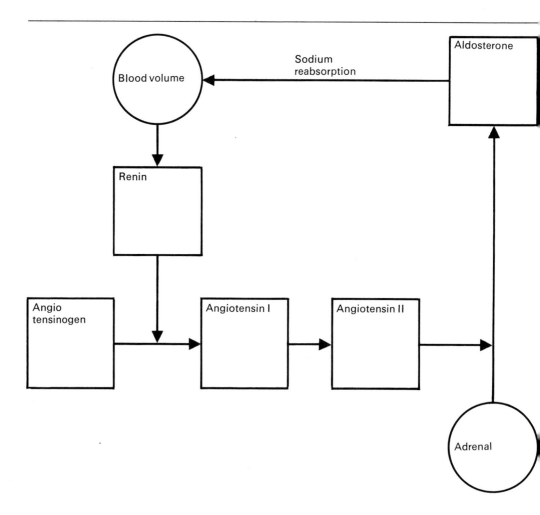

In the English prospective study, the incidence of hypertension was 2.6 times that of controls after 5 years of pill usage. Overall, 5 percent of pill users developed statistically significant hypertension after 5 years of pill usage. The frequency increased with duration of usage.

A puzzling finding in the English study was the failure to demonstrate a relationship to estrogen. In fact, an apparent correlation was demonstrated with the dose of progestin. It is possible that this correlation is related to the metabolism of the 19-nortestosterone compounds to estrogens within the body, since administration of 19-nortestosterone agents to patients affects the renin-angiotensin-aldosterone system in the same fashion as estrogen. Progesterone and 17-acetoxy progestational agents do not have this effect. It seems reasonable to believe that hypertension with the pill is an estrogen effect, due to the estrogenic contribution from both the estrogen and progestin components of the pill.

One must also consider the effects of oral contraceptives in patients with pre-existing hypertension or cardiac disease. Again a judgment is necessary as to the importance of 100% contraception. Pre-existing hypertension does not seem to be a contraindication as long as close follow-up is maintained. Close follow-up is also indicated in patients with a history of pre-existing renal disease, hypertension during pregnancy, and a family history of hypertension and its consequences. One consideration is the effect of the oral contraceptive on cardiac work. Significant increases in cardiac output, systolic blood pressure, and plasma volume have been recorded, probably a result of fluid retention. (26) Because of these changes, patients with marginal cardiac reserve should utilize other means of contraception.

Other Metabolic Effects

Gastrointestinal disorders, breast discomfort, and weight gain remain the most common disturbing effects. Fortunately, these are most intense in the first few months of use, and in most cases, gradually disappear. It should be emphasized that the weight gain which takes place usually responds to dietary restriction. For some patients, this is very difficult and fluid retention accentuates the problem.

Chloasma, an increase in facial pigment, was at one time found to occur in approximately 5% of pill users. It is our clinical impression that chloasma is now an infrequent problem, perhaps due to the increasing use of low dose oral contraceptives. Unfortunately, once chloasma appears, it fades gradually following discontinuance of the pill, and may never disappear completely. Skin blanching medications may be useful.

297

In the English prospective study (5) urinary tract infe
tions were increased by 20%, and a correlation w
noted with the estrogen dose. An increased incidence
cervicitis was reported, an effect related to the progest
dose. The incidence of cervicitis increased with the leng
of time the pill was used, from no higher after 6 montl
to 3 times higher by the 6th year of use. Though tl
difference was not quite significant, there seemed to be
trend toward an increased number of new cases of ej
lepsy.

Hematologic effects include an increased sedimentatic
rate due to increased levels of fibrinogen, increased tot
iron-binding capacity due to the increase in globulin
and a decrease in prothrombin time. The cyclic use of tl
pill may prevent the appearance of symptoms in porphyr
precipitated by menses. On the other hand porphyr
may be worsened.

In rare cases, mental depression is associated with or
contraceptives. In some cases, the effect is due to estroge
interference with the synthesis of tryptophan. The mec:
anism is unknown, but the effect is reversible. Thoug
infrequent, a reduction in libido is occasionally encou:
tered, and may be cause for seeking an alternative methc
of contraception.

Useful side effects include relief of dysmenorrhea in 90 ¹
of patients. Improvement may also be seen with preme:
strual tension, heavy bleeding and iron deficiency anemi
acne, and hirsutism.

**Postpill
Amenorrhea**

There are claims that postpill amenorrhea is a relative
common problem. However an etiologic role for the p
is by no means certain. Most women (80%) resun
normal function in 3 months after discontinuing the pi
and 95–98% are ovulating in 1 year. (27, 28)

The approximate incidence of postpill amenorrhea is 0
to 0.8%. (29, 30) If a cause and effect relationsh
exists, one would expect the incidence of postpill ame
orrhea to exceed that of spontaneous secondary amenc
rhea. Little information is available on the normal in
dence of secondary amenorrhea.

There is only one report in the literature which estimat
the incidence of spontaneous secondary amenorrhea.
retrospective postal survey of the female population
Uppsala County, Sweden, revealed an incidence of 0.7
of secondary amenorrhea of more than 6 months dur
tion. (31) This figure corresponds remarkably to tl
usual reported incidence of secondary amenorrhea
women who discontinue oral contraception.

If a cause and effect relationship exists between the p
and subsequent amenorrhea, one would expect the in
dence of infertility to be increased after a given populatic

298

discontinues use of the pill. In those women who discontinue the pill in order to get pregnant, 50% conceive by 3 months; and after 2 years, a maximum of 15% of nonparous women and 7% of parous women fail to conceive (5), figures comparable to those quoted as the prevalence of spontaneous infertility. Thus there appears to be no increase in the incidence of infertility in women discontinuing the pill. This argues against a cause and effect relationship between the pill and secondary amenorrhea. It is more likely that patients with this problem come more quickly to our attention because of the previous pill use and physician follow-up. Patients who have not resumed menstrual function within 6 months should be evaluated as any patient with secondary amenorrhea. Not all postpill amenorrheas are hormonally related and reversible. Other pathologic entities such as pituitary tumors arising during pill use must be excluded.

An important question is: should birth control pills be advised for a young girl with irregular menses and oligo-ovulation? The fear of subsequent infertility should not be a deterrent to providing appropriate contraception. Our clinical experience is that hypothalamic suppression is less of a risk to the patient than leaving her unprotected. The need for contraception should take precedence.

Evaluation of Patient and Choice of Pill

Absolute contraindications to the use of the pill:

1. Thrombophlebitis, thromboembolic disorders, cerebral vascular disease, coronary occlusion, or a past history of these conditions, or conditions predisposing to these problems.

2. Markedly impaired liver function.

3. Known or suspected carcinoma of the breast.

4. Known or suspected estrogen-dependent neoplasia.

5. Undiagnosed abnormal genital bleeding.

6. Known or suspected pregnancy.

7. Obstructive jaundice in pregnancy.

8. Congenital hyperlipidemia.

Relative contraindications requiring clinical judgment and informed consent by the patient:

1. Migraine headache.

2. Hypertension.

3. Uterine leiomyomata.

4. Epilepsy.

5. Varicose veins.

299

6. Gestational diabetes.

7. Elective Surgery.

Patients should be seen every 6 months for exclusion of contraindications by history, palpation of the liver, urinalysis for sugar and protein, and blood pressure. This can be performed reliably by appropriately trained paramedical personnel. Breast and pelvic examinations with PAP smear should be done yearly. A plasma triglyceride level may be indicated in selected cases.

The therapeutic principle remains: utilize the pill which gives effective contraception and the greatest margin of safety. The major side effects, those which are responsible for significant morbidity and mortality, are related to the estrogen component of the combination pill. The recent information reviewed above results in a compelling argument for a dose-related response between the incidence of thrombosis and the estrogen content of the pill. While there is no current evidence to support the view that there is greater safety with pills containing less than 50 μg of estrogen, it is reasonable for the physician to begin treatment with the new lower dose estrogen combination pills.

In our clinical experience, the 20 μg pill is associated with excessive breakthrough bleeding. The 30 μg pill, however, combines the possible safety of reduced estrogen levels with a tolerable level of problems. The breakthrough bleeding is not excessive and can be handled as outlined below. Contraceptive efficacy is not diminished with the 30 μg pill. (32)

There appears to be no advantage to using pills which contain 35 μg of estrogen, and there is no advantage clearly demonstrated for one brand over another. The overriding principle is to utilize a brand of 30 μg for its implied safety margin. The pharmacologic effects in animals of various birth control pills have been used as a basis for therapeutic recommendations in selecting the optimum oral contraceptive pill. (33, 34, 35, 36) All too often the physician prescribes a pill of excessive estrogen dosage with its attendant increased risk of serious side effects. This approach (tailor-making the pill to the patient) is not supported by appropriate controlled clinical trials. It is far more prudent to be guided by the principles of effectiveness and safety.

There is no rationale for recommending a pill-free interval. The serious side effects of greatest frequency (thromboembolic phenomena) are not related to duration of usage. Pill-free intervals all too often result in unwanted pregnancies.

Combination pill contraception can diminish lactation, but of greater concern is the potential hazard of the

300

crossover of steroids to the infant. Use should be deferred until lactation is discontinued.

What to do for Amenorrhea on the Pill

The lack of withdrawal bleeding on the pill is a common situation with the new low dose pills. The lower estrogen content, for many women, is not of sufficient potency to allow endometrial growth. Hence the endometrium is shallow, and atrophic, lacking sufficient tissue to produce a withdrawal bleed. The major problem with this development is the anxiety produced in the patient, since the lack of bleeding may be an early sign of pregnancy. Permanent atrophy of the endometrium does not occur, and resumption of normal ovarian function will restore endometrial growth and function.

Retrospective studies have indicated that exogenous hormone administered during pregnancy is associated with the following deformities: neural tube defects, abnormalities of the heart and great vessels, and limb reduction deformities. None of the reported deformities has occurred in the continuing English prospective survey (37) In fact, no adverse effects on subsequent births have been noted including the spontaneous abortion rate. Nevertheless, the first episode of amenorrhea deserves evaluation. Reassurance of the patient along with a basic education as to why there is no bleeding usually alleviates the concern. Alerting patients upon starting the pill to the possibility of no withdrawal bleeding may totally avoid subsequent anxiety. Some women cannot reconcile themselves to a lack of bleeding for a variety of reasons, and this is one of the indications for utilizing a pill with a higher estrogen dose (almost never greater than 50 μg).

What to do for Breakthrough Bleeding

There are two kinds of irregular bleeding with the new low dose pills. The first kind occurs in the first several months upon starting the 30 μg pill. This represents adjustment to the new dose of the pill, whether one is starting anew, or switching from a higher estrogen dose. Encouragement and reassurance generally suffice as the bleeding settles down and becomes regular. The second type of irregular bleeding is breakthrough bleeding occurring at any time during the pill cycle after a patient has been on the pill beyond several months.

Both kinds of irregular bleeding respond well to short courses of exogenous estrogen. Conjugated estrogens 2.5 mg or ethinyl estradiol 20 μg daily for 7 days can be administered when the bleeding is persistent, annoying, or heavy. Usually one course of exogenous estrogen will solve the problem. Occasionally repeat courses of estrogen are necessary. The treatment is effective no matter how long the patient has been on the pill. Any bleeding which is not handled by this routine requires investigation for the presence of pathology.

Responding to irregular bleeding by having the patie take two or three pills daily rather than one is n effective. The progestin component of the pill will alwa dominate, hence doubling the number of pills will al double the progestational stimulus. This increases t decidualizing, atrophic impact on the endometrium.

Should the Older Woman Use the Pill?

The retrospective studies on myocardial infarction a pulmonary embolism indicated an increasing risk wi increasing age, especially marked in pill users who smok Utilizing assumptions based on this data, Tietze (38 performed a computer simulation study which indicat the age-specific mortality which was associated with fert ity control.

Death due to the use of the pill is significantly lower tha the birth-related risk of death without fertility contro After the age of 30, the risk to life increases rapidly f pill users who smoke. After the age of 40, the death ra due to the pill in women who smoke is now actual higher than if no method of contraception were use Such a statistical analysis has led to the recommendatic that women over the age of 40 who smoke should u contraceptive methods other than the pill and rely upc therapeutic abortion for the occasional method failur Even more reasonable is to urge upon one of the partne a surgical sterilization.

Since the average age of menopause is 51.5, some mea of contraception may be necessary in most women un the age of 50. If an older woman (over 35) elects to utili oral contraception, she should be aware of the higher ris involved with increasing age, and that additional facto such as diabetes, smoking, hypertension, and obesity ad to the risk of death due to a variety of circulatory disease Very recent data have indicated that women who hav been taking the pill for more than 5 years also seem be at greater risk for death.

An Alternative to the Pill

A useful alternative to the pill, especially in those wome in whom estrogen is contraindicated, is Depo-Prover Two observations are important: first, it requires 6 to months for the drug to totally clear from the averag woman, and second, the effective contraception level maintained for 4 months. Therefore, 150 mg given intr muscularly every 3 months assures 100 percent contrace tion. (39)

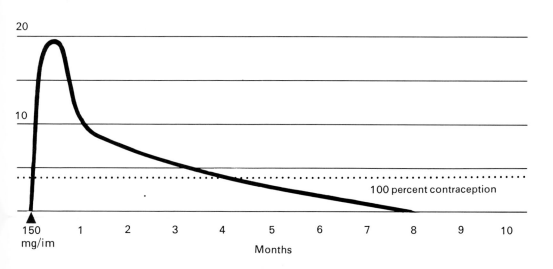

The progestin in depo form effectively blocks the LH surge, and in addition affects the endometrium and cervical mucus. The suppression of gonadotropins is not as complete as it is with the pill. This is an advantage, since follicular growth is maintained at a sufficient level to produce estrogen levels comparable to those in the follicular phase of a normal cycle. In other words, Depo-Provera does not produce a hypoestrogenic state.

This progestin, in large continuous doses, produced breast cancer in Beagle dogs. This appears to be an effect unique to the Beagle dog, and has not appeared in other animals, or in women after years of use. (39) Major problems with this drug are breakthrough bleeding, weight gain, and depression. (40) Breakthrough bleeding can be treated with exogenous estrogen as noted above. Serious weight gain and depression are not relieved until the drug clears 6 to 8 months after the last shot.

Depo-Provera has cortisol-like effects, and in large doses, suppresses adrenal function. (41) Although this does not appear to be a significant clinical problem in contraceptive doses, further investigation is warranted.

The major advantage to the use of Depo-Provera is its freedom from the side effects of estrogen. Hence it can be used in patients with congenital heart disease, sickle cell anemia, or patients with a previous history of thromboembolism. Another advantage is the finding that Depo-Provera increases the quantity of milk in nursing mothers, a direct contrast to the effect seen with the pill. (42) However the concentration of the drug in the breast milk and the effects of the drug on the child are unknown.

The belief that infertility with suppressed menstrual function may be caused by Depo-Provera is not borne out by the available data. The pregnancy rate in women ceasing the injections because of a desire to become pregnant is normal. However only 2 followup studies have been reported. (43, 44) Thus, although further documentation is necessary, it appears that suppressed menstrual function persisting beyond 8 months after the last injection is probably not due to the drug itself.

Other Methods

While the pill provides almost 100% contraception, many women still find even minor side effects intolerable. Even more important are some of the unanswered questions concerning long-term use. For these reasons, a search for better contraception continues.

The minipill is the continuous daily use of a low dose of a potent progestational agent. The contraceptive effect is more dependent upon endometrial and cervical mucus effects, since luteinizing hormone is not consistently suppressed. (45) Tubal physiology may also be affected. The main disadvantage is less than perfect contraception (2.5% failure). Another drawback is unexpected and irregular bleeding, to the point of extreme patient dissatisfaction with the method.

The use of cyclopentyl ether derivatives of ethinyl estradiol and progestins for once-a-month pills or injections depends upon fat storage with daily release for effect. Variability in body response is a problem, since large doses of hormones are given.

Steroids diffuse through the walls of Silastic capsules at a rate controlled by thickness of the walls and the surface area. A large dose of a potent progestin inside of a Silastic capsule implanted under the skin will give contraception for 1–2 years. However, the capsules must be removed through an incision. Bleeding problems are similar to use of the mini-pill, since the principle is the same. Another approach is the use of vaginal Silastic rings impregnated with progestational compounds. One advantage would be the possibility for patient insertion and removal on a monthly basis. The problem of side effects can be further reduced using low dose progestin-impregnated Silastic devices in the cervix. These could be contraceptive by changing cervical mucus and blocking sperm transport.

Postcoital Contraception

Estrogen in large doses is effective in preventing conception after midcycle coital exposure. (46) Diethylstilbestrol, 50 mg/day, is given for 5 days, within 72 hours after exposure, along with an antiemetic for control of gastrointestinal symptoms. The mechanism for this "morning after" technique remains to be determined, but its effectiveness has been confirmed in a large clinical study. (47) There is no reason to believe that other estrogens would not be as effective; however in the absence of documentation with clinical studies, no recommendations can be made as to proper dosage. Because of possible harmful effects to a fetus, an already existing pregnancy should be ruled out prior to use of diethylstilbestrol. Furthermore, the patient should agree to therapeutic abortion if the drug fails.

The Medicated IUD

The intrauterine device is relatively inexpensive, does not require continued motivation, and is easily reversible. There are significant drawbacks, however, including: bleeding, pain, expulsion of the device, perforation, increased risk of pelvic infection, and unplanned pregnancies, either with the device in situ or after unnoticed expulson or perforation. In addition the IUD does not protect against ectopic pregnancies. The newer IUDs have utilized hormones, copper, and different sizes and shapes in an effort to conform better to the endometrial cavity, thus causing minimal mechanical effects and reducing the incidence of side effects.

It is likely that the contraceptive effect of copper involves a direct metabolic effect upon endometrial cells. The copper T and the copper 7 have pregnancy rates from 1.5 to 3.0 per 100 women per year. Such devices are approved for up to 2 years of use, but investigational programs have continued through 3 and 4 years. It appears that adding more copper reduces the pregnancy rate, although proper insertion with placement high in the fundus continues to be essential for effective contraceptive action.

The combination of progesterone with the T device is the first hormonal device available in the U.S. (48) The continuous release of small amounts of the hormone is associated with a local uterine activity without systemic effects. Sustained continuous release allows the use of progesterone itself, rather than one of the synthetic progestins. Even though progesterone has a short half life, the steady release allows maintenance of a constant and effective local level of the hormone.

The mechanism of action is unknown, although it believed that the local effect of the progesterone on the endometrium (decidualization) renders it incapable of sustaining implantation. The local progesterone also affects the cervical mucus, thus making passage of sperm difficult. There has been a reduction in the incidence of cramping and bleeding. In addition, there may be beneficial effect of the local progesterone on dysmenorrhea and menorrhagia perhaps due to an inhibition of prostaglandin production by the endometrium. The pregnancy rates are approximately 1.9 and 2.5 per 100 woman-years in parous and nulliparous women respectively. (48) Currently, the device must be replaced yearly.

The risk of salpingitis is increased in women using intrauterine devices. (49) Although it has been suggested that copper may protect against gonorrhea, no such protective effect could be detected in a clinical study. (49) Because of these factors, we do not recommend an IUD until the patient understands that future fertility can be compromised.

References

1. **Goldzieher, JW, Maqueo M, Chenault CB, and Woutersz TB,** Comparative Studies of the Ethinyl Estrogens Used in Oral Contraceptives. I. Endometrial Response, Am Obstet Gynec 122:615, 1975.

2. **Goldzieher JW, De La Pena A, Chenault CB, and Woutersz TB,** Comparative Studies of the Ethinyl estrogens Used in Oral Contraceptives. II. Antiovulatory Potency, Am J Obstet Gynec 122:619, 1975.

3. **Goldzieher JW, De La Pena A, Chenault CB, and Cervantes A,** Comparative Studies of the Ethinyl Estrogens Used in Oral Contraceptives. III. Effect on Plasma Gonadotropins, Am J Obstet Gynec 122:625, 1975.

4. **Maqueo M, Azuela JC, Calderon JJ, and Goldzieher JW,** Morphology of the Cervix in Women Treated with Synthetic Progestins, Am J Obstet Gynec 96:994, 1966.

5. **Royal College of General Practitioners,** *Oral Contraceptives and Health,* Pitman Publishing Company, New York 1974.

6. **Boston Collaborative Drug Surveillance Program,** Oral Contraceptives and Venous Thromboembolic Disease, Surgically Confirmed Gallbladder Disease, and Breast Tumors, Lancet 1:1399, 1973.

7. **Boston Collaborative Drug Surveillance Program,** Surgically Confirmed Gallbladder Disease, Venous Thromboembolism, and Breast Tumors in Relation to Postmenopausal Estrogen Therapy, New Eng J Med 290:15, 1974.

8. **Fasal E, and Paffenbarger RS, Jr.,** Oral Contraceptives as Related to Cancer and Benign Lesions of the Breast, J Natl Cancer Inst 55:767, 1975.

9. **Feinleib M, and Garrison RJ,** Interpretation of the Vital Statistics of Breast Cancer, Cancer 24:1109, 1969.

10. **Vessey, MP, Doll, R. Fairnbairn, AS, and Glober, E,** Postoperative Thromboembolism and the use of Oral Contraceptives, Br Med J 2:123, 1970.

11. **Masi, AT, and Dugdale, M,** Cerebrovascular Diseases Associated with the Use of Oral Contraceptives, Ann Intern Med 72:111, 1970.

12. **Collaborative Group for the Study of Stroke in Young Women,** Oral Contraceptives and Stroke in Young Women, JAMA 231:718, 1975.

13. **Collaborative Group for the Study of Stroke in Young Women,** Oral Contraception and Increased Risk of Cerebral Ischemia or Thrombosis, New Eng J Med 288:871, 1973.

14. **Mann, JI, Vessey, MP, Thorogood, M, and Doll, R,** Myocardial Infarction in Young Women with Special Reference to Oral Contraceptive Practice, Br Med J 2:241, 1975.

15. **Mann, JI, and Inman, WHW,** Oral Contraceptives and Death from Myocardial Infarction, Br Med J 2:245, 1975.

16. **Burke, CW,** Biologically Active Cortisol in Plasma of Oestrogen-treated and Normal Subjects, Br Med J 2:798, 1969.

17. **Meikle, AW, Jubiz, W, Matsukura, KS, Harada, G, West, CD, and Tyler, FH,** Effect of Estrogen on the Metabolism of Metyrapone and Release of ACTH, J Clin Endocrinol Metab 30:259, 1970.

18. **Beck, P,** Effects of Gonadal Hormones and Contraceptive Steroids on Glucose and Insulin Metabolism, in Salhanick, HA, Kipnis, DM, and Vande Wiele, RL, eds, *Metabolic Effects of Gonadal Hormones and Contraceptive Steroids,* Plenum Press, New York, 1969, p. 97.

19. **Salhanick, HA, Kipnis, D M, and Vande Wiele, RL, eds,** *Metabolic Effects of Gonadal Hormones and Contraceptive Steroids,* Plenum Press, New York, 1969.

20. **Nissen, ED, Kent, Dr, and Nissen, SE,** Etiologic Factors in the Pathogenesis of Liver Tumors Associated with Oral Contraceptives, Am J Obstet Gynec 127:61, 1977

21. **Bennion, LJ, Ginsberg, RL, Garnick, MB, and Bennett, PH,** Effects of Oral Contraceptives on the Gallbladder Bile of Normal Women, New Eng J Med 294:189, 1976

22. **Brownrigg, GM,** Toxemia in Hormone-induced Pseudopregnancy, Can Med Assoc J 87:408, 1962.

23. **Laragh, JH, Sealey, JE, Ledingham, JGG, and Newton, MA,** Oral Contraceptives, Renin, Aldosterone, and High Blood Pressure, JAMA 201:918, 1967.

24. **Skinner, Sl, Lumbers, ER, and Symonds, EM,** Alteration by Oral Contraceptives of Normal Menstrual Changes in Plasma Renin Activity Concentration, and Substrate, Clin Sci 36:67, 1969.

25. **Crane, MG, Harris, JJ, and Winsor, W, III,** Hypertension, Oral Contraceptive Agents, and Conjugated Estrogens, Ann Intern Med 74:13, 1971.

26. **Walters, WAW, and Lim, YL,** Cardiovascular Dynamics in Women Receiving Oral Contraceptive Therapy, Lancet 2:879, 1969.

27. **Mears, E,** Pregnancy Following Antifertility Agents, Int J Fertil 13:340, 1968.

28. **Rice-Wray, E, Correu, S, Gorodovsky, J, Esquivel, J, and Goldzieher, JW,** Return of Ovulation after Discontinuance of Oral Contraceptives, Fertil Steril 18:212, 1967.

29. **Furuhjelm, M, and Carlstrom, K,** Amenorrhea Following Use of Combined Oral Contraceptives, Acta Obstet Gynec Scand 52:373, 1973.

30. **Shearman, RP, and Smith, ID,** Statistical Analysis of Relationship Between Oral Contraceptives, Secondary Amenorrhea and Galactorrhea, J Obstet Gynec Brit Comwlth 79:654, 1972.

31. **Pettersson, F, Fries, H. and Nillius, SJ,** Epidemiology of Secondary Amenorrhea. I. Incidence and Prevalence Rates, Am J Obstet Gynec 117:80, 1973.

32. **Woutersz, TB,** Three and One-half Years' Experience with a Lower-dose Combination Oral Contraceptive, J Reprod Med 16:338, 1976.

33. **Behrman, SJ,** Which "Pill" to Choose? Hospital Practice 4:34, 1969.

34. **Nelson, JH,** Selecting the Optimum Oral Contraceptive, J Reprod Med 11:135, 1973.

35. **Dickey, RP, and Stone, SC,** Progestational Potency of Oral Contraceptives, Obstet Gynec 47:106, 1976.

36. **Chihal, HJW, Peppler, RD, and Dickey, RP,** Estrogen Potency of Oral Contraceptive Pills, Am J Obstet Gynec 121:75, 1975.

37. **Royal College of General Practitioners,** The Outcome of Pregnancy in Former Oral Contraceptive Users, Br J Obstet Gynec 83:608, 1976.

38. **Tietze, C,** New Estimates of Mortality Associated With Family Control, Family Planning Prospectives 9:74, 1977.

39. **Nash, HA,** Depo-Provera: A Review, Contraception 12:377, 1975.

40. **Schwallie, PC, and Assenzo, JR,** Contraceptive Use-Efficacy Study Utilizing Medroxyprogesterone Acetate Administered as an Intramuscular Injection Once Every 90 Days, Fertil Steril 24:331, 1973.

41. **Hellman, L, Yoshida, K, Zumoff, B, Levin, J, Kream, J, and Fukushima, OK,** The Effect of Medroxyprogesterone Acetate on the Pituitary-Adrenal Axis, J Clin Endocrinol Metab 42:912, 1976.

42. **Schwallie, PC,** Experience with Depo-Provera as an Injectable Contraceptive, J Reprod Med 13:113, 1974.

43. **McDaniel, EB, and Pardthiasong, T,** Depo-Medroxyprogesterone Acetate as a Contraceptive Agent: Return of Fertility After Discontinuation of Use, Contraception 8:407, 1973.

44. **Schwallie, PC, and Assenzo, JR,** The Effect of Depomedroxyprogesterone Acetate on Pituitary and Ovarian Function and the Return of Fertility Following Discontinuation, A Review, Contraception 10:181, 1974.

45. **Taymor, ML, and Levesque, LA,** Levels of Serum Follicle-Stimulating Hormone, Luteinizing Hormone, and Plasma Progestin During Microdose Chlormadinone Treatment, Fertil Steril 22:1, 1971.

46. **Morris, J, McL, and van Wagenen, G,** Compounds Interfering with Ovum Implantation and Development. III. The Role of Estrogens, Am J Obstet Gynec 96:804, 1966.

47. **Kuchera, LK,** Postcoital Contraception with Diethylstilbestrol, Contraception 10:47, 1974.

48. **Pharriss, BB, Erickson, R, Bashaw, J, Hoff, S, Plac VA and Zaffaroni, A,** Progestasert: A Uterine Therape tic System for Long-term Contraception. I. Philosop and Clinical Efficacy, Fertil Steril 25:915, 1974.

49. **Westrom, L, Bengtsson, LP, and Mardh, P,** The Risk Pelvic Inflammatory Disease in Women Using Intraute ine Contraceptive Devices Compared to Non-users, La cet 2:221, 1976.

15

Investigation of the Infertile Couple

Infertility affects approximately 10% of couples, which makes it one of the more common problems for which people seek medical aid. In response to this need physicians should have three goals in mind:

1. The first is to seek out and to correct the causes of infertility. With proper evaluation and therapy, approximately 50% of couples attending an infertility clinic will become pregnant.

2. The second is to provide accurate information for the couple and to dispel the misinformation commonly gained from friends and mass media.

3. The third objective is to counsel the couple at what point to discontinue the investigation and to seek adoption as an alternative to conception. Unfortunately this option has been severely limited by the recent lack of children available for adoption.

Because of the shortage of adoptable babies, couples are more susceptible now to suggestions of therapy no matter how tenuous their rationale. Women should not be told that they are infertile because they are too nervous. Unless anxiety interferes with ovulation or coital frequency, there is no present evidence that infertility is caused by the usual anxieties besetting a couple attempting to conceive. (1) Despite many anecdotes to the contrary, adoption does not increase a couple's fertility. (2) The treatment of euthyroid infertile women with thyroid has repeatedly been shown to be worthless. (3, 4). A dilatation and curettage (D and C) is not a legitimate part of a routine infertility investigation. It provides minimal information beyond that obtained by endometrial biopsy and is both expensive and potentially hazardous because it subjects the woman to the risk of general anesthesia. There is also no evidence to support the old belief that a woman becomes more fertile following D and C. If a woman has menstrual bleeding that indicates patency of the canal, then dilatation of the cervix for "stenosis" will not improve fertility.

Unfortunately, uterine suspensions are still being performed as a primary treatment for infertility. In a study by Carter et al, it was shown that patients with retroversion of the uterus, unassociated with pelvic adhesions, who were subjected to suspension operations, had a lower pregnancy rate than women with retroversion who had no surgery. (5) Uterine suspension is helpful only when it is secondary to operation for other indications such as endometriosis or pelvic adhesions.

The uterus has a tremendous capacity for expansion, given the proper stimulus, and this holds true for every size uterus. Therefore, we do not believe that the so called "infantile" or "hypoplastic" uterus should ever be blamed for infertility. Many young women have been psychologically traumatized because a physician told them that their uterus was too small for pregnancy.

Equally ill advised in the investigation of infertility is the routine ordering of laboratory tests such as skull x-rays, urinary determinations of 17-ketosteroids, and gonadotropins not indicated by clinical judgment. These may be of value in selected cases but certainly not in every case.

The philosophy should not be "try it, it might just work." We have seen too many disillusioned couples who, without any indication, have been given clomiphene, Provera, and low dose estrogen, and then have been treated with husband inseminations. The goals of the practitioner should be to accomplish a thorough investigation, to treat any abnormalities that are uncovered, to educate the couple in the working of the reproductive system, and to give the couple some estimate of their fertility potential. If these goals are achieved by a sympathetic, understanding physician they will satisfy most couples who suffer from infertility.

Knowledge of the interactions that take place between sperm and the female reproductive tract can aid the physician to make rational clinical judgments. *Therefore prior to reviewing the clinical problems of infertility, this chapter will briefly examine the mechanisms involved in fertilization.*

Mechanisms in Fertilization

Sperm Transport

Semen forms a gel almost immediately following ejaculation but then is liquefied in 20–30 minutes by enzymes derived from the prostate gland. The alkaline pH of semen provides protection for the sperm from the acid pH of the vagina. This protection is transient and most sperm left in the vagina are immobilized within 2 hours. The more fortunate sperm by their own motility gain entrance into the tongues of cervical mucus which layer over the ectocervix. Sperm have been found in mucus within 90 seconds of ejaculation. (6) Bedford demonstrated that destruction of all sperm in the vagina 5 minutes after ejaculation does not interfere with fertilization in the rabbit which further attests to the rapidity of transport. (7) Uterine contractions propel the sperm upward and in the human they can be found in the tube 5 minutes after insemination. (8) It is possible that the first sperm to enter the tube are at a disadvantage. In the rabbit these early sperm have only poor motility and there is frequent disruption of the head membranes. (9) Therefore, sperm temporarily held in the cervical mucus, then released into the uterus, may be critical for fertilization.

The attrition of sperm numbers from vagina to tube is substantial. Of an average of 200,000,000 to 300,000,000 sperm deposited in the vagina, less than 200 achieve proximity to the egg. (8, 10) The major loss occurs in the vagina with expulsion of semen from the introitus playing an important role. Other causes for loss are digestion of sperm by vaginal enzymes, phagocytosis of sperm all along the reproductive tract and, to a limited extent, movement of sperm through the fallopian tube into the peritoneal cavity. (11, 12) There are also reports of sperm burrowing into or being engulfed by endometrial cells.

Sperm Capacitation

The discovery in 1951 that mammalian spermatozoa must spend some hours in the female tract before acquiring the capacity to penetrate ova stimulated intensive research efforts to delineate the environmental conditions required for this sperm capacitation. (13, 14) Attention was focused on the hormonal and time requirements, the potential for *in vitro* capacitation, and the identification of a substance in seminal fluid which, when added to capacitated sperm, rendered them decapacitated. (15, 16) An important finding was that capacitation changes the surface characteristics of sperm as exemplified by

313

modification of their surface charge. (16, 17) These changes, which cannot be identified morphologically, result in decreased stability of the plasma membrane and the membrane lying immediately under it, the outer acrosomal membrane. The membranes undergo further more striking modification, when capacitated sperm reach the vicinity of an ovum or when they are incubated in follicular fluid. There is a breakdown and merging of the plasma membrane and the outer acrosomal membrane (16) This allows egress of the enzyme contents of the acrosome, the cap-like structure which covers the sperm nucleus. These enzymes, hyaluronidase, a neuraminidase like factor, corona dispersing enzyme, and a protease called acrosin, are all thought to play roles in sperm penetration of the egg investments. (15, 18)

Capacitation which has been carefully elucidated in the rabbit and identified in a number of other species may have little relevance to human reproduction. Human sperm, as well as that of the mouse, after incubation in a defined medium are capable of fertilizing an ovum. (19) A period of residence in the female reproductive tract is not required.

Speculation concerning the use of the seminal fluid constituent that decapacitates sperm as a contraceptive agent was stimulated by its successful use in rabbits. Consideration of the amounts of material needed and the requirements for a delivery system indicated that, at least for the human, decapacitation factor is not a realistic contraceptive.

Egg Transport
And
Fertilization

The egg is ovulated surrounded by follicular cells. These adhere together to the ovarian surface until picked up by the fimbria of the Fallopian tube. The cilia of the fimbria move the cumulus mass into the tube. If the ovum is freed from the follicular cells the cilia are unable to move the egg effectively. The follicular cells thus provide the contact vital to the initial transport of the ovum. In addition, processes from the follicular cells extend through the zona pellucida to make contact with the vitelline membrane of the egg and this could be a mechanism for the transfer of nutrients. On occasion follicular cells have been found to migrate through the zona and Zamboni has demonstrated that the egg has the ability to ingest these cells. (20) The vast majority of follicular cells, however, are removed from the surface of the zona by the action of tubal fluid. (21)

Fertilization normally takes place in the ampulla of the tube. The initial adherence of the sperm to the egg is followed by rapid passage through the zona. The post acrosomal cap region of the sperm then establishes contact with the vitelline membrane. (22, 23) Enzymes have been localized in this area and these may mediate the cell membrane fusion that allows the egg to engulf the sperm

Once the process is completed the chromosomes contained in the sperm head become less condensed and the male pronucleus is formed.

When the sperm penetrates the egg, meoisis is completed by extrusion of the second polar body. At the same time the zona becomes impervious to penetration by a second sperm. This change in surface characteristics is associated with the breakdown and disappearance of the cortical granules which lie just below the vitelline membrane. Extracts of cortical granule material when added to unfertilized eggs prevent their penetration by sperm. (24)

The phase of egg transport from the fimbria to the ampullary isthmic junction can occur in minutes or a few hours, and is accomplished by segmental contractions of the tubal musculature. The cilia appear to play a minor role in this stage of egg transport. The rapidity of egg transport in the tube is species dependent. In the human the egg passes from the tube into the uterus 60–70 hours after ovulation while in dogs this may require as long as 8–10 days. (25) While thought of as floating free in the uterine cavity for 2–3 days prior to implantation, the egg may be in fairly intimate contact with the endometrium.

Early studies of egg transport in the rabbit suggested that low doses of estrogen accelerated egg transport while higher doses caused tube locking of ova. Progesterone also caused accelerated transport. These observations have been modified only slightly by a large number of subsequent investigations. However, because of differences in species, timing of hormone administration, hormone concentrations, and types of hormones used in different studies it's difficult to form a coherent picture which encompasses all the effects of hormone administration on egg transport. There must be fine tuning of the system, for early or late entry of eggs into the uterus results in significant reproductive loss. High levels of estrogen present at the time of ovulation could contribute to maintaining eggs in the tube until the endometrium is advanced into a secretory state. (26) The postovulatory rise in progesterone found in most species could trigger release of the ova into the uterus at the same time it causes the appropriate change in endometrial morphology.

In most animals the egg resides in the tube for at least a short period of time following fertilization to insure successful development. In the rabbit, eggs can be fertilized in the uterus but they perish unless they are transferred to the tube within 3 hours of fertilization. (27) Similar observations have been made in the hamster. (28) Surprisingly the human seems to be an exception and there are a number of reports, almost all in the older literature, detailing successful pregnancy following an Estes procedure. (29) In this and related procedures the ovary is transposed to a position in the uterine wall which allows ovulation to occur into the endometrial cavity.

315

The isthmic portion of the tube is richly endowed with adrenergic fibers, and hormone effects can be mediated through the sympathetic nervous system. (30) The functional importance of this system is open to question because denervation of the tube does not interfere with egg tranport. (31) Equally uncertain is the role of prostaglandins in egg transport. $PGF_{2\alpha}$ may stimulate closure of the isthmus of the tube and prevent premature passage of eggs into the uterus while PGE produces an opposite effect. (32)

The portrayal of the egg as a passive participant in the reproductive process, being propelled by tubal contractions and penetrated by the sperm, does it an injustice. From early in the cleavage stages and even prior to ovulation there is active protein synthesis. (33, 34) Interference with RNA synthesis in the preimplantation stage for even brief periods of time diminishes the chances for implantation and further development. (35, 36) It has been hypothesized that this effect occurs by interference with the production of a protein or other product by the embryo which could be the signal to the uterus to initiate the implantation process. There is some evidence that the blastocyst does provide a signal, and that this signal may be carbon dioxide. (37) This coincides with a suggestion by Böving that CO_2 blowoff leads to an alkaline reaction which makes the trophoblast sticky. (38) It has been suggested that trophoblast adhesion and penetration of the epithelium occur only over a vessel. Work *in vitro* however, indicates that trophoblast has the ability to adhere even to plastic surfaces. (39) Thus, at least the process of adhesion does not require the participation of maternal tissues.

In Vitro
Fertilization

In vitro fertilization has been accomplished in a number of species and a number of laboratories have reported live births following transfer of *in vitro* fertilized ova to pseudopregnant recipients. (40, 41) Steptoe and Edwards have reported successful *in vitro* fertilization of human ova obtained by aspiration of follicles at the time of laparoscopy. (19) A number of attempts to continue the pregnancies by transcervical instillation of the embryo into the uterus has produced only one pregnancy and that in the Fallopian tube. (42) Steptoe and Edwards hypothesized that in this latter case the high placement of the embryo in the fundus of the uterus resulted in retrograde migration through the uterotubal junction. Despite these failures the success of embryo transfer in other species suggests that it can be achieved eventually in the human.

In vitro fertilization in rabbits and rats can result on occasion in abnormal development, and for this reason some workers have maintained that work in the human is premature. (43, 44) Because of the difficulties in recovering ova from nonhuman primates, the diminished financial support for basic research in reproduction, and the demands of patients with infertility due to tubal disease it can be anticipated that experimental work in the human will continue.

Infertility

A couple complaining of infertility deserves a systematic examination of all aspects of the reproductive tract to rule out pathology. Infertility is usually defined as 1 year of unprotected coitus without pregnancy. It is estimated that the male factor is implicated in 40% of infertility problems, failure of ovulation will account for another 10–15%, 20–30% will be caused by tubal pathology, and in 5% a cervical factor is associated with the infertility. The remaining 10–20% of couples will have no known cause for their infertility.

There are many advantages to having the male present during the initial interview. He may contribute valuable historical information. It also gives the physician the opportunity to emphasize that both husband and wife are involved in the infertility investigation. A husband who has been acquainted at its inception with the physician's treatment of the infertility problem will be less reluctant, as time progresses, to ask for clarification of any aspect of the testing. This can prevent misunderstandings engendered when the husband's only source of information is his wife. Early in the physician-couple interaction frequency of coitus and possible sexual problems should be ascertained.

The examination of the husband's semen should be the first diagnostic step of the investigation (see Chapter 18). It is still all too common to find the wife subjected to an operative procedure before it was determined that her husband was azospermic. If the semen characteristics, and the initial examination of the wife are normal, attention can be directed to demonstrating the adequacy of cervical mucus, ovulation, and tubal patency. Tests for all these factors need to be scheduled at specific times of the menstrual cycle.

317

Postcoital Test

Cervical mucus is a hydrogel and under the influence of the peak estrogen levels present at ovulation, the water content of mucus increases to approximately 95–98%. The mucus at this time should be clear, watery, and often so abundant as to be noted by the woman. When dried on a slide it should form a distinct fern pattern. Earlier in the cycle when estrogen output is lower and starting 2 to 3 days after ovulation when progesterone secretion increases, the water content drops to approximately 89% and the mucus is thick, viscid, and opaque. Cervical mucus contains chains of glycoproteins which line up in parallel at midcycle to create channels through which sperm can migrate. Davajan, Nakamura and Kharma have published an excellent review of the biophysics and biochemistry of cervical mucus. (45)

Fern Pattern

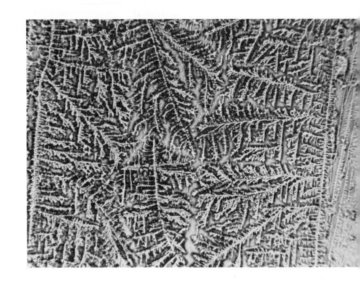

Lack of Fern

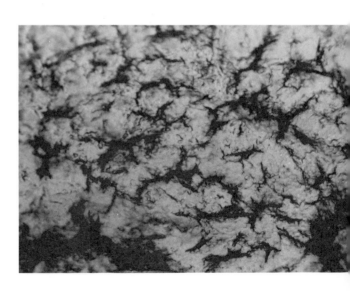

The postcoital test provides information about both male and female factors. The couple should abstain from intercourse for 48 hours prior to the test which is performed around the time of expected ovulation as determined by previous basal body temperature charts or by the length of prior cycles. Cervical mucus is removed with a nasal polyp forcep and examined for macroscopic and microscopic characteristics. The optimal time interval between coitus and examination of the mucus has not been determined. While a study by Gibor and associates indicated no drop in the number of sperm at any time during the first 24 hours, there are reports that the number of sperm does decrease after 8 hours. (46, 47) This is similar to our experience and we suggest that, if possible, the couple have coitus in the morning and that the test be performed early in the afternoon at the latest. If the fractional postcoital test, to be described below, is used, the time interval should be $2^1/_2$ hours or less.

If the mucus is thick rather than thin, opaque instead of clear, the proximity of the test to ovulation should be determined by the onset of the next period (or by the temperature chart if one is being taken during that cycle). If poor mucus quality is related to inaccurate timing, the test should be repeated in the subsequent cycle. Poor mucus at ovulation time is a physical barrier critically diminishing sperm penetration and requiring alteration to enhance fertility. Buxton and Southam found that 33% of women who had good mucus became pregnant while only 14.5% of women with repeatedly poor mucus achieved a pregnancy. (48) In our clinic, 53.8% with good mucus became pregnant while 37% with poor mucus became pregnant, a statistically significant difference. In all likelihood some of these poor tests are reflections of inaccurate timing. It also points out that poor mucus is not an absolute bar to pregnancy but only indicates a poorer prognosis.

Treatment of poor mucus is best accomplished by low dose estrogen (e.g. conjugated estrogens 0.625 mg or 1.25 mg) daily for 8 or 9 days preceding the expected time of ovulation. In a 28-day cycle that would be between days 5 and 13. There is no advantage to continuing the hormone treatment through the luteal phase of the cycle. If there is evidence of chronic cervicitis with thick yellowish mucus, systemic or local antibiotics are used initially. If this is not successful the cervix is treated with electrocautery or cryosurgery.

Another tactic to overcome the barrier of thick cervical mucus is intrauterine insemination of sperm. (49) This is accomplished using a tuberculin syringe with an attached thin, sterilized polyethylene tube (#16 Intercath) which is threaded through the cervix. Normally after coitus only the sperm enter the uterine cavity and semen remains in the vagina. Intrauterine insemination of even small

319

amounts of semen may stimulate strong uterine contrac
tions and produce an anaphylactic type reaction. Fo
this reason no more than 0.3 cc of semen should be
introduced. The intrauterine method allows direct intro
duction of bacteria into the uterus, and a few cases o
tubal infection have been reported following this proce
dure.

The postcoital test also gives information concerning the
male. Absence of sperm requires a review of the couple':
coital technique. Repeated cancellations of appointment:
for the postcoital test may be a clue that there are sexua
problems that have not been uncovered by the interview
More important, absence of sperm necessitates a detailed
review of the semen specimen.

What constitutes a normal number of sperm in a postcoita
test has been a matter of dispute. The estimates range
from 1 to over 20/high power field (HPF). More critica
than controversy over theoretical normal values is the
question of what prognostic value the postcoital test has
for the infertile couple. In a study by Buxton and Southam
good sperm migration in the postcoital test yielded a
pregnancy rate of 48.9%, while with poor sperm migra
tion the conception rate was 31.6%. (48) The poo
category included tests in which no sperm, only dead
sperm, or rare motile sperm were found. The good
classification included those tests in which a few or more
motile sperm were found in each HPF. A study from ou
clinic showed that there was a statistically significan
increase in the percentage of pregnancies when there
were more than 20 sperm/HPF. (50) There was no
statistically significant difference in percentage of preg
nancies between groups having 0, 1–5, 6–10, or 11–20
sperm/HPF. It would obscure the issue to call a postcoita
test with 21 or more sperm/HPF "normal," suggesting
that less than 21 is somehow abnormal. The former give:
a better prognosis for pregnancy, but a substantial number
of pregnancies occur even when no sperm are found in
the postcoital test. If only immotile sperm are found in
the mucus the percentage of pregnancies is significantly
lower than when motile sperm are found.

Fractional postcoital tests have been advocated as a more
sophisticated means of assessing sperm mucus interaction
In this technique the mucus is collected in a polyethylene
tube by aspiration with a syringe. The tube is cut in
segments and the contents of each segment assessed
individually. This allows identification of the mucus from
different levels of the cervical canal. A normal specimen
should have at least 5 motile sperm in the upper segment
A recent publication did not provide data which would
warrant making the more laborious fractional postcoita
test a routine procedure. (51) Fractional tests were per
formed in 143 infertile couples, of whom 51 had had
abnormal routine postcoital tests and 92 normal routine

postcoital tests. Of the 92 women who had normal routine tests, 16 had abnormal fractional postcoital tests. All 16 were treated with low dose diethylstilbestrol, and 3 became pregnant. However, all 3 had poor spinnbarkeit, a result that should have been apparent also with a routine test. In summary, 143 fractional postcoital tests were performed for a questionable gain of 3 pregnancies. Unless it can be shown more convincingly that the 16 woman categorized by the fractional postcoital test are a unique population and can be helped by specific therapy, we see no reason to use the fractional test in clinical practice.

Tredway et al. have shown that a normal fractional postcoital test is sufficient evidence of a normal male factor and the need for a semen analysis is obviated. (52) A similar claim has been made for the routine postcoital test if there are more than 20 motile sperm per HPF. (53)

One of the most difficult problems in infertility is the postcoital test which repeatedly shows only dead sperm or absence of sperm despite good mucus and a normal semen analysis. The patient should be cautioned that lubricants such as K-Y Jelly and Surgilube have a spermicidal effect *in vitro* and should not be used by infertile couples. If lubrication is necessary, olive, peanut or safflower oil or glycerin can be used without interfering with sperm movement. (54) Re-examination of the husband's semen to check sperm motility is an absolute necessity. Following this, the pH of the cervical mucus is determined at midcycle. If it is below 7, treatment with a precoital alkaline douche (Proception, Milex) may be helpful. This must be an extremely rare finding. Thirdly, sperm antibody testing is in order. A possible therapeutic approach is the use of intrauterine inseminations. (49)

In summary, what useful information can be gleaned from the postcoital test? If sperm are found in the mucus it is reasonable assurance that coital technique is adequate. This precludes the need for the woman to flex her thighs following intercourse or to place a pillow under her hips as a means of keeping sperm in the vagina. During normal intercourse sperm rapidly leave the semen pool and enter the cervical mucus. The semen is lost through the vaginal introitus or is broken down by vaginal enzymes. Women should be told that loss of semen is the normal occurrence and not a cause for infertility. If live sperm are found in the cervical mucus the pH is not hostile and the pregnancy rate is higher than if the sperm are all immotile. If there are more than 20 sperm/HPF, the male, in all likelihood, has a sperm count above 20 million/cc and the couple has a significantly better chance for pregnancy than if the post coital test contains less than 20 sperm/HPF. If the mucus is clear and abundant with good spinnbarkeit, the patient has a better chance for pregnancy than if it is thick and sparse. Beyond this basic information little more can be obtained from the postcoital test. There is little advantage in having, for example, 10 sperm/HPF compared to having 1 sperm/HPF. If one or more motile sperm/HPF are found and the mucus is good there is no purpose in repeating the test in hope of finding a greater number of sperm.

We do not consider a postcoital test to be a substitute for a semen analysis. While 21 or more sperm/HPF is almost always associated with a sperm count above 20 million/cc, the postcoital test gives little information concerning the morphology of sperm in the ejaculate. There are considerably fewer abnormal forms in the cervical mucus compared to the ejaculate. This may represent a filtering effect of the cervical mucus or may indicate that abnormal forms do not have the motility to penetrate the cervical mucus.

Tests of Tubal Patency

A history of pelvic inflammatory disease, septic abortion, ruptured appendix, or ectopic pregnancy alerts the physician to the possibility of tubal damage. One-half of patients however, who are eventually found to have tubal damage and/or pelvic adhesions have no history of antecedent disease. There have been a few reports of damaged tubes showing histologic evidence suggestive of viral infection which could explain the absence of traditional causes for tubal damage. In cases of tubal damage of unknown etiology, we have found it both honest and helpful for the patient's peace of mind to emphasize the possibility that a viral infection in childhood may have caused the problem.

If there is a history of pelvic inflammatory disease a sedimentation rate is first obtained and, if elevated, antibiotic therapy is given. The test for tubal patency is then scheduled for 2 to 3 months in the future. Shortly before, a repeat sedimentation rate is obtained. If this is still elevated or if masses or tenderness are revealed by the pelvic examination consideration should be given to bypassing the hysterosalpingogram and to evaluating the pelvis by laparoscopy.

The convenience of performing a Rubin's test with CO_2 in the office, and the avoidance of irradiation have been outweighed by the discomfort of the test and the high percentage of false readings which suggest tubal occlusion. This may result from tubal spasm initiated by the gas. In our practice hysterosalpingography (HSG) has replaced the Rubin's test except in women who give a history suggestive of dye allergy. The x-ray study is performed 2 to 6 days after cessation of a menstrual flow. This preovulatory testing decreases the possibility of flushing a fertilized egg out of the tube into the peritoneal cavity.

HSG should be done under image intensification fluoroscopy and a minimum number of films taken. Only three films are usually required—a preliminary before dye is injected, a film showing spill of dye from one or both tubes, and a delayed film to show spread of dye through the peritoneal cavity. There is no need to take films from all angles as additional pictures rarely add information beyond that provided by the three basic films and it unnecessarily increases radiation dosage.

The dye can be injected using a classic Jarcho cannula with a single tooth tenaculum, or alternatively a suction apparatus can be appended to the cervix and dye injected through a contained cannula. This latter device eliminates the discomfort associated with application of the tenaculum. In either case the cannula should be bubble-free. A third technique is to insert a foley catheter into the uterus. When Ethiodol, an oil dye, is used there is no need to premedicate the patient or to restrict her to a liquid diet the day of examination. Bowel evacuation by enema is not required. In short, the patient needs no preparation and most certainly does not require an anesthetic.

The dye should be injected slowly so that abnormalities of the uterine cavity are not obscured. Usually no more than 3-6 cc of dye are required to fill the uterus and tubes. If the patient complains of cramping, the injection of dye should be stopped for a few minutes and fluoroscopy temporarily discontinued. Spasm is rare with Ethiodol, our preferred medium, but if it does occur, slow injection with pauses may be helpful. If the tubes fill but dye droplets do not spill from the ends of the tubes, the uterus should be pushed up in the abdomen by means of the tenaculum or suction cup. This puts the tubes on stretch and may help to release dye from the fimbriated end. The droplets seen coming from the tube are the result of mixing of the oil dye and peritoneal fluid. On occasion, injection of dye into a hydrosalpinx will produce a similar pattern, and the 24 hour film is crucial in differentiating this condition from normal spill.

Much has been written concerning the need to have multiple tests suggesting nonpatency of the tubes before the patient has exploratory surgery. Buxton and Southam reported that 8 of 71 women having tubal closure demonstrated by hysterosalpingography, but not treated surgically, became pregnant. (48) Despite these false results, there is no need for repetitive x-rays because the results of hysterosalpingography can be checked by injection of dye at laparoscopy.

323

If the 24-hour film shows good distribution of dye with only an occasional small loculation of dye, the loculations are probably not significant. On the other hand, if the tubes fill with dye but the 24-hour film shows only 2 large dye globules at the end of the tubes without spillage of dye into the peritoneal cavity, the prognosis is very poor.

In viewing films it is important not to overlook the proximal portion of the tube. Salpingitis isthmica nodosum can be diagnosed by a speckled appearance of dye around the tube near its insertion into the uterus.

If dye goes through one tube rapidly and fails to fill the other tube, it usually means that the dye-containing tube presents the path of least resistance. In this situation the nonfilling tube is usually normal. When both tubes were patent on x-ray, the pregnancy rate in our own series was only slightly higher (58%) than when there was unilateral patency (50%). (55) This finding, though, is at variance with an earlier study of Wahby et al. in which only 23% (11 of 48) of women conceived with unilateral patency on Lipiodol hysterosalpingography. (56) With bilateral patency their pregnancy rate was 36%.

While the diagnostic usefulness of hysterosalpingography is unquestioned, its value as a therapeutic procedure in infertility is a subject of some controversy. Whitelaw et al. found no increase in the pregnancy rate following hysterosalpingography. (57) Palmer, though, reported that 75% of patients having a hysterosalpingogram showing tubal patency and whose husbands had normal sperm counts became pregnant within 1 year of the procedure. (58) This was three times the pregnancy rate found by the same author among patients who had not had a hysterosalpingogram. Speculation concerning the precise mode of therapeutic action of the procedure has included the following:

1. It may effect a mechanical lavage of the tubes, dislodging mucus plugs.

2. It may straighten the tubes and thus break down peritoneal adhesions.

3. It may provide a stimulatory effect for the cilia of the tube.

4. It may improve the cervical mucus.

5. The iodine may exert a bacteriostatic effect on the mucus membranes.

If hysterosalpingography does enhance fertility, is the effect seen with both oil- and water-soluble dyes? Gillespie reported a conception rate of 41.3% within 1 year of hysterosalpingography with oil media, while the rate was only 27.3% when water-soluble agents were employed. (59) This is in accord with the experience at the Yale Infertility Clinic. (55) Three groups of infertile patients were compared. One had hysterosalpingograms done with Ethiodol, another had hysterosalpingograms with Salpix, a water dye, and the third had no hysterosalpingograms. Within 1 year of the termination of their infertility workup the group which had Ethiodol hysterosalpingograms had a significantly higher percentage of pregnancies, the great majority of which followed within 7 months of the x-rays. (see Table) There was no difference between the groups having hysterosalpingography with Salpix and those who did not have x-rays. In addition to its value in enhancing fertility, Ethiodol produces a better film image and a lower incidence of pain on injection compared to water-soluble dyes.

Conception Rate

	Percent Pregnant	
No Hysterogram	43	
		$p < 0.01$
Ethiodol HSG	55	
		$p < 0.02$
Salpix	40	

The use of an oil medium has been criticized on grounds that it is only slowly absorbed and may cause granuloma formation on the peritoneum or in the tube. Granulomas probably do not form in normal tubes. It is only the abnormal tube with increased sequestration of dye which is prone to granuloma formation. Granulomas also have been reported following hysterosalpingography with Salpix. An additional fear with oil dye is embolization, a complication which has never occurred in our series. When fluoroscopy is used venous or lymphatic intravasation can be detected immediately and injection of dye halted. In his monograph, Siegler reported nine deaths attributable to HSG. (60) Lipiodol, an oil medium, was used in six of these cases, the last occurring in 1947. Since that time there was only one fatality, which occurred in 1959 after embolization of a water-soluble dye.

Disorders of Ovulation

Disorders of ovulation account for approximately 15% of all infertility problems. These may be anovulation or severe oligo-ovulation. In the latter cases, even though ovulation does occur, its relative infrequency diminishes the woman's chances for pregnancy. If she has periods only every 3 or 4 months, for practical purposes it matters little whether these are ovulatory or anovulatory. She should be treated with clomiphene to increase the frequency of or to initiate ovulation (see Chapter 19) and this can be started immediately, even before other areas have been investigated.

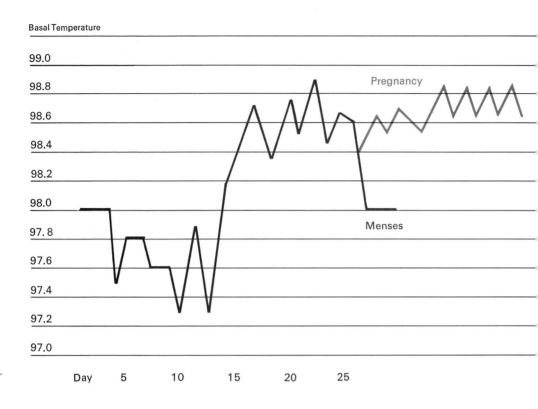

Basal Temperature

99.0	
98.8	Pregnancy
98.6	
98.4	
98.2	
98.0	
97.8	Menses
97.6	
97.4	
97.2	
97.0	

Day   5   10   15   20   25

Basal Body Temperature. Women who have menstrual periods at monthly intervals marked by premenstrual symptoms and dysmenorrhea are almost always ovulatory. Indirect confirmatory evidence of ovulation is obtained by use of basal body temperature (BBT) charts. The temperature can be taken either orally or rectally with a regular thermometer or with special instruments that show a range of only a few degrees and thus are easier to read. It is worth emphasizing that the temperature must be taken immediately upon awakening and before any activity. It may be surprising to find that the basal temperatures are substantially lower than the usual 98.6°. Characteristically, prior to ovulation they are in the 97.2°–97.4° range, and after ovulation the basal temperature is over 98°. Days when intercourse take place should be noted on the chart and this may give the physician an indication that coital frequency is a problem.

Even using temperature charts, no one can pinpoint the exact day of ovulation. A significant increase in temperature is not noted usually until 2 days after the luteinizing hormone (LH) peak coinciding with a rise in peripheral levels of progesterone to greater than 4 ng/ml. (61) In a recent report 22 of 27 cycles were marked by an LH surge on the same day or within one day of the BBT nadir. However in 2 cycles it was 2 days after the nadir and in 1 cycle 3 days before the nadir. (62) Despite this variability, physical release of the ovum probably occurs on the day prior to the time of the first temperature elevation. This may or may not be marked by a dip in the temperature to the lowest level of the cycle. The temperature rise should be sustained for 10 to 16 days (average 14) and the reading will then drop at the time of the subsequent menstrual period. If an approximate time of ovulation can be determined by temperature charts, a sensible schedule for coitus is every other day in a period encompassed by 3 to 4 days prior to and including 2 to 3 days after expected ovulation. While this would be ideal, it is unwise to demand rigid adherence to a schedule. This may produce psychologic stress sufficient to inhibit sexual relations.

In discussing coital timing the patient will usually want to know the fertilizable life of the sperm and the egg. The information on human gametes is speculative. Cases have been reported when isolated coitus even up to 7 days prior to the rise in basal body temperature has resulted in pregnancy, but this probably represents the limits of biologic variation. Estimates have been made that sperm retain their ability to fertilize for 24 to 48 hours and that the human egg is fertilizable for 12 to 24 hours. In a study of 22 women Ahlgren could not find sperm in the Fallopian tube 86 hours after coitus. (10)

Endometrial Biopsy. This is performed 2 or 3 days prior to the expected period and the histology is read by the criteria outlined by Noyes, Hertig, and Rock. (63) While premenstrual biopsy may present the possibility of interrupting a pregnancy if performed in a conception cycle, the danger is minimal. Buxton and Olson, in their study of biopsies done during the conception cycle, found that only 2 of 26 patients aborted. (64) We have found the Meig's curette (Codman and Shurtleff, Inc.) very suitable for obtaining a small strip of tissue from high on the anterior wall. It is slightly smaller than the usual suction endometrial biopsy instruments.

Inadequate Luteal Phase. Inadequate luteal phase is often an ambiguous diagnosis, and many times it has been invoked as an excuse to warrant the use of clomiphene or other hormones. Moreover, there is considerable confusion surrounding both the diagnosis and treatment of the inadequate luteal phase. The questions that need answering are:

1. What is an inadequate luteal phase?

2. What means should be used to establish the diagnosis?

3. How frequently is it seen in infertile couples?

4. What is the correct treatment?

327

The term inadequate luteal phase suggests inadequate production of progesterone by the corpus luteum. The diagnosis is established if the histologic dating of the endometrium is more than 2 days behind the cycle day determined by the onset of the subsequent menstrual flow. There must be more than a 2-day lag in the endometrium, for Tredway et al., using the LH surge to pinpoint ovulation, found that 5 of 11 normally ovulating women had biopsies 2 days out of synchrony with the day of the menstrual cycle. (65) There are obvious difficulties in establishing a diagnosis using the histologic criterion. There can be variations in the interpretations of the same biopsy by different observers. The same endometrium can show varying patterns, and there can be discrepancies between the maturation of the glands and that of the stroma. Despite these drawbacks, biopsy remains the classical way of diagnosing an inadequate luteal phase.

If the basal temperature chart shows a rise which is sustained for less than 10 days this too can be considered evidence of an inadequate luteal phase. Concern is often expressed when the temperature shows a very slow rise though it remains elevated for the normal length of time. This is of doubtful significance but should be checked by endometrial biopsy.

Serum progesterone levels have been used to confirm the presence of ovulation. Israel et al. found that a single luteal phase serum progesterone of 3 ng/ml or more provided presumptive evidence of ovulation. (66) Abraham et al. suggested that if the sum of three plasma progesterone determinations, taken between 4 and 11 days prior to menses, were equal to 15 ng/ml, ovulation had occurred and there was normal corpus luteum function. (67) However, these levels can be exceeded in cases where the endometrial biopsy shows a lag of 3 days or more. (68) While groups of women with inadequate luteal phase have lower levels of progesterone than do women with normal function, there is an overlap of values.

Many women will have isolated cycles characteristic of the inadequate luteal phase and they do not require treatment. Estimates are that less than 4% of infertile women have repeated cycles with this deficiency, and demonstration of its occurrence in more than one cycle is required before therapy is warranted. (69)

Jones and co-workers at Johns Hopkins have achieved a high conception rate by using progesterone vaginal suppositories (50 mg) daily following the midcycle rise in temperature. (68, 70) The suppositories are not available commercially and must be compounded by a pharmacy. Another tactic is to give injections of human chorionic gonadotropin (HCG) in varying doses 2 to 3 days after the rise in temperature. Either 10,000 international units (IU) can be given at that time as the sole treatment, or smaller doses (2,500–5,000 IU) can be given every 2 to 3 days for four injections. The injection of HCG can delay the onset of menses for up to 7 days. Other treatments include clomiphene and human menopausal gonadotropin. The latter has been used because of evidence that an inadequate luteal phase can result from a deficiency of follicle-stimulating hormone in the proliferative phase of the cycle. (71) Evaluation of any therapy is difficult because a significant number of conceptions occur without treatment. One group of drugs which has been widely used for treatment of the inadequate luteal phase, but which may in fact be deleterious, is the synthetic progestins. Provera, in higher doses than those used in the inadequate luteal phase cases, depresses progesterone levels when given after ovulation. (72)

Mycoplasma

Mycoplasma, a pleuropneumonia-like organism, has been implicated as a possible cause of habitual abortions and salpingitis. Gnarpe and Friberg from Uppsala, Sweden, reported that infertile couples had a markedly higher prevalence of T mycoplasma in cervical mucus and semen than did a group of fertile women and men. Treatment with doxycycline decreased the numbers of couples with mycoplasma and also was associated with pregnancy in 15 of 52 couples (29%), all of whom had had primary infertility of at least 5 years duration. (73) However a series of reports from England agreed with these findings in only one respect. They confirmed that treatment with doxycycline could eliminate mycoplasma from the genital tract of the majority of individuals. In this study there was no difference in the frequency of either T strain or mycoplasma hominis between infertile and fertile couples. (74) In a double blind study, treatment with doxycycline for 28 days had no effect on the rate of conception, and the English group suggested that culturing for mycoplasma in the routine investigation of infertility was unrewarding. (75)

Sperm Allergy

In 1964, Franklin and Dukes reported that in couples with no demonstrable cause for infertility, 72% had evidence of circulating antibodies to sperm. (76) A smaller number (5.7%) of fertile women, however, also had sperm agglutinins in their serum. Sexual abstinence or use of condom by the husband for a period of 2–6 months was used to lower the antibody titer. Ten of 13 patients in the initial series showed a decline and pregnancy occurred in 9 of the 10. Not only must condoms be used during intercourse, but all contact of sperm with the woman, for example through oral genital contact, must be interdicted. In 1968, Franklin's group reported their total experience in which 48% of women with no known cause for infertility had circulating sperm agglutinins. (77) The positive rate for fertile women was now 13%. Of 61 infertile women with positive reactions, 41 used condom therapy and 24 (58.6%) became pregnant. Twenty couples refused condom therapy and two women (10%) became pregnant.

In our clinic, only 20% of women with unexplained infertility had positive tests for agglutinating antibodies. (78) In positive cases we suggest that condom therapy be used for 3 months, at the end of which time a retest is done. If it is still positive, the condom is used for a further 3 months. In general, we have not encouraged couples to continue condom use beyond 9–12 months. On two occasions we have seen women whose sperm agglutination tests remained positive after 9 and 11 months of condom therapy, yet both became pregnant within 1 month of discontinuing condom use. When the test becomes negative or at the end of the 9–12 months of condom treatment, condom use is still maintained early and late in the cycle but is discontinued during the week around expected ovulation time. About 35% of women become pregnant after this treatment. Avoidance of contact with sperm is the only known therapy.

Despite the many studies that have appeared in the years since the first publication of Franklin and Dukes, the basic question of whether circulating antibodies in the female interfere with fertility remains unanswered.

Among the reasons for this uncertainty are the following: In many cases the serum component responsible for sperm agglutination is not a γ-globulin but rather a β-globulin, possibly attached to a steroid hormone. (79) In addition, some women with sperm-agglutinating antibodies will become pregnant without treatment. This does not necessarily negate the importance of the agglutinating antibodies, because their activity *in vivo* may depend on the vigor of the sperm population that they face. Some sperm are more readily incapacitated by the same antibody than are others. (80) This could explain the presence of sperm-agglutinating antibodies in women of known fertility.

In infertile women a sperm immobilization test gives a lower percentage of positive tests compared to the agglutination reaction (approximately 5 to 10%), but positive reactions in fertile women are almost nonexistent. (81) The serum component involved appears to be a gamma-globulin. Condom therapy does not seem to overcome this antibody, as it does in 35% of women with positive sperm-agglutinating tests. (78)

While many physicians now order testing for sperm allergy only in couples who have a poor postcoital test, it should be recognized that sperm antibodies can be present despite a postcoital test showing adequate numbers of moving sperm. Testing of serum to uncover the reaction may not be the best approach. There are cytotoxic antibodies in the cervical mucus which may not be present in the serum. (82) In addition, there may be tissue-fixed antibodies in the cervical and endometrial tissue which may not be mirrored by circulating antibody. (83)

Certainly, it would be advantageous to study cervical mucus and cervical tissue for antibodies not found in the serum. For clinical purposes this is impractical.

The evidence for an infertility effect of sperm antibodies in men seems more firmly established than it is in women. Higher titers in males are correlated with diminished chances for conception. (84) Other than clearing genitourinary tract infections, there is no known therapy.

Many workers in the field of infertility feel that sperm-agglutinating antibodies are nonspecific and unrelated to infertility. Some believe that tests for immobilizing antibodies provide the better estimate of immunologic reactions against sperm, while others feel that this test also is meaningless. It is our impression that there are a few men and women who are infertile on the basis of an immunologic reaction. It may still be worthwhile to try to uncover these cases by testing both the male and the female for agglutinating and immobilizing antibodies.

Culdoscopy and Laparoscopy

Culdoscopy or laparoscopy is the final diagnostic procedure in any infertility investigation. If the hysterosalpingogram is normal the endoscopic procedure is done after an interval of at least 6 months. This allows time for the fertility-enhancing effect of the x-ray procedure. Obviously if the hysterosalpingogram shows tubal occlusion no such delay is necessary.

Because of the better view it affords of the cul-de-sac laparoscopy is preferred. The anesthesia department should be aware of the problems of ventilation that can arise from CO_2 insufflation of the abdominal cavity, use of muscle relaxants and Trendelenburg position. Endotracheal intubation and support of respiration are essential.

Approximately 20% of women will have pelvic pathology unsuspected prior to endoscopy. While risks of laparoscopy are small and complications limited they do exist. Subcutaneous dissection of CO_2, perforation of a viscus, intra-abdominal hemorrhage, and cardiac arrhythmias have all been reported.

For detailed information on endoscopy the reader is referred to the monographs by Decker and Steptoe. (85, 86)

Hormonal Treatment for Recurrent Abortion

Abortion is defined as the termination of pregnancy prior to achieving a fetal weight or maturity compatible with survival. In specific terms this is below 20 weeks of gestation or below 500 g fetal weight. Approximately 15% of all pregnancies between 4 and 20 weeks of gestation will undergo spontaneous abortion. (87, 88) It may well be that the true abortion rate is closer to 25%, because the rate of abortion in the weeks after conception (2–4 weeks of gestation) is uncertain.

Habitual abortion has been classically defined as three or more consecutive abortions. In 1938, Malpas, using theoretical calculations, stated that a woman with a history of three consecutive abortions had a 73% chance of aborting in the next pregnancy. (89) In 1946, Eastman presented statistical calculations indicating that after three abortions, the risk was 83.6%. (90) These early papers propagated the notion that the chance of a subsequent abortion increases with each successive abortion. Despite data to the contrary, this discouraging dictum has survived to plague patients and physicians facing the problem.

Recent studies have indicated that the risk of abortion after three successive abortions, is, in fact, only 25 to 30% (88). The original projections by Malpas and Eastmen were theoretical exercises which were not confirmed when appropriate data were collected. With this new information, it is not surprising that treatment with a wide range of approaches, including vitamins and psychotherapy, produced successful pregnancies in over 70% of women with histories of habitual abortion. These cures were not due to the therapy, but rather the claims of success were based on a comparison to the early, now discredited statistics of Malpas and Eastman.

Nevertheless, hormonal treatment for recurrent abortion is still in obstetric vogue in many parts of the world. Various forms of treatment (mostly the use of progestational agents) have yielded salvage rates of 65–80%, and thus have gained an undeserved reputation. Undeserved, because claims of success were impressive for the simple reason that results of treatment were compared once again with Malpas' original theoretical and incorrect figures. The spontaneous "cure rate" in patients with recurrent abortions is 70–80%, no matter what form of treatment is used.

The utilization of various indices to reveal low progesterone levels cannot be depended upon to select patients for treatment. It has been demonstrated that spontaneous restoration of abnormally low urinary pregnanediol excretion to normal levels occurs in 80% of patients with eventual continuation and achievement of full-term pregnancy (91, 92). Furthermore, the demonstration of a hormonal deficiency does not categorically mean that abortion is inevitable. Even if a hormonal deficiency is uncovered, it may not be an etiologic factor, but rather the result of fetal and trophoblastic morbidity. A pregnancy doomed to abort because of defective germ tissue may display low progesterone secretion, a condition which is obviously not amenable to hormone treatment.

Beyond these theoretical considerations, we believe the empiric use of progestins in patients with recurrent abortions should be discontinued on the basis of the following studies. Warburton and Fraser (88), in an analysis of

332

clinical data, found that the risk of abortion after one abortion is approximately 25 to 30% in each successive pregnancy. Three double-blind controlled studies of prophylactic progestin treatment have been carried out each using a different progestin, and each concluding that the rate of abortion in the treated group was no different than that in the control or placebo group. (91–93) For emphasis, it should be repeated that there has been no advantage demonstrated for progestin therapy in recurrent abortion. We should also state that the use of thyroid medication is indicated only in properly dignosed hypothyroidism.

The patient with recurrent abortions usually represents an anxious frustrated individual on the verge of despair. Evaluation should be spaced over several visits, allowing the physician to establish communication and rapport with the patient. Except in the rare specific problem (infection, anatomical abnormalities, chromosomal translocation), an approach utilizing psychologic support and routine medical evaluation is sufficient. It must be remembered that the cure rate is 70–80%, no matter what form of treatment is used.

Placebo treatment may be useful in maintaining a physician-patient relationship from which the patient derives needed psychologic sustenance. It seems to us, however, that the use of a hormonal substance for a placebo effect on the basis of no known harmful response denies the important lesson learned in the discovery of the relationship between diethylstilbestrol treatment and vaginal neoplasia in progeny. Reputed harmlessness is a potentially dangerous approach based on negative data.

**When Should
Adoption be
Advised?**

The practitioner must keep in mind that 10–20% of couples will have a problem that cannot be diagnosed by the currently known tests. Eventually, after a thorough investigation, it may be necessary to tell them that there is no known cause for their infertility and that further testing and treatment offer little chance for improving fertility. Despite the absence of pathology, couples with 4 or more years of infertility have a poor prognosis, and the physician should encourage consideration of adoption.

When local resources have been explored and a scarcity of available children requires a long waiting period, international adoptions may be investigated through the following agencies:

Holt Adoption Program
PO Box 2420
Eugene, Oregon 97420

Families for Children, Inc.
10 Bowling Green
Pointe Claire 720
Quebec, Canada

Counseling and support for infertile couples are available from the following organization:

RESOLVE, Inc.
PO Box 474
Belmont, Massachusettes 02178

References

1. **Noyes, RW, and Chapnick, EM,** Literature on Psychology and Infertility: A Critical Analysis, Fertil Steril 15:543, 1964.

2. **Rock, J, Tietze, C, and McLaughlin, HB,** Effect of Adoption on Infertility, Fertil Steril 16:305, 1965.

3. **Tyler, ET,** The Thyroid Myth in Infertility, Fertil Steril 4:218, 1953.

4. **Buxton, CL, and Herrmann, WL,** Effect of Thyroid Therapy on Menstrual Disorders and Sterility, JAMA 155:1035, 1954.

5. **Carter, B, Turner, V, Davis, CD, and Hamblen, ED,** Evaluation of Gynecologic Surgery in Therapy of Infertility, JAMA 148:995, 1952.

6. **Sobrero, AJ, and MacLeod, J,** The Immediate Postcoital Test, Fertil Steril 13:184, 1962.

7. **Bedford, JM,** The Rate of Sperm Passage into the Cervix after Coitus in the Rabbit, J Reprod Fertil 25:211, 1971.

8. **Settlage, DSF, Motoshima, M, and Tredway, DR,** Sperm Transport from the External Cervical Os to the Fallopian Tubes in Women: A Time and Quantitation Study, Fertil Steril 24:655, 1973.

9. **Overstreet, JW, and Cooper, GW,** Rabbit Sperm Do Not Survive Rapid Transport Through the Female Reproductive Tract, Abstract Presented at the Ninth Annual Meeting of the Society for the Study of Reproduction, Philadelphia, Pennsylvania, August 10–13, 1976.

10. **Ahlgren, M,** Sperm Transport to and Survival in the Human Fallopian Tube, Gynec Invest 6:206, 1975.

11. **Horne, HW Jr, and Thibault, JP,** Sperm Migration Through the Human Female Reproductive Tract, Fertil Steril 13:135, 1962.

12. **Moyer, DL, Legoretta, G, Maruta, H, and Henderson, V,** Elimination of Homologous Spermatozoa in the Female Genital Tract of the Rabbit: A Light and Electron-microscope Study, J Path Bacteriol 94:345, 1967.

13. **Austin, CR,** Observation on the Penetration of the Sperm into the Mammalian Egg, Aust J Sci Res B 4:581, 1951.

14. **Chang, MC,** Fertilizing Capacity of Spermatozoa Deposited into the Fallopian Tubes, Nature 168:697, 1951.

15. **Williams, WL,** Biochemistry of Capacitation of Spermatozoa, in Moghissi, KS, and Hafez, ESE, eds, *Biology of Mammalian Fertilization and Implantation,* Charles C. Thomas, Springfield, 1972.

16. **Bedford, JM,** Sperm Capacitation and Fertilization i Mammals, Biol Reprod Suppl 2:128, 1970.

17. **Vaidya, RA, Glass, RH, Dandekar, P, and Johnson, K** Decrease in the Electrophoretic Mobility of Rabbit Spermatozoa Following Intra-Uterine Incubation, J Repro Fertil 24:299, 1971.

18. **Zaneveld, LJD, and Williams, WL,** A Sperm Enzym that Disperses the Corona Radiata and Its Inhibition b Decapacitation Factor, Biol Reprod 2:363, 1970.

19. **Edwards, RG, Steptoe, PC, and Purdy, JM,** Fertilizatio and Cleavage In Vitro of Preovulatory Human Oocytes Nature 227:1307, 1970.

20. **Zamboni, L, Moore Smith, D, and Thompson, RS** Migration of Follicle Cells Through the Zona Pellucid and their Sequestration by Human Oocytes In Vitro, Exp Zool 181:319, 1972.

21. **Mastroianni, L, Jr, and Komins, J,** Capacitation, Ovur Maturation, Fertilization and Preimplantation Develop ment in the Oviduct, Gynec Invest 6:226, 1975.

22. **Yanagimachi, R, and Noda, YD,** Physiological Change in the Postnuclear Cap Region of Mammalian Spermato zoa: Necessary Preliminary to the Membrane Fusio between Sperm and Egg Cells, J Ultrastruct Res 31:486 1970.

23. **Gordon, M,** Observations on the Postacrosomal Regio and the Neck Membranes of Rabbit Spermatozoa Staine En Bloc with Uranyl Acetate, Z Zellforsch 131:15, 1972

24. **Barros, C, and Yanagimachi, R,** Induction of Zon Reaction in Golden Hamster Eggs by Cortical Granul Material, Nature 233:2368, 1971.

25. **Croxatto, HB, and Ortiz, MS,** Egg Transport in th Fallopian Tube, Gynec Invest 6:215, 1975.

26. **Greenwald, GS,** A Study of the Transport of Ov Through the Rabbit Oviduct, Fertil Steril 12:80, 1961.

27. **Glass, RH,** Fate of Rabbit Eggs Fertilized in the Uterus J Reprod Fertil 31:139, 1972.

28. **Hunter, RHF,** Attempted Fertilization of Hamster Egg Following Transplantation into the Uterus, J Exp Zoo 168:511, 1968.

29. **Estes, WL, Jr,** Ovarian Implantation, Surg Gynec Obste 38:394, 1924.

30. **Coutinho, EM, de Mattos, CER, and da Silva, AR,** The Effect of Ovarian Hormones on the Adrenergic Stimulation of the Fallopian Tube, Fertil Steril 22:311, 1971.

31. **Hodgson, BJ, and Eddy, CA,** The Autonomic Nervous System and Its Relationship to Tubal Ovum Transport— A Reappraisal, Gynec Invest 6:162, 1975.

32. **Spilman, CH, and Harper, MJK,** Effects of Prostaglandins on Oviductal Motility and Egg Transport, Gynec Invest 6:186, 1975.

33. **Mintz, B,** Synthetic Processes and Early Development in the Mammalian Egg, J Exp Zool 157:85, 1964.

34. **Piko, L,** Synthesis of Macromolecules in Early Mouse Embryos Cultured In Vitro: RNA, DNA, and a Polysaccharide Component, Devel Biol 21:757, 1970.

35. **Bell, PS, and Glass, RH,** Development of the Mouse Blastocyst after Actinomycin D Treatment, Fertil Steril 26:449, 1975.

36. **Glass, RH, Spindle, AI, and Pedersen, RA,** Differential Inhibition of Trophoblast Outgrowth and Inner Cell Mass Growth By Actinomycin D in Cultured Mouse Embryos, J Reprod Fertil 48:443, 1976.

37. **Hetherington, CM,** Induction of Deciduomata in the Mouse by Carbon Dioxide, Nature 219:863, 1968.

38. **Böving, BG, and Larsen, JF,** Implantation, in Hafez, ESE, and Evans, TN, eds, *Human Reproduction,* Harper and Row, Hagerstown, Maryland, 1973, pp 133.

39. **Spindle, AI, and Pedersen, RA,** Hatching, Attachment, and Outgrowth of Mouse Blastocysts In Vitro: Fixed Nitrogen Requirements, J Exp Zool 186:305, 1973.

40. **Chang, MC,** Fertilization of Rabbit Ova In Vitro, Nature 184:466, 1959.

41. **Mukherjee, AB, and Cohen, MM,** Development of Normal Mice by an In Vitro Fertilization, Nature 228:472, 1970.

42. **Steptoe, PC, and Edwards, RG,** Reimplantation of A Human Embryo with Subsequent Tubal Pregnancy, Lancet 1:880, 1976.

43. **Toyoda, Y, and Chang, MJ,** Fertilization of Rat Eggs In Vitro by Epididymal Spermatozoa and the Development of Eggs Following Transfer, J Reprod Fertil 36:9, 1974.

44. **Barnes, RD,** In Vitro Fertilization, Lancet 1:1016, 1976.

337

45. **Davajan, V, Nakamura, RM, and Kharma, K,** Spermatozoan Transport in Cervical Mucus, Obstet Gynec Surv 25:1, 1970.

46. **Gibor, Y, Garcia, CJ, Cohen, MR, and Scommegna, A,** The Cyclical Changes in the Physical Properties of the Cervical Mucus and the Results of the Postcoital Test, Fertil Steril 21:20, 1970.

47. **Danezis, J, Sujan, S, and Sobrero, AJ,** Evaluation of the Postcoital Test, Fertil Steril 13:559, 1962.

48. **Buxton, CL, and Southam, AL,** *Human Infertility,* Hoeber-Harper, New York, 1958.

49. **White, RM, and Glass, RH,** Intrauterine Insemination of Husband's Sperm, Obstet Gynec 47:119, 1976.

50. **Jette, NT, and Glass, RH,** Prognostic Value of the Postcoital Test, Fertil Steril 23:29, 1972.

51. **Moran, J, Davajan, V, and Nakamura, R,** Comparison of the Fractional Postcoital Test with the Sims Huhner Postcoital Test, Int J Fertil 19:93, 1974.

52. **Tredway, DR, Settlage, DSF, Nakamura, R, Motoshima, M, Umezaki, CO, and Mishell, DR, Jr.,** Significance of Timing for the Postcoital Evaluation of Cervical Mucus, Am J Obstet Gynec 121:387, 1975.

53. **Glass, RH, and Mroueh, A,** The Postcoital Test and Semen Analysis, Fertil Steril 18:314, 1967.

54. **Goldenberg, R, and White, R,** The Effect of Vaginal Lubricants on Sperm Motility in Vitro, Fertil Steril 26:872, 1975.

55. **Mackey, RA, Glass, RH, Olson, L, and Vaidya, RA,** Pregnancy Following Hysterosalpingography with Oil and Water Soluble Dye, Fertil Steril 22:504, 1971.

56. **Wahby, O, Sobrero, AJ, and Epstein, JA,** Hysterosalpingography in Relation to Pregnancy and its Outcome in Infertile Women, Fertil Steril 17:520, 1966.

57. **Whitelaw, MJ, Foster, TN, and Graham, WH,** Hysterosalpingography and Insufflation, J Reprod Med 4:56, 1970.

58. **Palmer, A,** Ethiodol Hysterosalpingography for the Treatment of Infertility, Fertil Steril 11:311, 1960.

59. **Gillespie, HW,** The Therapeutic Aspect of Hysterosalpingography, Brit J Radiol 38:301, 1965.

60. **Siegler, AM,** *Hysterosalpingography,* Medcom Press, 1974.

61. **Moghissi, KS, Syner, FN, and Evans, TN,** A Composite Picture of the Menstrual Cycle, Am J Obstet Gynec 114:405, 1972.

62. **Morris, NM, Underwood, LE, and Easterling, W,** Temporal Relationship Between Basal Body Temperature Nadir and Luteinizing Hormone Surge in Normal Women, Fertil Steril 27:780, 1976.

63. **Noyes, RW, Hertig, AT, and Rock, J,** Dating the Endometrial Biopsy, Fertil Steril 1:3, 1950.

64. **Buxton, CL, and Olson, LE,** Endometrial Biopsy Inadvertently Taken During Conception Cycle, Am J Obstet Gynec 105:702, 1969.

65. **Tredway, Dr, Mishell, DR, Jr, and Moyer, DL,** Correlation of Endometrial Dating with Luteinizing Hormone Peak, Am J Obstet Gynec 117:1030, 1973.

66. **Israel, R, Mishell, DR, Jr, Stone, SC, Thorneycroft, IH, and Moyer, DL,** Single Luteal Phase Serum Progesterone Assay as an Indicator of Ovulation, Am J Obstet Gynec 112:1043, 1972.

67. **Abraham, GE, Maroulis, GB, and Marshall, JR,** Evaluation of Ovulation and Corpus Luteum Function Using Measurements of Plasma Progesterone, Obstet Gynec 44:522, 1974.

68. **Jones, GS, Aksel, S, and Wentz, AC,** Serum Progesterone Values in the Luteal Phase Defects, Obstet Gynec 44:26, 1974.

69. **Murthy, YS, Arronet, GH, and Parekh, MC,** Luteal Phase Inadequacy, Obstet Gynec 36:758, 1970.

70. **Jones, GS,** Luteal Phase Defects in Behrman, SJ, and Kistner, RW, eds., *Progress in Infertility,* Little, Brown, Boston, 1975, 2nd edition.

71. **Strott, CA, Cargille, CM, Ross, GT, and Lipsett, MB,** The Short Luteal Phase, J Clin Endocrin Metab 30:246, 1970.

72. **Johansson, EDB,** Depression of the Progesterone Levels in Women Treated with Synthetic Gestagens after Ovulation, Acta Endocrin 68:779, 1971.

73. **Gnarpe, H, and Friberg, J,** T-Mycoplasmas as a Possible Cause for Reproductive Failure, Nature 242:120, 1973.

74. **de Louvois, J, Blades, M, Harrison, RF, Hurley, R, and Stanley, VC,** Frequency of Mycoplasma in Fertile and Infertile Couples, Lancet 1:1073, 1974.

75. **Harrison, RF, de Louvois, J, Blades, M, and Hurley, R** Doxycycline Treatment and Human Infertility, Lancet 1:605, 1975.

76. **Franklin, RR, and Dukes, CD,** Further Studies on Sperm Agglutinating Antibody and Unexplained Infertility, JAMA 190:682, 1964.

77. **Malinak, LR, Mumford, DN, and Franklin, RR,** An Expanded Study of Sperm Agglutinating Antibodies in Fertile and Infertile Couples, Presented at the 24th Annual Meeting of the American Fertility Society, San Francisco, 1968.

78. **Glass, RH, and Vaidya, RA,** Sperm Agglutinating Antibodies in Infertile Women, Fertil Steril 21:657, 1970.

79. **Boettcher, B, and Kay, DJ,** Agglutination of Spermatozoa by Human Sera with Added Steroids, Andrologie 5:265, 1973.

80. **Fjallbränt, B,** Cervical Mucus Penetration by Human Spermatozoa Treated with Anti-Spermatozoal Antibodies from Rabbits and Man, Acta Obstet Gynec Scand 48:71, 1969.

81. **Isojima S, Li, T, and Ashitaka, Y,** Immunologic Analysis of Sperm Immobilizing Factor Found in Sera of Women with Unexplained Sterility, Am J Obstet Gynec 101:677, 1968.

82. **Parish, WE, Caron-Brown, JA, and Richards, CB,** The Detection of Antibodies to Spermatozoa and the Blood Group Antigens in Cervical Mucus, J Reprod Fertil 13:469, 1967.

83. **Schwimmer, WB, Ustay, KA, and Behrman, SJ,** Sperm Agglutinating Antibodies and Decreased Fertility in Prostitutes, Obstet Gynec 30:192, 1967.

84. **Rumke, P, Van Amstel, N, Messer, EN, and Bezemer, PD,** Prognosis of Fertility of Men with Sperm Agglutinins in the Serum, Fertil Steril 25:393, 1974.

85. **Decker, A,** *Culdoscopy*, FA, Davis, Philadelphia, 1967.

86. **Steptoe, PC,** *Laparoscopy in Gynecology*, E and S Livingstone, Edinburgh and London, 1967.

87. **French, FE, and Bierman, JM,** Probabilities of Fetal Mortality, Public Health Rep 77:835, 1962

88. **Warburton, D, and Fraser, FS,** Spontaneous Abortion Risks in Man: Data from Reproductive Histories Collected in a Medical Genetic Unit. Am J Hum Genet 16:1, 1964.

89. **Malpas, R,** Study of Abortion Sequences, J Obstet Gynaec Br Commonw 45:932, 1938.

90. **Eastman, NJ,** Habitual Abortion, in Meigs, MV, and Sturgis, SJ, ed, *Progress in Gynecology*, Grune & Stratton, New York, 1946.

91. **Goldzieher, JW,** Double-blind Trial of Progestin in Habitual Abortion, JAMA 188:561, 1964.

92. **Shearman, RP, and Garrett, WJ,** Double-blind Study of Effect of 17-Hydroxy-Progesterone Caproate on Abortion Rate, Br Med J 1:292, 1963.

93. **Klopper, A, Macnaughton, MD,** Hormones in Recurrent Abortion, J Obstet Gynaec Brit Commonw 72:1022, 1965.

Tubal Surgery

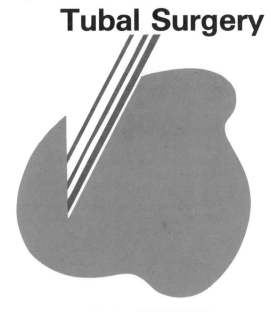

16

Tubal pathology is responsible for 20–30% of infertility. The current epidemic of venereal disease suggests that this figure may be even higher in the future, thereby increasing the demand for tubal surgery. Given the need for surgery, what can the physician do to enhance the results? Foremost is the proper selection of cases. Couples who have other infertility problems, for example, oligospermia or anovulation, constitute a group where surgery offers less than a normal chance for success and should rarely be used. Each case requires individual evaluation. Preoperative selection of patients for surgery based on hysterosalpingography findings will be discussed later in this chapter. Laparoscopy or culdoscopy can be used not only to ascertain the need for surgery but they also can be useful in eliminating cases with a hopeless prognosis. When both tubes are large hydrosalpinges it is unwise to attempt reparative surgery. Similarly, tubes which are occluded both at the cornua and at the fimbriated end offer minimal chances for success. Fertility is diminished after 35 in the normal woman and serious thought must be given before undertaking tubal surgery in this age group.

Tubal surgery should be performed by an experienced infertility surgeon. Gentle handling of tissues with fine instruments, the use of delicate sutures, for example 6-0 to 10-0, and avoidance of rubbing the tube with gauze sponges are all important aspects of surgical technique. The operative area on the tube can be kept free of obscuring blood by jets of saline from an asepto syringe.

343

Lysis of Adhesions (Salpingolysis)

If the tubes are intrinsically normal but motility i hindered by adhesions, lysis of these adhesions offers a 40–50% chance of subsequent pregnancy. Uterine sus pension is useful as a means of preventing the tubes from falling back on raw denuded areas in the cul-de-sac and this is an important adjunct to the surgery. Every effor should be directed to covering the raw areas on the peritoneum. A piece of free omentum can be laid over these raw areas and held in place by a few interrupted 4 0 plain sutures.

Salpingostomy or Fimbrioplasty

The degree of success with this type of surgery is largely dependent on the extent of the tubal disease. If the fimbria are normal and the only pathology is a few bands across the end of the tube the prognosis is very good. If the tubes are completely occluded and no fimbria are present the chances for subsequent pregnancy are slim The variability of the pathology is a major reason why it is almost impossible to compare results from different centers when cases are lumped together under headings such as "salpingostomy" or "fimbrioplasty."

In a series from Lebanon there were no pregnancies in 46 patients who underwent bilateral salpingostomies. (1) Crane and Woodruff from Johns Hopkins reported 34 salpingostomies with only three women achieving a live birth. (2) In a series from our clinic 24 women had bilateral salpingostomies, resulting in one full term and one ectopic pregnancy. (3)

Israel and March have provided important information on the results of tubal evaluation and surgery in a clinic population prone to pelvic inflammatory disease. (4) Laparoscopy revealed extensive tubal disease in 28 of 155 patients and further therapy was not attempted in this group. No patient became pregnant over the 7 to 46 month follow-up period. Twenty seven women with lesser degrees of damage were treated by salpingostomy and seven conceived a total of 10 pregnancies. Only two pregnancies, however, went to term. There were 6 ectopic pregnancies and 2 spontaneous abortions. Given these results, the authors question whether salpingostomy is warranted in similar clinic populations.

The value of Silastic hoods in this type of surgery is doubtful. A major liability is the need for a second laparotomy to remove the prosthesis. Mulligan had a pregnancy rate of 36% in cases of bilateral fimbrial occlusion when Silastic hoods were used. (5) In compari son, an earlier group of his patients who were treated without hoods achieved only a 14% pregnancy rate. Interestingly, when Mulligan's group used hoods in a series of clinic patients the pregnancy rate was only 16.7%. (6) In a series from Montreal in which hoods were not used, surgery for distal occlusion produced a 25% pregnancy rate. (7) In another group, reported

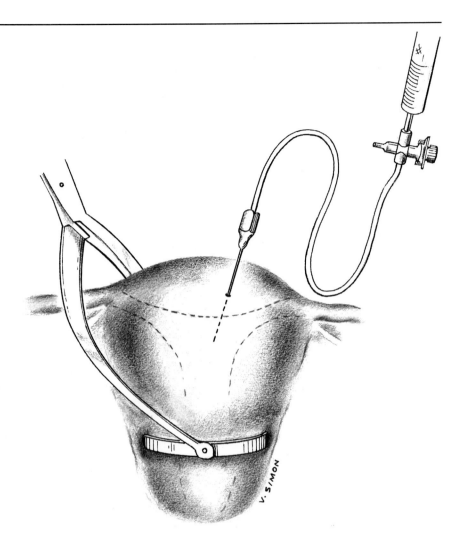

from Australia, again without hoods, Grant achieved a
41% pregnancy rate. (8) He stressed the importance of
frequent postoperative hydrotubation with chymotrypsin.
It appears, therefore, that equally good results can be
achieved without Silastic hoods. Case selection and surgical technique are the more crucial factors.

A coil prosthesis has also been used as a mechanism for
maintaining tubal patency in the postoperative period.
(9, 10) The end of the device is buried subcutaneously
for removal under local anesthesia at a later date. Its
value has not been established and in one case it was
thought to play a role in a bowel obstruction that followed
tubal surgery.

If the diagnosis of distal occlusion is confirmed at laparoscopy or laparotomy it is wise to test immediately for
proximal patency. If both ends of the tube are blocked,
surgery offers little hope. At laparotomy the cervix can

be occluded by the Buxton clamp devised for this purpose. Indigo carmine is injected with a No. 20 needle through the fundus into the uterus. A lowering of resistance is felt as the needle enters the uterine cavity. The injected dye can be seen filling the tube if cornual obstruction is not present. After removing the syringe the needle should be left in place with a closed stopcock to occlude the lumen. This provides a means for flushing the tubes free of adherent blood clot after reparative surgery.

Adhesions are first removed by sharp and blunt dissection. This can be particularly difficult when the distal one-third of the tube is densely adherent to the ovary. The dividing line between adhesions and mesosalpinx is often obscure. The dissection will produce bleeding in this area and bleeding points should be grasped with fine mosquito clamps and tied with nylon or fulgurated with needle cautery.

Often the distally occluded tube will have a slight indentation at the site where the lumen was located. A small X-shaped incision just through the serosa should be placed over this area. A Kelly clamp can then be bluntly inserted into the lumen and gently opened. Entry is signified by release of indigo carmine dye. This method will often permit uncovering of fimbria without bleeding. If this opening is too small the serosa can be cut back approximately 1/2 cm. The distal end of the tube is then everted and either sutured back to the serosa or left free.

Postoperative hydrotubation is useful for flushing out blood clots and keeping fimbria nonadherent. However, it should not be done in the presence of uterine bleeding. For that reason surgery should be scheduled for after a menstrual flow. Flushing of endometrial debris through the tubes and into the peritoneal cavity can produce endometriosis. Using a Jarcho apparatus we instill 20 ml sterile normal saline containing 100 mg hydrocortisone through the cervix on the 3rd and 5th postoperative days. The procedure is repeated once between the 14th and 20th days and once in the preovulatory period in the subsequent cycle. Grant uses lavages with hydrocortisone every 3 days for 2 weeks after surgery then switches to chymotrypsin. Arronet uses Elase (Parke, Davis), 1 vial in 10 cc normal saline at surgery. (11) Around day 8, washings are performed with a cortisone mixture. This is repeated 2–6 times at monthly intervals.

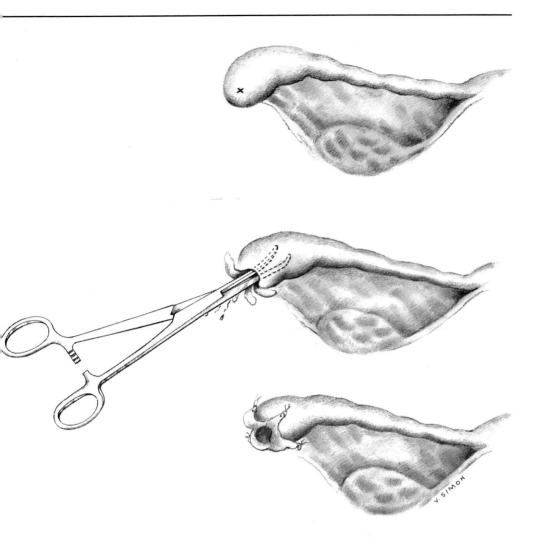

We do not use antibiotics in our flushing solutions nor do we feel that there is any evidence that routine use of antibiotics following tubal surgery improves the results.

An alternative approach to prevent closure of the tube and formation of adhesions is the use of steroids and promethazine. The aim of this treatment is to dissolv the fibrinous exudate and delay fibroblast proliferation. The drugs are given intra-muscularly and in separate syringes. The recommended dosage is 20 mg dexametha sone and 25 mg promethazine 2–3 hours preoperatively and every 4 hours for 12 doses starting 4 hours after surgery. In addition a similar dose separated by saline is instilled into the peritoneal cavity just prior to wound closure. It is suggested that permanent suture be used to close the fascia and that the skin stitches be left in place for 10 days. In a multicenter study 38% of women who had salpingostomies in association with the dexametha sone-promethazine treatment became pregnant and 24% went to term. (12) A study in monkeys, however, failed to show any beneficial effect of dexamethasone-prometh azine in preventing adhesions. (13)

Our current practice is to instill 500–1,000 mg of hydro cortisone into the cul de sac prior to closing the peritonea cavity, while we await further data on the dexamethasone promethazine therapy.

Tubal Implantation

O'Brien et al. reported a 43.3% intrauterine pregnancy rate following bilateral tubal implantation. (7) They stress the importance of not resecting the tube beyond the isthmus nor allowing the distal implanted part to be shorter than 1 inch. One added refinement of their technique is the removal of the serosal layer from the portion of the tube used for implantation, as an aid to tissue adherence.

Most other reports do not approach this success rate and a figure of 10–15% is more typical. Shirodkar has noted three principal causes for failure of the implantation operation (14):

1. Extrusion of the tube from the uterus. To prevent this occurrence the mesosalpinx should be fixed to the uterus by a figure of 8 suture.

2. Faulty placement of sutures from the tube to the uterus so that the tubal lumen faces markedly upward or down-ward. To avoid this problem, Shirodkar suggested that the uterine fundus be split from cornua to cornua. This allows a more precise removal of the occluded segments of the tube and more exact placement of the remaining tubal segments.

348

3. Growth of endometrium into the new tubal lumen. As a preventative the patient is placed on 3 months of cyclic combination contraceptive pills which will minimize endometrial growth. Hormonal therapy should be started after discharge from the hospital.

Before undertaking tubal reimplantation the diagnosis of cornual obstruction must be confirmed at laparoscopy and again at laparotomy. Transfundal injection of indigo carmine with the cervix occluded will produce distension of the uterus in the face of cornual obstruction. It is not a simple matter to determine the limits of the obstructed portion of the tube. Passing a probe through from the fimbriated end is unsatisfactory. The interstitial portion of the tube is often convoluted and defies passage of a straight probe. (15) The isthmus which begins from the uterotubal junction and extends distally for 2–3 cm is too narrow to allow atraumatic passage of a probe. A preferable technique is the injection of dye down the fimbriated end of the tube in order to stain the mucosa. The tube is transected close to the uterus and small slices are progressively taken toward the fimbriated end until a patent lumen or dye-stained mucosa is noted.

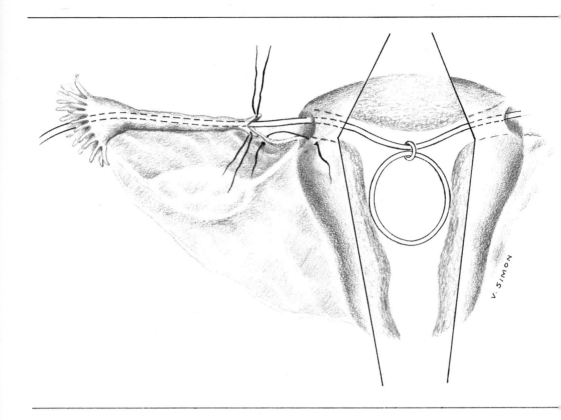

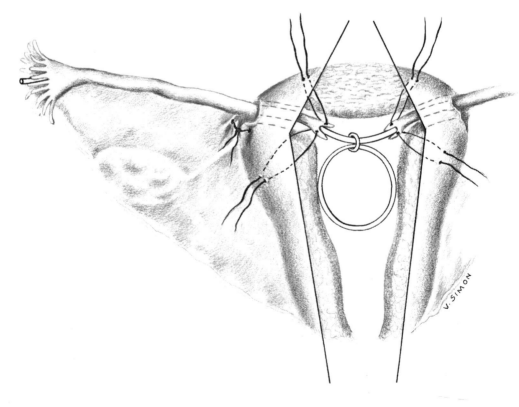

We do not use the technique of fundal splitting advocated by Shirodkar. The interstitial portion of the tube is removed using a cork borer or by scapel dissection with a No. 11 blade. The transected distal tube is split approximately $1/2$ cm at 3 and 9 o'clock. A 3-0 suture is placed and tied through each corner of the newly created flaps. These are left long. The looped portion of a Silastic prosthesis is inserted into the uterus through the cornual opening, aided by a Kelly clamp which is inserted through the contralateral cornual opening. The wings of the prosthesis are threaded out through the tubes and the distal ends of the prosthesis cut flush with the fimbria following tubal implantation. The sutures on the tubal flaps are then brought through the cornual opening and sutured through the myometrium. Each is tied on the serosal surface of the uterus after the tube is threaded through the cornual opening. A suture previously placed between the mesosalpinx and the uterus just beneath the cornua is now tied. A few interrupted sutures are placed between tubal serosa and myometrium. It is important that these do not angulate the tube. A few additional sutures may be required to close myometrial defects or for hemostasis. Care must be taken to ensure that these do not compromise the tubal lumen. Any defects in the broad ligament are then closed.

The prosthesis is left in place for 1 month. During this time the patient is on cyclic combination birth control pills to minimize endometrial growth. The device can be removed through the cervix with an IUD hook. In general this is done in the office, although on occasion cervical dilatation under anesthesia is required to effect removal.

End to End Anastomosis

There appears to be an increasing demand for reversal of tubal sterilization. Reanastomosis following Pomeroy ligation can be accomplished by the method of Williams outlined below. A pregnancy rate of 25–40% can be anticipated. Success rates of 60–70% have been reported with microscopic visualization.

In cases requiring tubal reanastomosis Williams has used a technique that is on occasion also applicable in cases of isthmic occlusion. (16) Those cases suitable for the procedure are diagnosed at the time of laparotomy when transfundal injection of dye fills a short portion of the proximal tube. Alternatively, if the tube does not fill at all thin slices can be cut from the cornua until the patent interstitial portion of the tube is reached. After the occluded segment is removed approximately 20 cm of a #1 nylon thread is passed through the proximal portion of the tube into the uterus. To aid placement of the nylon the proximal tube is first lifted forward in the direction of the round ligament and then, as the nylon is continuously threaded toward the uterus, the tube is lifted in an upward direction. The other end of the nylon is threaded through the distal portion of the tube and out the fimbriated end. The reanastomosis is performed over the nylon splint by bringing together the cut ends with 3 interrupted mattress sutures of 5-0 or 6-0 nylon or Dexon. These bring together serosa and muscularis but do not go through the mucosa. The nylon splint is removed either immediately or with a crochet hook on the 5th postoperative day.

Women who have had laparoscopic fulguration of the tubes are among those requesting repair. The extensive destruction of the tube accomplished by fulguration has made us hesitant to undertake surgery in these cases. There is a recent report, however, indicating a few pregnancies following reimplantation of fulgurated tubes. (17) Laparoscopic evaluation of the remaining structures may avoid an unnecessary laparotomy.

In all cases of tubal surgery a hysterosalpingogram should be performed if pregnancy does not occur within 6 months of exposure. High rates of patency are seen often despite poor conception rates. Thus obtaining an open tube does not insure normal function. Of the pregnancies that do occur, the majority are within 12–24 months of exposure. One of our patients, though, conceived 8 years following lysis of adhesions and release of agglutinated fimbria.

Ectopic Pregnancies

Ectopic pregnancies follow tubal surgery in some 12% of cases and patients should be warned of this danger and its symptoms. If the patient has one badly damaged tube and one that can be repaired more easily, it is best to remove the bad tube. It holds little potential for normal pregnancy but an increased possibility for tubal pregnancy.

Selection of Cases

A marked improvement in the results obtained by tubal surgery could occur through a better selection of cases. In a small series, failure of a 24-hour hysterosalpingogram (using the oil dye Ethiodol) to show peritoneal spill of dye was associated with failure of surgery to establish fertility. (3) (This included only cases of distal occlusion and not cornual obstruction.) Conversely, 9 of 20 patients showing peritoneal spill became pregnant following surgery. Ozaras noted a better prognosis when tubal rugae were visualized on hysterosalpingography with water-soluble dye. (18)

Surgery under microscopic visualization is being used at a number of centers. There is preliminary evidence at this time that it improves the outcome in cases of tubal reanastomosis (19). Operating loupes which provide a magnification of only 2.5× are helpful in identifying the lumen of the tube for passage of splints. This compares to the magnification of 4–20× achieved with a microscope.

Estes Procedure

While the results of tubal surgery are discouraging, attempts to bypass damaged tubes are no more promising. In the Estes procedure the cut surface of the ovary is attached to the uterine cornua after excision of the tube. (20, 21) In a variant of the original technique the ovary, still attached to the mesovarium, is inserted into the uterine cavity through an incision in the posterior wall of the uterus. (22) Ikle reviewed the literature on ovarian implantation and found 28 pregnancies reported after 269 operations. (23) It is our impression that the general experience is much less favorable, reflecting a tendency to report only success. Even if pregnancy is achieved the abortion rate is high.

References

1. **Mroueh, A, and Hajj, SN,** Tubal Plastic Surgery, Int J Fertil 13:215, 1968.

2. **Crane, M, and Woodruff, JD,** Factors Influencing the Success of Tuboplastic Procedures, Fertil Steril 19:810, 1968.

3. **Glass, RH, McCarthy, CPN, and Buxton, CL,** Prognosis in Tubal Plastic Surgery, Fertil Steril 20:919, 1969.

4. **Israel, R, and March, CM,** Diagnostic Laparoscopy: A Prognostic Aid in the Surgical Management of Infertility, Am J Obstet Gynec 125:96, 1976.

5. **Mulligan, WJ,** Results of Salpingostomy, Int J Fertil 11:424, 1966.

6. **Young, PE, Egan, JE, Barlow, JJ, and Mulligan, WJ,** Reconstructive Surgery for Infertility at the Boston Hospital for Women, Am J Obstet Gynec 108:1092, 1970.

7. **O'Brien, JR, Arronet, GH, and Eduljee, SY,** Operative Treatment of Fallopian Tube Pathology in Human Fertility, Am J Obstet Gynec 103:520, 1969.

8. **Grant, A,** Infertility Surgery of the Oviduct, Fertil Steril 22:496, 1971.

9. **Roland, M, and Leisten, D,** Tuboplasty in 130 Patients, Obstet Gynec 39:57, 1972.

10. **Yamaguchi, R,** A New Instrument for Salpingostomy, Obstet Gynec 31:429, 1968.

11. **Arronet, GH, Eduljee, SY, and O'Brien, JR,** A Nine Year Study of Fallopian Tube Dysfunction in Human Infertility, Fertil Steril 20:903, 1969.

12. **Horne, HW, Clyman, M, Debrovner, C, Griggs, G, Kistner, RW, Kosasa, T, Stevenson, CS, and Taymor, M,** The Prevention of Postoperative Pelvic Adhesions Following Conservative Operative Treatment for Human Infertility, Int J Fertil 18:109, 1973.

13. **Seitz, HM, Jr., Schenker, JG, Epstein, S, and Garcia, CR,** Postoperative Intraperitoneal Adhesions: A Double Blind Assessment of Their Prevention in the Monkey, Fertil Steril 24:935, 1973.

14. **Shirodkar, VN,** Further Experiences in Tuboplasty, Aust NZ J Obstet Gynec 5:1, 1965.

15. **Sweeney, WJ,** The Interstitial Portion of the Uterine Tube — Its Gross Anatomy, Course and Length, Obstet Gynec 19:3, 1962.

16. **Williams, EA,** "Aspects of Fallopian Tube Surgery," in *Recent Advances in Obstetrics and Gynecology,* editors J Stallworthy and G Bourne, Churchill Livingston. Edinburgh, 1977, p 219.

17. **Peterson, EP, Musich, JR, and Behrman, SJ,** Uterotubal Implantation and Obstetric Outcome After Previous Sterilization, Am J Obstet Gynec 128:662, 1977.

18. **Ozaras, H,** The Value of Plastic Operations on the Fallopian Tubes in the Treatment of Female Infertility, Acta Obstet Gynec Scand 47:489, 1968.

19. **Gomel, V,** Tubal Reanastomosis by Microsurgery, Fertil Steril 28:59, 1977.

20. **Estes, WL, Jr.,** Ovarian Implantation, Surg Gynec Obstet 39:394, 1924.

21. **Estes, WL, Jr., and Heitmeyer, PL,** Incidence of Pregnancy Following Ovarian Implantation, Am J Surg 24:563, 1934.

22. **Preston, PG,** Transplantation of the Ovary into the Uterine Cavity for the Treatment of Sterility in Women, J Obstet Gynec Br. Commonw 60:862, 1953.

23. **Ikle, FA,** Pregnancy After Implantation of the Ovary into the Uterus, Gynaecologia 151:95, 1961.

17 Endometriosis and Infertility

Endometriosis is both a common disease and a frequent cause of infertility. Gray was able to make a diagnosis of endometriosis in 13–17% of 761 consecutive new gynecologic patients. (1) Other investigators have estimated that 6–15% of infertile patients have endometriosis as the sole responsible factor for their problem. (2)

The most attractive theory concerning the etiology of endometriosis is that retrograde menstrual flow causes a spread of endometrial cells into the pelvis where they implant or where they set up irritative foci which stimulate differentation of peritoneal lining cells into endometrial type tissue. This theory has been supported by the following observations:

1. The cervix of monkeys was transposed so that menstrual flow emptied into the peritoneal cavity. After a number of months endometrial implants were noted. (3)

2. Endometrial cells injected under abdominal skin can grow and form endometrial implants. (4)

3. In some women blood can be seen regurgitating through the end of the Fallopian tube at the time of menstruation.

Endometriosis at distant sites may be due to vascular or lymphatic transport of endometrial fragments. Still another possibility is the transformation of coelomic epithelium into endometrial type glands as a result of unspecified stimulation. (5)

Diagnosis of Endometriosis

For the clinician, the major problems are establishing the diagnosis and choosing suitable treatment for the individual patient. While the complaint of infertility should be sufficient to alert the physician to the possibility of endometriosis, the index of suspicion is elevated if the women has progressively severe dysmenorrhea, dyspareunia, or pain on defecation. Dysmenorrhea is even more suggestive of endometriosis if it begins after years of relatively pain-free menses.

The pain of endometriosis is most severe during the menses but may also be present throughout the month. Pain is probably secondary to stretching of peritoneal or fibrous bands following bleeding into cavities created by the endometrial implants. Frequently the degree of pain is disproportionate to the pathology. Women with large endometriomas may be symptom-free, while minimal endometriosis may cause severe discomfort. It is probably of little value to attempt to characterize the pain of endometriosis in terms of location or radiation. Rather, dysmenorrhea or pelvic pain of any type should raise a suspicion of its presence. Low back pain, too, may be due to endometriosis.

An association of myomas with endometriosis has been reported and this may account for the increased menstrual flow seen in some patients.

The pelvic examination may be normal in the presence of minimal endometriosis while more extensive disease will often produce enlargement of the ovaries. They may be stuck in the pelvis and frequently are associated with a fixed retroverted uterus. Beading, nodularity, and tenderness of the uterosacral ligaments are characteristic of endometriosis. This can best be appreciated on rectovaginal examination.

Treatment of Endometriosis

Minimal findings such as slight beading of the uterosacral ligaments in the young, single, asymptomatic patient can be treated by observation or by combination contraceptive pills in low dosages on a continuous basis. By causing some degree of endometrial atrophy, the hormonal therapy diminishes menstrual flow and lessens the chance for reflux through the tube into the peritoneal cavity. One drawback to treating such patients is the possibility that the minimal physical findings are, in fact, not endometriosis. For that reason, patients with minimal symptoms and physical signs should be carefully followed without therapy.

356

If symptoms are more severe or if there is slight ovarian enlargement with fixation of a retroverted uterus and nodular tender uterosacral ligaments, specific steps toward therapy are indicated. If infertility is the major complaint, a normal sperm count and evidence of ovulatory function should be obtained. If a hysterosalpingogram done with Ethiodol shows tubal patency and there is no gross ovarian enlargement, we prefer to wait 6 months, because of the fertility enhancing effect seen after this procedure, before proceeding with laparoscopy. This is, in fact, the same course of action that is followed in our cases of infertility, even if there is no suspicion of endometriosis.

If laparoscopy reveals endometriomas or pelvic adhesions involving the adnexae, then surgery is indicated. Surgery is also advised if the signs and symptoms suggest endometriosis and there is significant ovarian enlargement.

While the preoperative use of hormones has been suggested to accomplish decidualization and softening of endometrial implants some surgeons feel that this treatment increases intraoperative bleeding and obscures tissue planes, and that it should not be used. This has not been our experience. If the signs and symptoms suggest endometriosis, and there is also significant ovarian enlargement, conservative surgery is undertaken following 6–8 weeks of noncyclic hormonal therapy with one of a number of oral contraceptive pills. Surgery is not delayed beyond this time because of the possibility that the ovarian enlargement may signify malignant disease rather than endometriosis. Hormones are not used in the immediate postoperative period because such use has not been shown to increase the chances for pregnancy. In addition, this time is the most opportune for achieving pregnancy and it should not be compromised by contraception.

Conservative surgery for infertility can be a tedious time-consuming procedure. Adhesions are lysed, endometriomas excised, implants of endometriosis fulgurated or excised, the uterus suspended, peritonealization performed (if necessary, using omental grafts), and the appendix removed. Presacral neurectomy is often recommended when there is severe dysmenorrhea. The primary surgical procedure itself, however, may cure the dysmenorrhea without incurring the possible liabilities of bladder and bowel dysfunction which can follow presacral neurectomy. The suggestion that presacral neurectomy enhances fertility is open to question.

Endometriosis often involves portions of the bowel. These usually consist of brownish puckered areas which can at times be excised without entering the lumen of the bowel. Uterine myomas, if present, should be excised.

The goal of conservative surgery is to preserve and to enhance reproductive function. When endometriomas are removed a vigorous attempt should be made to leave behind any normal ovarian tissue. Even one tenth of an ovary may be enough to preserve function and fertility. A superficial incision is made through the capsule of the ovarian cyst which is then shelled out. Invariably the cyst will rupture during the removal but this does not compromise fertility if the spilled chocolate type material is absorbed by sponges and the pelvis irrigated with saline.

Conversely, of nine women who experienced spontaneous rupture of an endometrioma prior to surgery, only one had a subsequent pregnancy (6). This would indicate that more prolonged contact of the peritoneum with the cyst material sets up irritative foci which can be sites for adhesion formation.

The majority of reports indicate that conception rates of 50% can be expected from conservative surgery (2). Ranney, however, reported pregnancies in 42 of 48 women who had conservative surgery for endometriosis and who had no other infertility problem (7). The average time to conception was 7.3 months and the longest was just over 2 years. The younger patient has a better prognosis in terms of pregnancy. The extent of the disease also has an effect on results. Petersohn found a 79% pregnancy rate if only simple endometrial cysts were found at the time of surgery compared to a 40% pregnancy rate if the cysts were accompanied by adhesions (8). A correlation between the extent of the disease and the success of surgery has been reported also by Acosta and his co-workers (9).

In most series the recurrence of endometriosis following conservative surgery is surprisingly low. Green reported it to be 7%, and in a series from The Johns Hopkins Hospital, only 13 of 101 women required additional operations because of endometriosis. (2, 6) Moreover, 5 of these 13 had conceived after their original operation, and had thus derived benefit from that procedure. Others have reported higher rates of recurrence. (10).

The majority of pregnancies following conservative surgery for endometriosis occur within 3 years of operation. If the patient is not pregnant within 2 years it is wise to encourage the couple to investigate the possibilities for adoption.

It is worth emphasizing that endometriosis with periovarian and peritubal adhesions associated with infertility is best treated surgically. On the other hand, when limited areas of endometriosis are identified by laparoscopy in the cul de sac, on the uterosacral ligaments, or the surface of the ovary, hormonal therapy can be utilized. We recommend continuous non-cyclic use of contraceptive pills for 6–9 months for those women who are infertile and who have moderate degrees of surface ovarian endometriosis. A pregnancy rate of 40% can be anticipated, when a variety of contraceptive pills such as Ovral are used. Depo Provera (150 mg every 3 months) can be prescribed when there is a need to avoid the estrogen component of the birth control pills. Oral Provera in a dose of 30 mg daily is also effective. (11) Hormonal therapy should not be used when there are myomas present. There are no figures available detailing the value of pseudopregnancy when a few small implants are noted only in the cul de sac, and the tubes and ovaries are free of endometriosis and adhesions. In these cases we choose to initiate and maintain pseudopregnancy for 3 to 6 months, a practice which seems reasonable but whose efficacy is not substantiated. It is not known how minimal endometriosis interferes with fertility nor has it been established what percentage of women can achieve pregnancy without treatment when there is minimal endometriosis in the pelvis.

Testosterone or methyltestosterone, 5 or 10 mg sublingual daily, is effective in reducing pelvic pain and dyspareunia when it is associated with endometriosis. Even smaller doses can be effective thus minimizing side effects. The latter are usually weight gain, acne, and occasionally depression. Ovulation is not eliminated and pregnancy can occur while the drug is being taken. While relief of symptoms is often impressive cure of infertility is less successful.

Danazol, a synthetic steroid which is an isoxazol derivative of ethisterone, has antigonadotropin and slight androgenic activities. In doses of 800 mg daily taken for 3 to 9 months it is effective in reducing the symptoms of endometriosis. It is thought that suppression of gonadotropins diminishes steroid hormone stimulation of endometriosis, allowing atrophy and spontaneous healing to occur. Side effects can be related to the antigonadotropin effect which produces lower estrogen levels and to the androgenic properties of the drug. Thus there are amenorrhea and hot flushes in some patients as well as weight gain, acne, and an increase in oiliness of the skin.

It is too early to assess the effects of Danazol on infertility. Friedlander indicated that 19 of 24 patients desiring pregnancy were successful following treatment with Danazol, while Dmowski and Scommegna reported 12 pregnancies in 24 women within six months of therapy. (12, 13)

There are two disturbing aspects to the reports on Danazol, in addition to the previously cited side effects. A few authors have noted rapid return of symptoms and pelvic abnormalities after the medication is discontinued. In the laparoscopy controlled study by Dmowski and Cohen, periovarian adhesions were noted in many cases following laparoscopic biopsy and Danazol. (14) If these are a byproduct of Danazol they could be a bar to fertility. If they are a reaction to biopsy it would be advisable to avoid this procedure when doing laparoscopy, prior to treatment with Danazol.

Long-Term Hormonal Therapy

Long-term (12–24 months) pseudopregnancy without surgery is useful in unmarried patients with severe symptoms but with little in the way of palpable findings. Before undertaking prolonged therapy, diagnosis should be established by laparoscopy. Prolonged therapy is also indicated if symptoms recur after conservative surgery.

When an endometrioma is unexpectedly discovered at surgery in a young woman without other evidence of endometriosis, post-operative use of cyclic combination birth control pills should be used to provide protection against further disease.

Prevention of Endometriosis

Numerous suggestions have been made concerning the prevention of endometriosis. The most reasonable is avoidance of tubal insufflation, hysterosalpingography, and cervical dilatation during a menstrual flow so that endometrial cells will not be forced out through the tubes into the peritoneal cavity. While pregnancy at an early age may possibly help to prevent endometriosis, this unproven course of action has social and economic drawbacks. More objectionable is the use of cervical dilatation for "stenosis" as a means of preventing retrograde menstrual flow. Many normal women have been subjected to dilatation and insertion of polyethylene cervical devices without evidence that this is of any benefit. If the cervical canal is patent for the menstrual flow, who is to say that the cervical canal is too small? Against the dubious benefit of dilatation is the risk of anesthesia and the expense of hospitalization and physician's fees. Equally unwarranted and of no proven value is the use of uterine suspension operations to prevent retrograde flow.

The most logical approach to the prevention of endometriosis would be the use of progestin contraception with its protective effect of decidualization.

References

1. **Gray, LA,** The Management of Endometriosis Involving the Bowel, Clin Obstet Gynec 9:309, 1966.

2. **Spangler, DB, Jones, GS, and Jones, HW, Jr.,** Infertility Due to Endometriosis, Am J Obstet Gynec 109:850, 1971.

3. **Scott, RB, TeLinde, RW, and Wharton, LR, Jr.,** Further Studies on Experimental Endometriosis, Am J Obstet Gynec 66:1082, 1953.

4. **Ridley, JH, and Edwards, IK,** Experimental Endometriosis in the Human, Am J Obstet Gynec 76:783, 1958.

5. **Merrill, JA,** Endometrial Induction of Endometriosis Across Millipore Filters, Am J Obstet Gynec 94:780, 1966.

6. **Green, TH,** Conservative Surgical Treatment of Endometriosis, Clin Obstet Gynec 9:293, 1966.

7. **Ranney, B,** Endometriosis, I. Conservative Operations, Am J Obstet Gynec 107:743, 1970.

8. **Petersohn, L,** Fertility in Patients with Ovarian Endometriosis Before and After Treatment, Acta Obstet Gynec Scand 49:331, 1970.

9. **Acosta, AA, Buttram, VC, Besch, PK, Malinak, R, Franklin, RR, and Vanderheyden, JD,** A Proposed Classification of Pelvic Endometriosis, Obstet Gynec 42:19, 1973.

10. **Andrews, WC, and Larsen, GD,** Endometriosis: Treatment with Hormonal Pseudopregnancy and/or Operation, Am J Obstet Gynec 118:643, 1974.

11. **Moghissi, KS, and Boyce, CR,** Management of Endometriosis with Oral Medroxyprogesterone Acetate, Obstet Gynec 47:265, 1976.

12. **Friedlander, RL,** Experiences with Danazol in Therapy of Endometriosis, Excerpta Medica International Congress Series No. 368, p 100, 1976.

13. **Dmowski, WP, and Scommegna, A,** The Rationale for Treatment of Endometriosis with Danazol, Excerpta Medica International Congress Series No. 368, p 87, 1976.

14. **Dmowski, WP, and Cohen, MR,** Treatment of Endometriosis with an Antigonadotropin, Danazol, Obstet Gynec 46:147, 1975.

Male Infertility

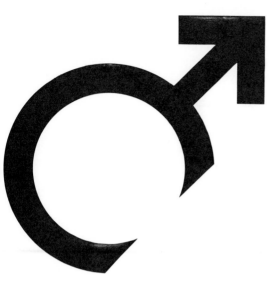

With 40–50% of infertility wholly or partially attributable to a male factor, it is important for the gynecologist to be knowledgeable in this area. After the initial semen analysis, it is his responsibility to determine whether urologic consultation is required. *This chapter will detail the analysis of semen, indicate factors responsible for abnormal semen, and consider available treatment for problems of male infertility, including artificial insemination.*

Semen Analysis

There are specific and important guidelines for the collection and analysis of semen. The specimen should be collected by masturbation into a clean glass jar, protected from cold, and brought to the laboratory within two hours of collection. Abstinence of 48 to 72 hours prior to ejaculation is recommended. The specimen should not be collected by withdrawal, because the sperm-rich fraction may be lost, nor should it be collected in a condom. The latter contain spermicidal agents. If the male cannot collect a specimen by masturbation he can be supplied with a special sheath, manufactured by the Milex Company, which does not contain a spermicide.

Interpretation of the semen analysis is often hampered by the erroneous "normal values" printed on data sheets supplied by many commercial laboratories. It is still common to see these laboratories quote the lower limits of normal as 60,000,000/cc, 80,000,000/cc or even 100,000,000/cc. The work of MacLeod has established that the percentage of pregnancies decreases when the sperm count drops below 20,000,000/cc, and this is the currently accepted lower limit of normal. (1, 2) Because of the errors inherent in doing a sperm count we usually prefer the count to be 30,000,000/cc or higher. It should be pointed out that pregnancies do occur even with counts below 20,000,000/cc, and this has been emphasized by recent reports of sperm counts in fertile males prior to vasectomy. (3) Of 386 men undergoing elective vasectomy, all of whom had at least one child, 20% had sperm counts less than 20,000,000/cc. (4)

While the sperm count requires proper dilution of semen and placement of the diluted specimen on a hemocytometer chamber for counting, sperm motility determination is less rigorous and can be performed in any office equipped with a microscope and glass slides. A drop of semen is placed on the slide (or, ideally, on a coverslip which is then placed over a depression slide to make a hanging drop preparation) and looked at initially without a coverslip at 100× magnification. A rough estimate is made of both the percentage of motile sperm and the percentage of sperm that show *progressive* motility across the field. At least 50% of the sperm should show the latter quality, and this can be confirmed by placing a coverslip on the specimen and using 400× magnification. In order to compare specimens it should be standard procedure to evaluate motility 2 hours after ejaculation; there is no evidence that checking *in vitro* at more prolonged intervals (e.g. 24 hours) gives any useful information concerning the male's fertility potential.

There are simple staining methods which can be done in the office to evaluate sperm morphology but in general we rely on the clinical laboratory for this evaluation. Normal human semen specimens contain a greater number and variety of abnormal sperm shapes than most mammalian species. In general up to 40% of sperm may show abnormal morphology without being a basis for infertility. MacLeod has emphasized that abnormal morphology is more important in a diagnostic sense than in its questionable affect on fertility. A high percentage of tapering forms and spermatids is often a clue to the presence of a varicocele. (2)

The usual ejaculate volume is between 3 and 5 cc (range 1–7 cc) and it is influenced by the frequency of ejaculation. Low volumes in association with absence of sperm in the postcoital test suggest the possible need for artificial insemination with the husband's sperm. Higher than normal volumes associated with a low concentration of sperm can be treated by the use of split ejaculate inseminations, a technique which will be discussed later in this chapter.

Other abnormalities in the semen which can contribute to infertility are: (1) Infection, manifested by the presence of white blood cells. Almost all semen specimens contain some of these cells, and it is important for each laboratory to establish its own range for a normal reading. (2) Failure of the semen to liquefy. Semen is ejaculated in liquid form; it quickly becomes a gel which again liquifies within 20 minutes. If a thick, viscid specimen is associated with a poor postcoital test, the semen can be liquefied by running it back and forth through a #19 hypodermic needle and then using it for insemination. Enzyme digestion of semen has also been used to overcome this problem. (5)

(3) Agglutination of sperm. Spontaneous agglutination of sperm in semen is often an isolated event which does not recur. Persistent agglutination can be caused by *Escherichia coli* infections or sperm antibodies. The former, which may be signified by white cells in the semen, can be diagnosed by urologic examination and treated with antibiotics. Agglutination due to sperm autoimmunity is seen rarely and there is no effective treatment, though treatment of infection may be helpful. It is most common in men who have had testicular injury or who have had vas ligation followed by a reanastomosis.

Abnormal Semen Follow-up

If the laboratory report on the initial semen analysis is abnormal we prefer to personally examine a second specimen before forwarding it to the laboratory. If the semen characteristics are again abnormal inquiry is made concerning the presence of the following factors, any of which may produce abnormal sperm quality and quantity:

1. History of testicular injury, surgery, mumps, or venereal disease.

2. Heat. A small rise in scrotal temperature can adversely affect spermatogenesis, and a febrile illness may produce striking changes in sperm count and motility. The effect of the illness can still be seen in the sperm count and motility 2 to 3 months later. This reflects the 70–74 days it requires for a spermatozoon to be generated from a primary germ cell. Environmental sources of heat (such as the use of jockey shorts instead of boxer shorts, excessively hot baths, frequent use of a sauna or steam bath, or occupations that require long hours of sitting, such as long distance truck driving) may all diminish fertility potential.

3. Severe allergic reactions with systemic effects. (6)

4. Exposure to radiation.

5. Use of certain drugs such as Furadantin. The effect, if any, of marijuana on spermatogenesis is still uncertain, but there is some preliminary evidence that it can depress androgen levels, and thus it could decrease spermatogenesis.

6. Coital timing. Counts at the lower level of the normal range may be depressed to below normal levels by ejaculations occurring daily or more frequently. Conversely, abstinence for 5–7 days or more "to save up sperm" is counterproductive because the minimal gain in numbers is offset by the lower motility produced by the increased proportion of older sperm. For most couples coitus every other day around the time of ovulation will give the optimal chance for pregnancy.

7. Cigarettes, alcohol, and hard work. While all three have been cited as causes of abnormal semen, there is very little evidence to either confirm or deny their connection. Alcohol can depress the level of testosterone in the serum. (7) Working hours and alcohol are probably of more importance in infertility as a cause of impotence or decreased libido. A small proportion of alcoholics who are impotent will remain so even after discontinuing alcoholic intake. (8) The deleterious effect of nicotine on so many aspects of health certainly raises a suspicion that it can also depress semen quality.

Urological Evaluation

If none of these problems pertain to the couple under investigation, then referral is made to a urologist in order to look for an anatomic abnormality, an infection, a varicocele, or an endocrine disorder.

Examination may reveal a physical impairment, such as a marked hypospadias which can cause sperm to be deposited outside the vagina. In rare cases of diabetes, in neurologic disease, or following prostatectomy there can be retrograde ejaculation into the bladder. Pregnancies have been reported after insemination of sperm obtained by catheterization of the bladder or by post-ejaculation voiding. (9, 10) Emptying of the bladder and instillation of a buffer glucose solution prior to ejaculation will aid sperm survival. More recently, therapy utilizing ephedrine or Ornade has been used with limited success in cases of retrograde ejaculation. (11, 12) Retrograde ejaculation may be only partial, and some men with this condition may have small amounts of ejaculate emitted from the urethra.

In a series of infertile males reported by Dubin and Amelar, 7.4% of the cases comprised some form of ductal obstruction. (13) The most common finding was epididymal obstruction due to gonorrhea or tuberculosis. A rarer finding was congenital absence of the duct system. If the ducts are congenitally absent, fructose will not be found in the semen because it is normally produced in the seminal vesicles.

Testicular damage may be found following mumps orchiditis and cryptorchidism. Finally, men with Klinefelter's syndrome usually have small testes and azospermia.

If the physical examination of the male does not uncover an abnormality, testicular biopsy may reveal the cause of the infertility. Azospermia associated with normal spermatogenesis indicates ductal obstruction. If the biopsy reveals complete hyalinization and fibrosis of the seminiferous tubules, there is almost no chance for fertility. Some who feel that hormonal therapy of male infertility is of value use testicular biopsy as a means of selecting those men who have the greatest chance of responding to drugs. (14, 15)

If the urologist finds infection in the genitourinary tract it can be cleared with antibiotics and possibly prostatic massage.

A small percentage of males with azospermia or severe oligospermia will have chromosomal abnormalities.

Hormonal Therapy

Endocrine disorders are an uncommon cause of male infertility. It is worthwhile, however, to test for abnormalities of TSH, FSH, LH and testosterone. Prolactin should also be measured and if elevated, further diagnostic tests are indicated to determine if a pituitary tumor is present.

At the present time there seems to be no reason to use hormonal therapy unless there is evidence of deficiency. This viewpoint is contrary to current urologic practice. Cytomel is almost automatically prescribed, even when evidence of thyroid dysfunction is lacking. This treatment continues despite its condemnation by the urologists with the greatest experience in problems of male infertility. (16)

While treatment of males with low counts with clomiphene has on occasion raised sperm numbers, a double blind study using 100 mg daily for 3- to 10-day periods at monthly intervals revealed no consistent changes in sperm density. (17, 18) One recent report indicated a marked increase in sperm count when clomiphene was given at a dose of 25 mg for 25 days of each month. This improvement was transient and only 2 pregnancies were achieved by the 22 males who were treated. (19) The same disappointing results have been found after therapy with human menopausal gonadotropins in men with normal levels of follicle-stimulating hormone and luteinizing hormone. (20) Injections of human chorionic gonadotropin (HCG) have been reported, in a few cases, to increase sperm motility. The usual dosage is 2,500 to 3,000 international units (IU) intramuscularly every 5 days. Substantial evidence is lacking for its clinical usefulness, though there is a suggestion that it may have specific benefit in cases where there is no response to varicocele ligation. In a study by Maddock and Nelson, injection of normal males with 5,000 IU of HCG three times a week for $1\frac{1}{2}$ to 2 months resulted in severe damage to the seminiferous tubules. (21)

367

Testosterone rebound therapy has a long history. Two to three months of testosterone, 30 mg daily, results in a marked depression of sperm count. In successful cases 2 to 3 months after therapy is discontinued the sperm count is elevated above the pretreatment level. Urologic literature would suggest that these successes are a small minority. Two additional drawbacks are the short duration of the improved sperm count and the occasional cases where the oligospermic male becomes permanently azospermic as a result of therapy.

Infusion of gonadotropin releasing factors can stimulate secretion of gonadotropins. There have been isolated reports of its usefulness in male infertility. (22) Because the evidence is, at the moment, equivocal, releasing factors should only be used in investigational studies.

In a review of the management of male infertility de Kretser pointed out that many different medications have been claimed to exert a beneficial effect on sperm, but that in the majority of cases claims have not been substantiated. Empirical therapy with vitamins and thyroid is condemned. (23)

Varicocele

One of the most striking advances in the field of male infertility was the discovery of the importance of varicocele in influencing semen quality. Approximately 25% of infertile males will have a varicocele of the left internal spermatic vein. (It has also been noted in approximately 10% of men under age 20, many of whom have poor sperm counts or motility.) One study from Denmark showed that a number of males with improved spermatogenesis after surgery for varicocele had a small drop in left testicular temperature postoperatively, indicating that increased temperature could be the mechanism through which a varicocele exerts its deleterious effects. (24) Elevated catecholamine levels also have been suggested as mediators of the antifertility effects of varicocele. (25) Whatever the reason for the infertility associated with varicocele, ligation of the left internal spermatic vein in men with a varicocele results in a 40–55% pregnancy rate. (26) The most striking improvement after operation is in sperm motility. MacLeod noted that 35% of the pregnancies occurred despite a sperm count remaining at 10,000,000/cc or under. (27) The stress pattern of sperm morphology, characteristic of varicoceles, with tapering forms predominating, often remained after ligation.

Every infertile male requires a careful examination. Even small varicoceles may significantly affect semen quality. A varicocele may empty in the recumbent position, and the urologist must be alert to the need to examine the patient in the upright position. Dubin and Amelar also stress the importance of doing the examination while the patient performs a Valsalva maneuver. (26) A recent European report stated that ligation of the left internal spermatic vein, even without a demonstrable varicocele, improved the pregnancy rate. (28)

Frequency of Exposure

A major question in the minds of the infertile couple concerns the optimal frequency of exposure to achieve pregnancy. It is true that the frequency of sexual relations may have an important bearing on fertility. In males with borderline sperm numbers, daily ejaculation may depress the count to a level where chances for pregnancy are diminished. Relations every other day during the week that encompasses the fertile period (if this can be defined) would seem to offer the best chance for conception. However, attempts to have the couple adhere to a rigid schedule are unwise and may provoke sexual difficulty in an already troubled couple. Persistence of infrequent coitus or premature ejaculation may require sexual counseling. These problems are now far more amenable to therapy utilizing the approach of Masters and Johnson. (29)

Artificial Insemination Husband (AIH)

If the urologist is unable to find an anatomic abnormality, an infection, a varicocele, or an endocrine deficiency, we prefer to work on the ejaculate rather than subject the male to non-specific endocrine therapy.

Insemination with husband's whole semen in cases of poor motility or decreased count does not increase the chances for pregnancy. (30)

On the other hand, husband inseminations using whole ejaculates are of value in refractory premature ejaculation, retrograde ejaculation, and cases where the male cannot ejaculate in the vagina but can give a specimen by masturbation. Freezing and thawing depresses, to some extent, sperm motility. Therefore a specimen with low motility will not survive freezing. Moreover specimens with a low count also do not tolerate freezing. There is little advantage in freezing and pooling specimens.

There have been a few reports of increased sperm motility following *in vitro* incubation with caffeine. (31, 32) Caffeine is mutagenic in bacteria, and its use to treat sperm seems highly questionable.

Ericsson and coworkers have layered sperm on columns of liquid albumin as a means of separating out Y-bearing sperm. (33) While the success of this technique is still disputed, the albumin column does allow separation of the most vigorous sperm from the dead and poorly moving sperm. (33, 34) Also removed are the debris and round cells often found in seminal plasma. The vigorously moving sperm suspended in physiologic solutions can be used for intrauterine inseminations. This technique is being studied in cases of male infertility in a number of clinics throughout the United States and Europe. Preliminary results have been disappointing, and only a few pregnancies have been achieved.

The Split Ejaculate

It is evident that in some males seminal fluid may be harmful to sperm. The first portion of the ejaculate contains the sperm-rich fraction and prostatic fluid. The remainder of the ejaculate originates in the seminal vesicles. Separating the two fractions by use of a split ejaculate can provide a specimen for insemination which has a greater concentration of sperm and improved motility. In this technique the first few drops of the ejaculate are collected in one jar and the rest in a second jar. Collection can be facilitated by taping the two jars together. Both must be checked, for while the first jar contains the superior specimen in 90% of cases the second is better in 5%. (In 5% there is no difference between the two.) If one of the specimens is not substantially better than the whole ejaculate there is no reason for doing inseminations. Amelar and Hotchkiss reported a series of couples in which split ejaculates were used and 22 of 39 (56%) achieved pregnancies. (35) However, males with very poor counts were largely excluded and some of the treated couples had counts and motilities in the whole ejaculates which now would be considered within the normal range. This should not detract from the possible usefulness of the technique, which can increase sperm concentration and motility and also provide a specimen with less viscosity. In cases where split ejaculates are advisable the couple can also use an *in vivo* technique: the husband withdraws as soon as he feels that ejaculation is starting. Amelar and Dubin have reported 33 pregnancies in couples using this method. (36)

Artificial Insemination Donor (AID)

The combined problems of male infertility and decreased availability of adoptable babies has increased the interest and demand for AID. Thousands of babies are born each year in this country as a result of AID.

Four points are worth emphasizing: (1) Donor inseminations do not guarantee pregnancy. The success rate is about 70% (50% with frozen semen). (2) The couple should give some thought to their feelings should the child be born with a congenital anomaly. This will occur in perhaps 4–5% of all pregnancies, irrespective of whether they follow normal intercourse or artificial insemination. (3). Venereal disease has been transmitted on occasion by donor insemination. (4) It is a wise precaution to have both the man and the woman sign a consent form. (37) The procedure is covered by law in only a few states. In California, once the husband signs the consent form he is the legal father of the baby conceived through AID. In other areas it would be worthwhile for the physician to know the legal status of AID in his/her state so that correct information can be conveyed to patients.

If the state has no law governing AID then the physician who does the inseminations should not be the obstetrician for that pregnancy. An obstetrician unaware of the inseminations can in clear conscience sign the birth certificate stating that the husband is the father of the child.

The donor should be unknown to the couple. His health must be excellent and there should be no family history of genetic diseases. The donor will not be a mirror image of the husband, but an attempt should be made to match physical characteristics. Use of RhoGAM makes Rh compatibility between the donor and the wife a less crucial issue today, though we still try to use Rh negative sperm donors for Rh negative women. AID is a private matter between the physician and the couple. Discussions with friends or relatives should be firmly discouraged. Use of friends or relatives as donors raises the potential for emotional problems in the future and should not be allowed. Similarly, requests to mix the husband's sperm with the donor's signifies that the couple may not have made the emotional adjustment to the thought of donor insemination. The husband's semen may also be deleterious to the donor's sperm.

Donor inseminations are useful in azospermia, severe oligospermia, or necrospermia refractory to treatment. They are also useful if the woman has a long history of fetal loss due to Rh sensitization. Here an Rh negative donor would be used. Genetic diseases may on occasion be an indication for donor insemination.

The basal body temperature chart is a most useful guide to the approximate time of ovulation. Initially, an attempt is made to inseminate on the day just before (or 2 days before) the temperature rise based on reviewing 2 months of charts. Usually one to three inseminations are done each month. Approximately 50% of the successful cases will occur within the first 2 months. If pregnancy has not occurred by that time, a hysterosalpingogram is performed. Approximately 90% of pregnancies that will occur happen within 6 months.

Inseminations can be placed in the uterus, cervix, or vagina. A cervical cap, used by some physicians, does not appear to enhance the success rate. Intrauterine inseminations run the potential risks of infection and of severe pain due to uterine cramping. For those reasons intrauterine insemination with donor semen should not be performed.

We prefer to inject at the entrance to the cervical canal by means of a polyethylene catheter (Milex Company). The major portion of the semen overflows into the posterior fornix. The overflow collects on the posterior blade of the speculum, and the cervical os is allowed to dip into the pool while the woman rests for 20 minutes with her hips elevated.

Physicians will be faced with requests for AID by single women and lesbian couples. In these cases evaluation by a social worker or a psychiatrist is a wise precaution.

Prostaglandins

Bygdeman showed that there was less prostaglandin E in the semen of males from functionally infertile marriages compared to males of proven fertility. (38) Hawkins found a relationship between levels of prostaglandins and conceptions in oligospermic males. (39)

It has not yet been demonstrated that addition of prostaglandin to semen would enhance fertility.

References

1. **MacLeod, J, and Gold, RZ,** The Male Factor in Fertility and Infertility II. Spermatozoon Counts in 1000 Men of Known Fertility and in 1000 Cases of Infertile Marriages, J Urol 66:436. 1951.

2. **MacLeod, J,** Human Male Infertility, Obstet Gynecol Survey 26:335, 1971.

3. **Derrick, FC, and Johnson, J,** Reexamination of "Normal" Sperm Count, Urologie 3:99, 1974.

4. **Nelson, CMK, and Bunge, RG,** Semen Analysis: Evidence for Changing Parameters of Male Fertility Potential, Fertil Steril 25:503, 1974.

5. **Wilson, VB, and Bunge, RG,** Infertility and Semen Nonliquefaction, J Urol 113:509, 1975.

6. **MacLeod, J,** A Testicular Response during and following Severe Allergic Reaction, Fertil Steril 13:531, 1962.

7. **Gordon, GG, Altman, K, Southern, AL, Rubin, E, and Lieber, CS,** Effect of Alcohol (Ethanol) Administration on Sex Hormone Metabolism in Normal Men, New Engl J Med 295:293, 1976.

8. **Lemere, F, and Smith, JW,** Alcohol Induced Sexual Impotence, Am J Psych 130:212, 1973.

9. **Bourne, RB, Kretzchmer, WA, and Esser, JR,** Successful Artificial Insemination in a Diabetic with Retrograde Ejaculation, Fertil Steril 22:275, 1971.

10. **Glezerman, M, Lunenfeld, B, Potashnik, G, Oelsner, G, and Beer, R,** Retrograde Ejaculation: Pathophysiologic Aspects and Report of Two Successfully Treated Cases, Fertil Steril 27:796, 1976.

11. **Stewart, BH, and Bergant, JA,** Correction of Retrograde Ejaculation by Sympathomimetic Medication: Preliminary Report, Fertil Steril 25:1073, 1974.

12. **Stockamp, K, Schreiter, F, and Altwein, JR,** α Adrenergic Drugs in Retrograde Ejaculation, Fertil Steril 25:817, 1974.

13. **Dubin, L, and Amelar, RD,** Etiologic Factors in 1294 Consecutive Cases of Male Infertility, Fertil Steril 22:469, 1971.

14. **Meinhard, E, McRae, CU, and Chisholm, GD,** Testicular Biopsy in Evaluation of Male Infertility, Br Med J 3:577, 1973.

15. **Schwartzstein, L,** Human Menopausal Gonadotropins in the Treatment of Patients with Oligospermia, Fertil Steril 25:813, 1974.

16. **Charney, CW,** Treatment of Male Infertility, in Behrman, SJ, and Kistner, RW, eds., *Progress in Infertility,* Little, Brown, Boston, 1968.

17. **Mellinger, RC, and Thompson, RJ,** The Effect of Clomiphene Citrate in Male Infertility, Fertil Steril 17:94, 1966.

18. **Foss, GL, Tindall, VR, and Birkett, JP,** The Treatment of Subfertile Men with Clomiphene Citrate, J Reprod Fertil 32:167, 1973.

19. **Paulson, DR, Wacksman, J, Hammond, CB, and Wiebe, HR,** Hypofertility and Clomiphene Citrate Therapy, Fertil Steril 26:982, 1975.

20. **Sherins, RJ,** Clinical Aspects of Treatment of Male Infertility with Gonadotropins: Testicular Response of Some Men Given HCG with and without Pergonal, in Mancini, RE, and Martini, L, eds., *Male Infertility and Sterility,* Academic Press, New York, 1974.

21. **Maddock, WO, and Nelson, WO,** The Effects of Chorionic Gonadotropin in Adult Men: Increased Estrogen and 17-Ketosteroid Excretion, Gynecomastia, Leydig Cell Stimulation and Seminiferous Tubule Damage, J Clin Endocrinol Metab 12:985, 1952.

22. **Schwarzstein, K, Aparicio, NJ, Turner, D, Calamera, JC, Mancini, R, and Schally, AV,** Use of Synthetic Luteinizing Hormone Releasing Hormone in Treatment of Oligo-Spermic Men, Fertil Steril 26:331, 1975.

23. **de Kretser, DM,** The Management of the Infertile Male, Clin Obstet Gynaec 1:409, 1974.

24. **Agger, P,** Scrotal and Testicular Temperature: Its Relation to Sperm Count before and after Operation for Varicocele, Fertil Steril 22:286, 1971.

25. **Cohen, MS, Plaine, L, and Brown, JS,** The Role of Internal Spermatic Vein Plasma Catecholamine Determinations in Subfertile Men with Varicoceles, Fertil Steril 26:1243, 1975.

26. **Dubin, L, and Amelar, RD,** Varicocelectomy as Therapy in Male Infertility: A Study of 504 Cases, Fertil Steril 26:217, 1975.

27. **MacLeod, J,** Further Observations on the Role of Varicocele in Human Male Infertility, Fertil Steril 20:545, 1969.

28. **Fogh-Anderson, P, Nielsen, MC, Rebbe, H, and Stakemann, G,** The Effect on Fertility of Ligation of the Left Spermatic Vein in Men without Clinical Signs of Varicocele, Acta Obstet Gynec Scand 54:29, 1975.

29. **Masters, WH, and Johnson, VE,** Human Sexual Inadequacy, Little, Brown, Boston, 1970.

30. **Dixon, RE, Buttram, VC, and Schum, CW,** Artificial Insemination Using Homologous Semen: A Review of 158 Cases, Fertil Steril 27:647, 1976.

31. **Bunge, RG,** Caffeine Stimulation of Human Ejaculated Spermatozoa, Urologie 1:371, 1973.

32. **Schoenfeld, C, Amelar, RD, and Dubin, L,** Stimulation of Ejaculated Human Spermatozoa by Caffeine, Fertil Steril 26:158, 1975.

33. **Ericsson, RJ, Langevin, CH, Nishino, M,** Isolation of Fractions Rich in Human Y Sperm, Nature 246:421, 1973.

34. **Ross, A, Robinson, JA, and Evans, HJ,** Failure to Confirm Separation of X and Y Bearing Human Sperm Using BSA Gradients, Nature 253:354, 1975.

35. **Amelar, RD, and Hotchkiss, RS,** The Split Ejaculate, Fertil Steril 16:46, 1965.

36. **Amelar, RD, and Dubin, L,** A New Method of Promoting Fertility, Obstet Gynec 45:56, 1975.

37. **Kleegman, SJ,** Therapeutic Donor Insemination, Fertil Steril 5:7, 1954.

38. **Bygdeman, M,** Prostaglandins in Human Seminal Fluid and their Correlation to Fertility, Int J Fertil 14:228, 1961.

39. **Hawkins, DF,** Relevance of Prostaglandins to Problems of Human Subfertility, in Ramwell, PW, and Shaw, JE, eds, *Prostaglandin Symposium of the Worcester Foundation for Experimental Biology,* Interscience, New York, 1967.

9

Induction of Ovulation

There are two categories of anovulatory patients: (1) the anovulatory woman who has gonadotropin and estrogen production, but does not cycle; and (2) the anovulatory woman who is deficient in gonadotropins and estrogen and *cannot* cycle. Each category has a specific medical therapy and patients are fortunate that the physician today has available for general clinical use two pharmacologic preparations, clomiphene citrate (Clomid) and human menopausal gonadotropins (HMG).

The programs of clomiphene and HMG administration described in this chapter have evolved over the past decade. These methods have reduced side effects to a clinically acceptable frequency and retained a high success rate in terms of induced pregnancies. *This chapter will review the principles which guide the use of clomiphene and HMG, and consider the results and complications of the medical induction of ovulation. In addition, ovarian wedge resection will be examined, and mention will be made of the use of GnRH and ergot alkaloids.*

Despite the specificity of the therapy and the promise of successful results, it is incumbent upon the practitioner to perform the appropriate medical evaluation to ensure that a contraindication to therapy is not overlooked and that the patient is placed in the proper anovulatory category. The reader is referred to Chapter 6 and 7 for a consider-

ation of anovulation and hirsutism; Chapter 5 for th
evaluation of amenorrhea; and Chapter 9 for the diffe
ential diagnosis of galactorrhea.

Clomiphene
Citrate
(Clomid)

Clomiphene citrate is an orally active nonsteroidal agen
distantly related to diethystilbestrol. Its chemical name
2-[p-(2-chloro-1,2-diphenylvinyl)phenoxy]triethylamin
dihydrogen citrate. Clomiphene is available in 50-m
tablets under the trade name of Clomid, costing $2/table
In some countries, the preparation is available as *ci*
Clomid, the 10-mg tablet being approximately equivalen
to the 50-mg tablet sold in the United States.

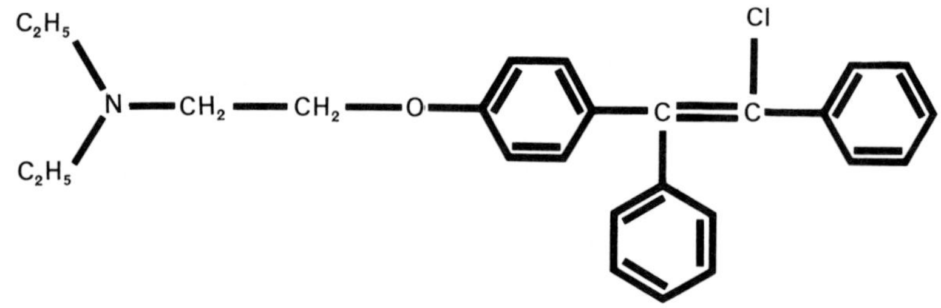

cis Clomiphene Citrate

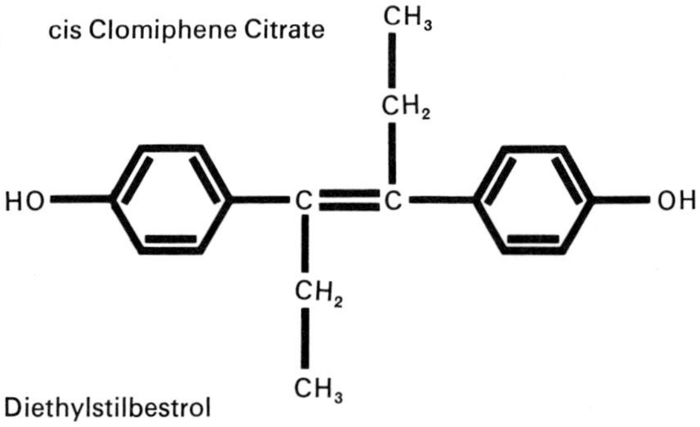

Diethylstilbestrol

The similarity of its structure to an estrogenic substance i
the clue to its mechanism of action. Clomiphene exert
only a very weak biologic estrogenic effect. The structura
similarity to estrogen is sufficient to achieve uptake an
binding in the hypothalamus by the estrogen receptor
Indeed, clomiphene does not competitively inhibit th
action of estrogen at the receptor level, but rather mod
fies hypothalamic activity by affecting the concentratio
of the intracellular estrogen receptors. Specifically th
concentration of cytoplasmic estrogen receptors is re
duced by inhibition of the process of receptor replenish
ment. (1) Therefore the hypothalamus cannot perceive o
act upon the true endogenous estrogen level in th
circulation. The homeostatic negative feedback relation
ship between estrogen and the gonadotropins is activated
Thinking that the estrogen level in the circulation is lov
because its perception is obscured, the hypothalmus sig
nals the pituitary gland to stimulate the ovarian follicula
apparatus. Releasing hormone is secreted into the porta
system, stimulating the pituitary to augment its secretion

of follicle-stimulating hormone (FSH) and luteinizing hormone (LH). During the period of clomiphene administration peripheral serum levels of FSH and LH rise. This rise in gonadotropins, especially that of FSH, can be compared to the initial rise in that gonadotropin occurring during menses in a normal cycle. As in the normal cycle, the rise in FSH stimulates a set of follicles to begin growth and maturation. The subsequent ovulation which occurs after clomiphene therapy is then a manifestation of the hormonal and morphologic changes produced by the growing follicles. Clomiphene therapy does not directly stimulate ovulation, but it initiates a sequence of events that are the physiologic features of a normal cycle. The effectiveness of the drug is restricted to its ability to cause an appropriate FSH discharge.

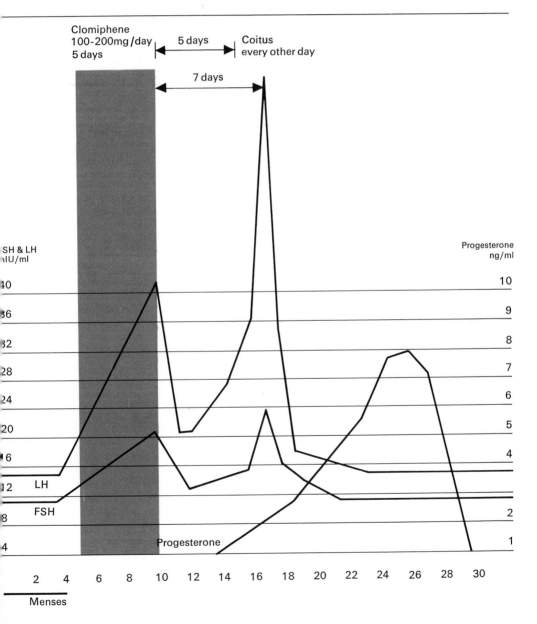

Clomiphene has no progestational, androgenic, or antiandrogenic effects. Clomiphene does not interfere with adrenal or thyroid function. In rats and rabbits, a dose dependent increase in the incidence of fetal malformations is seen when clomiphene is given during the period of organogenesis. Extremely high doses inhibit fetal development. Although clomiphene therapy should be withheld if there is any possibility of pregnancy, there has been no evidence that clomiphene is teratogenic in humans. Furthermore, infant survival and performance after delivery are normal.

Selection of Patients

Absent or infrequent ovulation is the chief indication for clomiphene therapy. It is the physician's responsibility to rule out nonreproductive disorders of pituitary, adrenal, and thyroid origin requiring specific treatment before initiating clomiphene therapy. A complete history and physical examination are mandatory, but only a minimum of laboratory procedures is necessary. The vast majority of patients are healthy women suffering only from infertility secondary to oligo-ovulation or anovulation.

While the effect of the drug is brief, only 51% of the oral dose is excreted after 5 days, and radioactivity from labeled clomiphene appears in the feces up to 6 weeks after administration. If history and physical examination findings suggest liver disease, liver function evaluation should precede clomiphene therapy.

If periods are infrequent it is not absolutely necessary to document infrequent or absent ovulation by basal body temperature records and endometrial biopsy. An endometrial biopsy is a wise precaution in a patient who has been anovulatory for a long period of time because of the tendency for these patients to develop adenomatous hyperplasia and even carcinoma of the endometrium. It is also wise to precede therapy with an evaluation of the semen, to avoid an unnecessary waste of time and effort in the presence of azoospermia. However, the remainder of the infertility workup in a patient with no previous medical or surgical problems is deferred until after a trial of clomiphene therapy. Because approximately 75% of pregnancies occur during the first 3 treatment cycles, the infertility workup is pursued only after the patient has responded with 3 months of ovulatory cycles and has not become pregnant.

Cases of ovarian failure are unresponsive to any form of ovulation induction. Therefore, the presence of ovarian tissue capable of responding to gonadotropins must be documented. This is only a problem in the patient with amenorrhea, since the presence of menstrual bleeding confirms the function (although perhaps limited) of the hypothalamic-pituitary-ovarian axis. The patient with amenorrhea who fails to produce a withdrawal bleed after a course of a progestational agent (Provera, 10 mg daily for 5 days) must be further evaluated (see Chapter 5). A case has been made by others for the usefulness of an ovarian biopsy, perhaps via the laparoscope, to establish the presence of competent ovarian tissue. It is our practice, however, to rely on the radioimmunoassay of gonadotropin levels and the response to Provera, thus avoiding unnecessary surgical and anesthetic risks, to accurately rule out hypergonadotropic hypogonadism (ovarian failure). Serum FSH levels in the postmenopausal or castrate range indicate an absence of estrogen-producing ovarian tissue. Attempts at medical induction of ovulation in these cases would be a waste of time and money.

The patients most likely to respond to clomiphene display some evidence of pituitary-ovarian activity as expressed in the biologic presence of estrogen (spontaneous or withdrawal menstrual bleeding). These are anovulatory women who have gonadotropin and estrogen production but do not cycle. The patient who is deficient in gonadotropin secretion and as a result is hypoestrogenic cannot be expected to respond to a further lowering of the estrogen signal, and thus should not respond to clomiphene. However, this principle is not completely applicable to clinical practice. An occasional patient who is by every criteria, hypoestrogenic, will respond. Therefore, any otherwise medically uncomplicated patient with infertility secondary to lack of ovulation is a candidate for clomiphene therapy. In addition, treatment is indicated in the patient who ovulates only occasionally in order to improve the timing and frequency of ovulation to enhance the possibilities of conception.

To our knowledge, the use of drugs for induction of ovulation does not improve the quality of the ovum, and the chance of pregnancy is not improved in women who ovulate regularly and spontaneously. There is one special instance where this restriction may not apply. Certain religious requirements, such as in orthodox Judaism, interfere with the normal reproductive process. In the devout orthodox Jewish couple, intercourse is prohibited in the presence of menstrual flow and for 7 days following its conclusion. In some women menstrual flow is prolonged or the follicular phase is shortened, so that coitus cannot take place until after ovulation. Clomiphene therapy can be utilized to defer ovulation. In the usual mode of treatment, medication is begun on day 5 of the cycle. Ovulation can be delayed to a more appropriate time by starting clomiphene later, usually on day 7 or 8 of the cycle. Ovulation can be expected in the interval 5–10 days after the last day of medication. This manipulation has its limitations. Administration too late in the cycle, beyond day 9, may have no effect.

The question is often asked whether the indications fo clomiphene therapy should be extended to include th initiation of cyclicity in the oligoamenorrheic patient wh does not seek fertility. In our opinion, this is an inappro priate use of clomiphene for several reasons: (1) th effectiveness of clomiphene is restricted to the cycle i which it is used and it should not be expected to induc cyclicity following the conclusion of treatment; (2) the us of clomiphene may aggravate the clinical problems o acne and hirsutism during the treatment cycle by increas ing LH stimulation of ovarian steroid production; and (3 the inability to induce cyclicity can be so discouraging t the patient that her acceptance of the drug will b impaired at some future date when it is legitimatel offered as a fertility agent for the induction of ovulation

How To Use Clomiphene

A program of clomiphene therapy is begun on the 5th da of a cycle following either spontaneous or induced bleed ing. The initial dose is 50 mg daily for 5 days. There is n advantage to beginning with a higher dose for the follow ing two reasons: (1). In a random distribution of patient begun with initial doses of either 50 mg or 100 mg daily the pregnancy rate was identical (2). The highest inci dence of side effects in our experience occurs at the 5 mg dose. Initial high doses should be approached with caution in those patients who experience side effects a the 50 mg level.

If ovulation is not achieved in the very first cycle o treatment, dosage is increased to 100 mg. Thereafter, i ovulation is not achieved in the first cycle, dosage i increased in a staircase fashion by 50 mg increments to maximum of 200 mg daily for 5 days. The highest dose i pursued for 3 to 4 months before considering the patien to be a clomiphene failure. The quantity of drug and th number of cycles go beyond those recommended by th manufacturer. However, in our experience those recom mendations are inappropriately limiting. We hav achieved a 15% pregnancy rate at the 150 mg and 200 mg dose levels. (2)

Following the 5 day course of clomiphene, the ovulator surge of gonadotropins may occur anywhere from 5 to 1 days after the last day of clomiphene administration. The patient is advised to have intercourse every other day fo 1 week beginning 5 days after the last day of medication

Prior to a treatment cycle the patient is evaluated for side effects, residual ovarian enlargement, and basal bod temperature changes. A basal body temperature record i necessary to follow the response. If an inadequate lutea phase is evident, the amount of clomiphene is increase to the next dose level. If the patient is already at th maximum level of 200 mg daily, HCG is added a discussed below. Maintenance of the temperature eleva tion beyond the expected time of menses is the earlies possible indication of success and pregnancy.

Some clinicians have decided that in reliable patients who keep meticulous temperature records and can be trusted to report any untoward symptoms or side effects, the monthly pelvic exam can be omitted. Obviously this liberty must be carried out only after very specific patient instruction and with frequent telephone contact.

Care should be taken to review with the patient and her husband the pathophysiology of her condition, the principles of treatment, the prolonged course of therapy which may be necessary, and possible complications. Repeated failures accumulate frustration and despair in the couple, making each successive cycle of treatment more difficult. The anxiety and stress may hinder coital performance, and it is not uncommon for a couple to have difficulty performing scheduled intercourse.

The additional use of human chorionic gonadotropin (HCG) is limited to those cases in which there is a failure to ovulate at the 200-mg dose level or when at that level a short luteal phase is demonstrated (5–6 days elevation of basal body temperature and menses occurring 6–9 days after the temperature rise). The rational is to improve on the midcycle LH surge, therefore 10,000 international units of HCG are given as a single intramuscular dose on the 7th–10th day after clomiphene when follicular maturation is at its peak. The precise timing of HCG administration is indicated by the biologic expression of estrogen production through cervical mucus changes (quantity and ferning). If HCG is administered in the morning, intercourse is advised for that night and for the next 2 days.

In the clinical management of infertility patients, treatment is monitored by the basal body temperature curve. Biphasic changes are taken as an indication of ovulation and success. It should be emphasized however that these changes can occur in the absence of the physical extrusion of the ovum. Luteinization of follicle cells without ovum release has been documented. This may be an explanation for the disparity between apparent ovulatory rates and pregnancy rates seen with clomiphene therapy. This disparity is not reduced by the use of more elaborate tests of progesterone production (secretory endometrium by biopsy, urinary pregnanediol levels, or plasma progesterone assays).

Results

In properly selected patients, 70% can be expected to ovulate, and approximately 40% become pregnant. The percent of pregnancies per induced ovulatory cycle is about 15%. The multiple pregnancy rate in accumulated national statistics is approximately 8%, almost entirely twins; there have been rare cases of quintuplet and sextuplet births. In our own experience in recent years, with standardization of therapy, the incidence of twins has approached normal. The abortion rate is not increased Most importantly, the incidence of congenital malformations is not increased, and infant survival and performance after delivery are no different from normal. (3).

Most of the pregnancies (75%) occur during the first 3 treatment cycles. With additional treatment cycles, the pregnancy rate diminishes although the ovulatory rate remains high. Approximately 15% of patients treated with the higher doses of 150 and 200 mg, will become pregnant. (2).

There is no evidence that the effect of clomiphene is long-lasting. A response is limited to that cycle in which the drug is used.

Complications

Side effects do not appear to be dose-related, occurring more frequently at the 50 mg dose. Patients requiring the high doses are probably less sensitive to the drug. The most common problems are vasomotor flushes (10%), abdominal distention, bloating, pain, or soreness (5.5%), breast discomfort (2%), nausea and vomiting (2.2%), visual symptoms (1.5%), headache (1.3%), and dryness or loss of hair (0.3%).

Visual symptoms include blurring of vision, scotoma (visual spots or flashes), or abnormal perception. The cause of these symptoms is unknown, but in every case studied thus far, the visual symptoms have disappeared upon discontinuation of the medication, and no permanent effects have been reported. Usually these symptoms disappear within a few days, but may take 1 or 2 weeks. In our opinion, the occurrence of visual symptoms is a contraindication to further use of the drug.

Significant ovarian enlargement is associated with longer periods of treatment, and is infrequent with the usual 5-day course. Maximal enlargement of the ovary usually occurs several days after discontinuing the clomiphene (in response to the increase in gonadotropins). If the patient is symptomatic, pelvic examination, intercourse, and undue physical exercise should be avoided because the enlarged ovaries are very fragile. Ovarian enlargement dissipates rapidly and only rarely is a subsequent treatment cycle delayed. Of course, if ovarian enlargement is encountered, clomiphene therapy should be withheld until normal size returns.

What to Do
With a
Clomiphene
Failure

Approximately 30% of patients who have evidence of estrogen production but fail to respond to clomiphene will become pregnant when treated with human menopausal gonadotropin. However, the decision to proceed with HMG therapy is not easily made. Evaluation of the patient is important since patients with persistent anovulation and polycystic ovaries demonstrate a low pregnancy rate with HMG. In the patient with persistent anovulation and polycystic ovaries who has failed to respond to a 9-month course of clomiphene up to the highest dose, we are faced with the probability of a poor response of HMG, plus the additional burden of the very great expense of that therapy. In this type of patient, we are inclined to offer the choice of an ovarian wedge resection.

Ovarian Wedge Resection

The purpose of wedge resection of the ovaries is to remove a significant amount of steroid-producing tissue. Documentation of hormonal changes following wedge resection indicates that the only important change is a sustained reduction in testosterone levels. (4) This suggests that the barrier to ovulation is the intraovarian, atresia-promoting effects of the high testosterone production. Removal of androgen-producing tissue effectively lowers this barrier, and ovulatory cycles may ensue.

The response to ovarian wedge resection is variable. Some patients resume ovulation permanently. However, most patients return to their anovulatory state. Some patients fail to respond at all. Furthermore the surgical procedure carries with it the potential problem of postoperative adhesion formation (estimated to be present in 14% of postoperative wedge resection patients who continue to be infertile) leading to another cause of infertility. (5)

The operative risk, the variable response, and the possiblity of postoperative adhesion formation are the liabilities of wedge resection. These must be weighed against the difficulties of HMG therapy. HMG treatment is expensive and the pregnancy rate may be lower in typical polycystic ovary patients. However the safety of HMG therapy, when monitored with estrogen measurements, is significantly improved in terms of multiple births and the hyperstimulation syndrome.

Human Menopausal Gonadotropins (HMG) (Pergonal)

HMG, human menopausal gonadotropins, is a purified preparation of gonadotropins extracted from the urine of postmenopausal women, available as Pergonal. The commercial preparation contains 75 units of FSH and 75 units of LH; the potency is expressed in terms of international units based on an international reference preparation. A significant factor in the use of HMG is its high cost, approximately $10–$15/ampule. Treatment may cost from $200–900/cycle for the drug alone. HMG is inactive orally and therefore must be given by intramuscular injection.

Selection of Patients

Not only because of its expense, but because of its greater complication rate, patients should not receive HMG without a very careful evaluation. An absolute requirement is the demonstration of ovarian competence. Abnormally high serum gonadotropins with a failure to demonstrate withdrawal bleeding indicate ovarian failure and preclude induction of ovulation.

A thorough infertility investigation must be performed. In addition to the demonstration of ovarian competence, tubal and uterine pathology should be ruled out, anovulation documented, and a semen analysis obtained. Nongynecologic endocrine problems must be treated. Hypogonadotropic function (low serum gonadotropins), including galactorrhea syndromes, requires evaluation for an intracranial lesion, with polytomography and measurement of prolactin levels. It is imperative to take all steps necessary to exclude treatable pathology to which anovulation is secondary.

In our practice we first offer a course of clomiphene, not only because of the cost and complications associated with HMG, but also because some apparently hypogonadotropic patients will unpredictably respond to clomiphene.

How to Use HMG

There are two commonly used techniques of HMG administration, the variable and the fixed dosage methods. Regardless of the technique employed the objective is to achieve follicular growth and maturation. Follicle stimulation is achieved by 7–14 days of continuous HMG, beginning with 2 ampules daily. Response is judged by the degree of estrogen produced by the growing follicles. Clinically, the quantity and quality of the cervical mucus are used as indicators of estrogen production. In addition, the patient is monitored periodically with the measurement of the 24-hour urinary excretion of total estrogens or the plasma estradiol level. The patient is seen on the 7th day of treatment and a decision is made to continue (fixed) or increase the dose (variable). After the 7th day, the patient is seen anywhere from daily to every 3rd day.

HMG comes as a dry powder in a sealed glass ampule, along with a second ampule containing 2 ml of diluent. One ampule of HMG requires 1 ml of diluent. When two ampules are to be administered, solution with 1 ml is accomplished in the first vial of HMG, and the solution is then deposited in the second vial. Thus when giving two ampules of HMG the contents of two vials are dissolved in a total of 1 ml of diluent. When 4 ampules are given, a total of 2 ml of diluent are used. Should 6 ampules of HMG be required, 3 ampules are dissolved in 1.5 ml of diluent and two injections are administered, each in the upper outer quadrant of each buttock. The HCG injection comes as a vial containing 10,000 units as a dry powder. One ml of the accompanying diluent is used for administration.

It cannot be emphasized too strongly that dosage administration and the judicious use of estrogen measurements depend upon the experience of the physician administering HMG. Clinically, when the cervical os opens and when cervical mucus changes (clarity, quantity, spinnbarkeit) comparable to a normal midcycle are achieved, the patient is ready to receive the ovulatory stimulus, 10,000 units of human chorionic gonadotropin given as a single dose intramuscularly. Because of its structural and biologic similarity to LH, HCG, readily available from human pregnancy urine and placental tissue, is used to simulate the midcycle LH ovulatory surge. The patient is advised to have intercourse the same day of the HCG injection and for the next 2 days. In view of the fragility of hyperstimulated ovaries, further intercourse as well as strenuous physical exercise should be avoided.

The use of estrogen measurements is necessary to prevent hyperstimulation and to choose the correct moment for administering the ovulatory dose of HCG. This is especially important in some patients who for unknown reasons fail to produce significant changes in cervical mucus, yet undergo impressive follicular growth and maturation. On day 7 of the therapeutic cycle the patient is examined and urine or blood is assayed for estrogen. Depending on the findings, the dosage of HMG is individualized for the duration of the cycle. With experience, the physician can avoid daily estrogen measurements, although sometimes this is necessary.

What should the urinary estrogen level be? Below 100 μg/24 hours, a significant but not maximal pregnancy rate may be achieved. Over 200 μg/24 hours, a significant rate of hyperstimulation is encountered. Between 100 and 200 μg/24 hours, hyperstimulation or multiple ovulation may be encountered, but also the maximal pregnancy rate is achieved. To project dosage requirements, a useful fact to keep in mind is that once the phase of rapidly increasing estrogen production is reached, the urinary estrogen level will approximately double each day.

What should the blood estrogen level be? We have accumulated less experience with this method, but the guiding principles appear to be similar to urinary estrogen. Measuring estradiol by radioimmunoassay, the optimum range appears to be between 1000 and 1500 pg/ml. As with the use of urinary estrogen, attempting to reproduce the normal midcycle levels of estrogen does not achieve a maximal pregnancy rate. In our experience levels between 1000 and 1500 pg/ml have not been associated with multiple births other than twins, and we have not experienced a single case of severe hyperstimulation. Due to the variability associated with random blood sampling, it does not appear that one can predict a doubling of values each day during the time period of rapid estrogen rise.

In some individuals, pregnancy will be achieved with the administration of 2 ampules/day for 7–12 days. In other individuals, presumably with extremely hyposensitive ovaries, adequate follicular stimulation requires doses up to 4, 6, and more ampules/day. In this group of amenorrheic women, there is a reduced chance of achieving success with a fixed dose regimen. Massive doses of gonadotropins are necessary, and with proper monitoring, pregnancy can be safely achieved. The range between the dose which does not induce ovulation and the dose which results in hyperstimulation is narrow. The situation is made even more difficult because the ovaries may react differently to essentially similar doses from month to month. Close supervision and experience in the use of HMG are necessary to avoid difficulties.

Instruction and counseling of the couple are essential. A thorough understanding of the need for daily treatment and observation is necessary prior to initiating therapy. As part of this instruction, the husband may be taught to administer injections. Daily recording of the basal body temperature and body weight is important for proper management. The couple should be told about the need for scheduled intercourse, the possibility that more than one course of treatment may be necessary, and the expense of the treatment. Above all, the patient must be prepared for the anguish that accompanies failure.

Results

The most significant aspect of this method of treatment is that it does achieve pregnancy in an otherwise untreatable situation. In general, more than 90% of patients with competent ovaries will ovulate in response to HMG-HCG, and a pregnancy rate of approximately 50–70% may be achieved. As with clomiphene, there is a normal incidence of congenital malformations, and the children born have a normal postnatal development. (6)

After the 10,000 units of HCG are given, the plasma level of HCG reaches a nadir level before the expected time of implantation. Therefore increased levels of HCG by radioimmunoassay 9 to 13 days after the injection of HCG represent gonadotropin production by the early pregnancy. (7) A beta-subunit assay of HCG at this time, or one of the more sensitive urine assays performed 2 to 4 weeks after the HCG injection, are reliable tests for pregnancy.

The multiple pregnancy rate has been reported as 20% (twins, 15%; 3 or more, 5%). The multiple pregnancies are secondary to multiple ovulations, and therefore the siblings are not identical. Fetal loss due to prematurity in the multiple pregnancies has been a serious problem. The abortion rate is approximately 20%. In view of the high rate of multiple pregnancies and the normal abortion rate, the overall fetal salvage rate has been diminished. Close monitoring with estrogen assays, however, should reduce the frequency of the large multiple births, and these figures should improve.

The likelihood of ovulation is dose-related, and complications are likewise dose-related. In general, 2–5 therapeutic cycles are required to achieve pregnancy. The rate of serious hyperstimulation has been 1%, but proper estrogen monitoring has reduced this complication to a rare happening.

Hyperstimulation
Syndrome (8)

Ovarian hyperstimulation may be life-threatening. In mild cases the syndrome includes ovarian enlargement, abdominal distension, and weight gain. In severe cases, a critical condition develops with ascites, pleural effusion, electrolyte imbalance, and hypovolemia with hypotension and oliguria. The ovaries are tremendously enlarged with multiple follicle cysts, stromal edema, and many corpora lutea.

The basic disturbance is a shift of fluid from the intravascular space into the abdominal cavity creating a massive third space. The resulting hypovolemia leads to circulatory and excretory problems. The genesis of the ascites is unclear. The very high level of estrogen secretion by the ovaries may be the primary factor, inducing increased local capillary permeability and leakage of fluid from the ovaries. The leakage of fluid is also critically related to the mass, volume, and surface area of the ovaries. Therefore, the larger the ovaries and the greater the steroid production, the more severe the condition.

The loss of fluid and protein into the abdominal cavity accounts for the hypovolemia and hemoconcentration. This in turn results in low blood pressure and decreased central venous pressure. The major clinical complications are increased coagulability and decreased renal perfusion. Blood loss as the cause of the clinical picture can be easily ruled out since a hematocrit will reveal hemoconcentration. The decreased renal perfusion leads to increased salt and water reabsorption in the proximal tubule producing oliguria and low urinary sodium excretion. With less sodium being presented to the distal tubule, there is a decrease in the exchange of hydrogen and potassium for sodium, resulting in hyperkalemic acidosis. A rise in the blood urea nitrogen is due to decreased perfusion and increased urea reabsorption. Because it is only filtered, creatinine does not increase as much as the BUN. Thus, the patient is hypovolemic, azotemic, and hyperkalemic.

Treatment is conservative and empiric. When a patient displays excessive weight gain (usually 20 or more pounds), hemoconcentration (Hct over 50%), oliguria, dyspnea, or postural hypotension, she should be hospitalized. Pelvic and abdominal examination are contraindicated in view of the extreme fragility of the enlarged ovaries. Ovarian rupture and hemorrhage are easily precipitated.

Upon admission, the patient is put on bed rest, with daily body weights, strict monitoring of intake and output, and frequent vital signs. Serial studies of the following are obtained: Hct, BUN, creatinine, electrolytes, total proteins with albumin-globulin ratio, coagulation studies, urinary sodium, and potassium. The electrocardiogram is utilized to follow and evaluate hyperkalemia. Intravenous fluids, plasma expanders, and albumin may be given as needed. Mannitol is used as necessary to maintain urinary output. Potassium exchange resins may also be necessary.

Diuretics are without effect, and indeed, may be disadvantageous. The fluid in the abdominal cavity is not responsive to diuretic treatment, and diuresis may further contract the intravascular volume and produce hypovolemic shock or thrombosis. Arterial thrombosis has been reported. One patient died due to an internal carotoid artery thrombosis, and one patient required a left leg amputation.

The possibility of ovarian rupture should always be considered, and serial hematocrits may be the only clue to intraperitoneal hemorrhage. Of course, a falling hematocrit *accompanied by diuresis* is an indication of resolution, not hemorrhage. Laparotomy should be avoided in these precarious patients. If surgery is necessary, only hemostatic measures should be undertaken and the ovaries should be conserved if possible, since a return to normal size is inevitable.

The key point is that the hyperstimulation syndrome will undergo gradual resolution with time. In a patient who is not pregnant, the syndrome will cover a period of approximately 7 days. In a patient who is pregnant and in whom the ovaries are restimulated by the emerging endogenous HCG production, the syndrome will last 10–20 days.

The syndrome will not develop unless the ovulatory dose of HCG is given. Thus, the major emphasis in recent years has been to utilize estrogen monitoring to avoid hyperstimulation. The general belief is that a 24-hour urinary excretion of more than 200 μg estrogen or a blood estradiol level greater than 2000 pg/ml makes the development of the syndrome a good possibility, and the ovulatory dose of HCG should be withheld. Current methodology permits urinary or blood estrogen measurement within 6 hours, and hence daily therapeutic projections are possible. *A severe case of hyperstimulation is not encountered unless the patient has ovulated.*

The relationship between estrogen levels and hyperstimulation is not a perfect one. Hyperstimulation has been found with relatively low estrogen levels, and high estrogen is not necessarily followed by hyperstimulation. Nevertheless, this is the only available deterrent to a potentially life-threatening situation. Estrogen measurement becomes especially important in the patient who responds to HMG with follicular maturation and estrogen production, but fails to produce appropriate cervical mucus. In such patients the only parameter for management is the assay of estrogen.

What to Do with the HMG Failure

The patient who has completed a course of HMG (2–5 drug cycles) and failed to achieve pregnancy has received the full range of therapy.

If funds and emotional reserves are sufficient, a repeat course of therapy is permissible after a review of the etiologic basis for infertility. Guidance to adoption services and emotional support continue to be part of the physician's obligation.

New Methods

Clomiphene-HMG Sequence

The combination of both clomiphene and HMG was explored in order to minimize the cost of HMG alone. As long as treatment is monitored with estrogen levels the side effects and complications should not be dissimilar to those with HMG alone. It has not been demonstrated that patients unresponsive to HMG alone would respond to the sequence method, and there is no logical reason to assume that this would be true.

The usual method of treatment is to administer clomiphene 100 mg for 5 to 7 days, then to immediately proceed with HMG beginning with 2 ampules per day. Estrogen levels are monitored as usual. This method may decrease the amount of HMG required by approximately 50%, however the same risks of multiple pregnancy and hyperstimulation can be expected. This reduced requirement for HMG is found only in those patients who demonstrate a positive withdrawal bleed following progestin medication or have spontaneous menses. (9)

Gonadotropin Releasing Hormone (GnRH)

The potential advantage in the utilization of GnRH lies in the short half life as compared to the long half life of HCG. Finer regulation of dosage may be possible and hyperstimulation avoided. However the short half life is also a disadvantage. In order to achieve follicular growth and ovulation, very frequent administration is necessary. Parenteral treatment is therefore impractical. The use of GnRH in the form of nasal drops may eventually solve this technical problem, especially if new longer acting analogues prove to be efficacious. Utilization of GnRH is limited currently to investigational studies necessary for clinical development.

Ergot Alkaloids

Ergot alkaloids, which directly inhibit pituitary secretion of prolactin, are effective in returning ovulatory function in patients with hyperprolactinemia. (Chapters 5 and 9) However, anovulatory patients with normal levels of prolactin may also respond to ergot alkaloid treatment with ovulation. (10) The mechanism is unclear although it is presumed that lowering of the 24 hour production rate of prolactin allows ovulation to resume. Response is relatively rapid; menses return in amenorrheic patients within 2 to 3 months. Because this method of treatment appears to be relatively uncomplicated, perhaps the attempts to induce ovulation and achieve pregnancy should begin with ergot alkaloid treatment, 2.5 mg bid or tid. Apparently there are no teratogenic effects when taken early in pregnancy; however, only a few cases have been reported (11)

References

1. **Clark, JH, Peck, EJ, and Anderson, JN,** Estrogen Receptors and Antagonism of Steroid Hormone Action. Nature 251:446, 1974.

2. **Gorlitsky, GA, Kase, NG, and Speroff, L,** Ovulation and Pregnancy Rates with Clomiphene Citrate, Obstet Gynec, March, 1978.

3. **Hack, M. Brish, M. Serr, DM, Insler, V, Salomy, M and Lunenfeld, B,** Outcome of Pregnancy after Induced Ovulation: Follow-up of Pregnancies and Children Born after Clomiphene Therapy, JAMA 220:1329, 1972.

4. **Judd, HL, Rigg, LA, Anderson, DC, and Yen, SSC,** The Effects of Ovarian Wedge Resection on Circulating Gonadotropin and Ovarian Steroid Levels in Patients with Polycystic Ovary Syndrome, J Clin Endocrinol Metab 43:347, 1976.

5. **Weinstein, D, and Polishuk, WZ,** The Role of Wedge Resection of the Ovary as a Cause for Mechanical Sterility, Surg Gynec and Obst 141:417, 1975.

6. **Hack, M, Brish, M, Serr, DM, Insler, V, Salomy, M, and Lunenfeld, B,** Outcome of Pregnancy after Induced Ovulation: Followup of Pregnancies and Children Born After Gonadotropin Therapy, JAMA 211:791, 1970.

7. **Catt, KJ, Dufau, ML, and Vaitukaitis, JL,** Appearance of HCG in Pregnancy Plasma Following the Initiation of Implantation of the Blastocyst, J Clin Endocrinol Metab 40:537, 1975.

8. **Engel, T, Jewelewicz, R, Dyrenfurth, I, Speroff, L, and Vande, Wiele, RL,** Ovarian Hyperstimulation Syndrome: Report of a Case with Notes on Pathogenesis and Treatment, Am J Obstet Gynec 112:1052, 1972.

9. **March, CM, Tredway, DR, and Mishell, DR, Jr,** Effect of Clomiphene Citrate Upon Amount and Duration of Human Menopausal Gonadotropin Therapy, Am J Obst Gynec 125:699, 1976.

10. **Seppala, M, Hirvonen, E, and Ranta, T,** Bromocriptine Treatment of Secondary Amenorrhea, Lancet 1:1154, 1976.

11. **Tyson, JE, Andreassen, B, Huth, J, Smith, B, and Zacur, H,** Neuro-endocrine Dysfunction with Psychogenic Implications in Postpill Galactorrhea-Amenorrhea, Obstet Gynec 46:1, 1975.

20 Clinical Assays

The purpose of this chapter is to review the laboratory assays which are commonly used in clinical gynecologic endocrinology. With this information, the clinician will have confidence in his selection of specific laboratory tests, and will be secure in his personal interpretation of the data returned to him.

Classically, hormones have been measured in blood by bioassays, i.e. dose-response measurements based upon organ responses in animals. Some of the principles fundamental to endocrinology were established by such methods. However, bioassay methods, although adequate for qualitative statements, are relatively imprecise, nonspecific, time-consuming, expensive and require too large an amount of the biologic sample in order to meet the quantitative requirements of modern research and clinical practice. Assays with far greater sensitivity and precision have been developed. These new methods depend upon the use of radioactive tracers and the delicate measurement of radioactivity. The most recent and popular techniques are the methods of saturation analysis.

**Saturation
Analysis
(Radio-
immunoassay,
Competitive
Protein
Binding)**

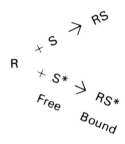

Basic Principles

The methods of saturation analysis yield greater simplicity, sensitivity, and precision. Reactions in saturation analysis follow the law of mass action. A protein or antibody (R) is mixed with a substance (S) for which it has specific binding sites, forming a complex, RS. The radioactive form of the substance (S*) also forms a complex, RS*. Since the number of binding sites on the protein or antibody are limited, the labeled and unlabeled compound, S and S*, will compete for binding sites in proportion to their concentrations. Since the binding reagent, R (protein or antibody), is kept constant, increasing the unlabeled compound, S, will displace more and more labeled tracer, S*. Plotting the change in either bound or unbound (free) tracer, S*, against the amount of unlabeled compound, S, added will produce a standard curve. The amount of radioactivity bound or free in the presence of an unknown level of compound will reveal the concentration of the compound when compared to the standard curve. The requirements for saturation analysis are, therefore, either a suitable binding protein, or an antibody, and a labeled pure form of the compound to be measured.

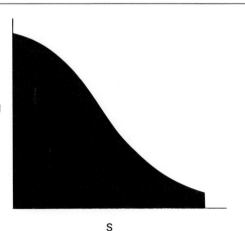

Percent Bound
RS*

S

Methodology

A purified, labeled amount of the substance to be measured is added to the biologic sample (e.g. plasma) to be assayed. The radioactive tracer equilibrates with the unlabeled and unknown amount of compound in the sample. The sample is now mixed with an appropriate solvent to extract the desired compound and tracer. The extraction process usually removes several compounds which may interfere with the assay, and separation (purification) of the desired substance is frequently necessary. A chromatographic separation utilizing thin layer chromatography or column chromatography is currently being used for most steroid assays.

The next step is to mix the extracted compound with a specific reagent. In the case of radioimmunoassay, this reagent is an antiserum, and in the case of competitive protein binding, this reagent is a protein which has affinity for the compound to be measured. The combination of the compound with this reagent (antiserum or specific protein) is called binding. Since the compound is in equilibrium with a small amount of labeled compound, the labeled compound will bind to the reagent in proportion to the amount of unlabeled compound present. This is the fundamental principle: the distribution of bound and unbound radioactivity is dependent upon the total concentration of the compound in the system. Measurement of the radioactivity, therefore, can be utilized to calculate the unknown amount of compound in the system.

In the case of polypeptide hormones (gonadotropins), radioimmunoassay techniques are based upon the use of antibodies prepared by injecting the protein hormone of one species into another. The protein hormones vary in their physicochemical characteristics and amino acid composition from species to species, and therefore, antibodies for use in radioimmunoassay are formed when protein hormones are administered cross-species. A highly specific antiserum may be produced to be utilized as the binding reagent. This specificity may make chromatographic separation that ordinarily follows extraction unnecessary.

Since steroid compounds are not antigenic, the production of a specific antiserum depends upon the linkage of a steroid to a large protein molecule. The protein molecule is antigenic in itself, but when combined with a steroid, the steroid-protein complex (hapten) stimulates a variety of antibodies, some of which recognize and are specific for the steroid. Thus, when the steroid-protein complex is injected into an animal the antiserum formed may be utilized as a reagent (R) for measurement of the steroid (S) in the technique of saturation analysis.

For example, a testosterone-bovine albumin conjugate may be formed by covalently linking testosterone to albumin at the 3 position via an oxime linkage to o-carboxymethyl hydroxylamine.

The cross-reactions to the antiserum produced with the above conjugate vary, and it is clear that this antiserum may be used to measure testosterone and dihydrotestosterone, and that testosterone and dihydrotestosterone must be separated by some chromatographic means.

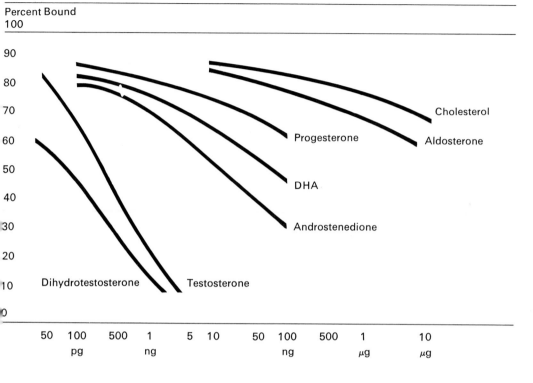

Percent Bound

Competitive Protein Binding. In competitive protein binding, the antiserum is replaced with a protein which has a high affinity for the steroid to be measured. For example, corticosteroid-binding globulin may be utilized to measure progesterone, with the corticosteroids separated by chromatography. Pregnancy plasma or estrogen-treated plasma is the source for this protein. Competitive protein-binding assays are currently being used for the thyroid hormones, steroid hormones, and vitamins.

Problems. These new methods are not without problems. Utmost precision and care in technique are necessary. An unknown variation in technique may completely disrupt an assay. The periodic appearance of the well-known laboratory "gremlin" may be traced to a simple thing like the water supply or a change in glassware-washing routine. The sensitivity of these ultramicromethods is such that large quantities of a steroid in a laboratory may interfere with the assay.

Measurement of Pituitary Gonadotropins

Pituitary gonadotropins may be measured by bioassay or by radioimmunoassay. The bioassay requires a 24-hour urine collection which is treated as follows. The urine is first acidified. Then the gonadotropins are absorbed onto kaolin, eluted at an alkaline pH, and precipitated with

397

acetone. The extract is injected into immature female mice, and the increase in the weight of the uterus is taken as the end point. This assay has commonly but erroneously been referred to as urinary follicle-stimulating hormone (FSH). It should be called a total urinary gonadotropin assay since uterine growth is the result of both FSH and luteinizing hormone (LH) stimulation of the ovaries and the resulting estrogen production. The greatest dilution of a 24-hour urine extract which will produce a 100% increase in uterine weight is the titer of gonadotropins, and is expressed as mouse uterine units per 24 hours (muu/24 hours). The normal adult level is 6–50 muu/24 hours. A prepubertal level and an adult hypogonadotropic level is less than 6 muu/24 hours. A castrate and postmenopausal level is greater than 200 muu/24 hours.

It should be emphasized that the bioassay of total gonadotropins is notoriously unreliable. When a series of 24-hour urines from normally cycling women were assayed, the total gonadotropin content was falsely pathologic in 1 out of 5 specimens. Therefore, our view is that the bioassay for total gonadotropins should be abandoned and the radioimmunoassay of serum gonadotropins utilized.

Normal serum levels for pituitary gonadotropins during the normal menstrual cycle are illustrated:

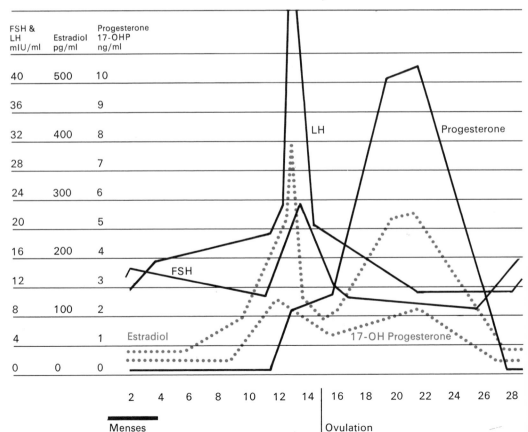

For clinical purposes, the following ranges are useful:

Clinical State	Serum FSH	Serum LH
Normal adult female	5–30 mIU/ml, with the ovulatory midcycle peak about 2 times the base level	5–20 mIU/ml with the ovulatory midcycle peak about 3 times the base level
Hypogonadotropic state: Prepubertal, Hypothalamic and Pituitary Dysfunction	Less than 5 mIU/ml	Less than 5 mIU/ml
Hypergonadotropic state: Postmenopausal, Castrate and Ovarian Failure	Greater than 40 mIU/ml	Greater than 25 mIU/ml

Measurement of Gonadal Steroids

The normal levels for total plasma estrogens or estradiol, and plasma progesterone during the normal menstrual cycle have been illustrated. Variation is seen from individual to individual, however, and the following ranges in gonadal steroids are normally reported:

	Total Estrogen or Estradiol	Progesterone	Testosterone
Follicular phase	25–75 pg/ml	Less than 1 ng/ml	0.2–0.8 ng/ml
Midcycle peak	200–600 pg/ml		0.2–0.8 ng/ml
Luteal phase	100–300 pg/ml	5–20 ng/ml	0.2–0.8 ng/ml
Pregnancy: 1st trimester	1–5 ng/ml	20–30 ng/ml	
Pregnancy: 2nd trimester	5–15 ng/ml	50–100 ng/ml	
Pregnancy: 3rd trimester	10–40 ng/ml	100–400 ng/ml	

Urinary Steroid Assays

The measurement of estrogen in a 24-hour urine collection is frequently utilized during administration of human menopausal gonadotropins (Pergonal).

Total Urinary Estrogen

Prepubertal	0–5 µg/24hrs
Follicular phase	10–25 µg/24hrs
Midcycle peak	35–100 µg/24hrs
Luteal phase	25–75 µg/24hrs
Postmenopausal	5–15 µg/24hrs

Pregnanediol is the main urinary metabolite of progesterone, although it accounts for only 7–20% of total progesterone production. Measurement of pregnanediol in a 24-hour urine has been used in the past to document pregnancy and especially the well-being of an early pregnancy. However, with the advent of the measurement of plasma progesterone, the use of urinary pregnanediol has waned.

Urinary Pregnanediol

Follicular phase	less than 1 mg/24hrs
Luteal phase	2–5 mg/24hrs
Pregnancy: 20 weeks	40 mg/24hrs
Pregnancy: 30 weeks	80 mg/24hrs
Pregnancy: 40 weeks	100 mg/24hrs

Pregnanetriol is the urinary metabolite of 17-hydroxyprogesterone, and is useful for the diagnosis of adrenal hyperplasia (the adrenogenital syndrome). Very little pregnanetriol is found in the urine of normal adults, but with the increased production of 17-hydroxyprogesterone due to an enzyme deficiency in the adrenal gland (adrenogenital syndrome), increased urinary excretion of pregnanetriol will occur.

Urinary Pregnanetriol

Children	Less than 0.5 mg/24 hours
Adults	0.2 to 2–4 mg/24 hours, the upper limit varying from lab to lab.

Measurement of Human Chorionic Gonadotropin

Secretion of human chorionic gonadotropin (HCG) by the syncytiotrophoblast cells of the placenta is predominantly into the maternal circulation. The assay of HCG in maternal urine has been the basis of pregnancy tests for many years. Aschheim and Zondek originated the bioassay pregnancy test in immature mice (the A–Z test) in the late 1920's.

The biologic tests for HCG depended upon the response of ovaries or testes in immature animals. This response was due to the gonadotropic properties of HCG and was measured either in terms of increased gonadal weight or hyperemia, or the secondary response in sex organs due to the increased gonadal steroidogenesis induced by the HCG. The expulsion of ova or sperm in amphibia was also widely utilized as end points for HCG. These biologic assays have now been succeeded by immunoassays for HCG in urine, commonly called urinary chorionic gonadotropin, hence the UCG test.

There are three general types of immunologic assays for HCG, utilizing specific antisera. The three are: hemagglutination-inhibition, complement-fixation, and radioimmunoassay. In the hemagglutination-inhibition reaction, the presence of HCG in maternal urine will inhibit an agglutination reaction between HCG-coated red cells and the antisera. This is the basic reaction in most commercial methods, with latex particles replacing the red cells in some methods. The rapid slide tests utilize latex particles and take 2 minutes to perform. The usual 2-hour test performed in a test tube is more sensitive and reliable. A first morning voided specimen is more concentrated than a random sample and this increases the chances of detecting HCG.

HCG is similar to LH in its structure and thus antibodies to one cross-react with the other. The sensitivity of most commercial assays is limited to approximately 1000 IU/liter in order to avoid false positive tests due to cross-reactivity with LH. Nevertheless, occasionally a urine specimen from an 80-year-old female patient is delivered to the wrong laboratory, and the ward is quite puzzled by the positive pregnancy test.

HCG can be detected in maternal urine from 9 to 16 days after ovulation. Because of the above limitation of sensitivity in most assays, the 2-hour pregnancy test is reliably positive approximately 38 days after the last menstrual period, and the 2-minute slide test, approximately 41 days after the last menstrual period.

Peak levels of HCG (aproximately 100,000 IU/liter) occur at 10 weeks gestation, declining and remaining at approximately 20,000 IU/liter by 12–14 weeks.

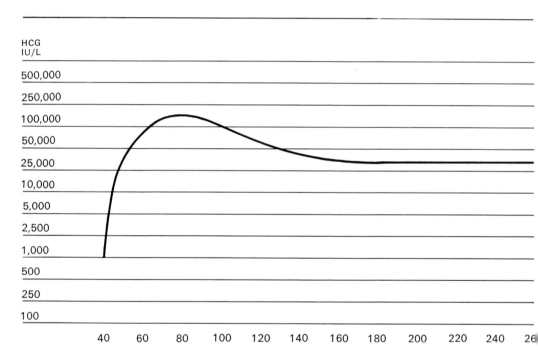

Days After Last Menstrual Period

Patients with hydatidiform moles generally have a urinary level of HCG around 300,000 IU/liter. Choriocarcinoma may be associated with levels in the millions; however the quantitative level of HCG is not absolutely diagnostic. It is well-known that multiple gestations also have high levels of HCG.

A quantitative estimation of HCG in a 24-hour urine may be helpful in the evaluation of a threatened abortion and ectopic pregnancy. A declining level of HCG indicates a poor prognosis for an intrauterine pregnancy, while a low level of HCG (below 5000 IU/liter) is usually, but not always, seen when the pregnancy test is positive with an ectopic pregnancy.

Evaluation of a patient following a spontaneous or therapeutic abortion is occasionally a difficult problem. The urinary pregnancy test can be reliably expected to be negative 3 weeks after abortion. Prior to 3 weeks, a positive pregnancy test may be encountered normally.

Measurement of 17-Ketosteroids, 17-Ketogenic Steroids, and 17-Hydroxycorticosteroids

These frequently used assays provide essential clinical information, yet misunderstanding of their meaning and limitations is still common. A basic appreciation for the methods and what they measure is necessary for the proper interpretation of these urinary assays.

A 24-hour urinary specimen is required to avoid the variations in steroid excretion which occur throughout a day. Refrigeration is essential to avoid degradation of metabolites. It is wise to obtain a urinary creatinine as a check of the validity of the 24-hour collection. Urinary creatinine excretion is a reflection of body muscle mass and remains relatively constant, approximately 1000 mg/24 hours.

The name "17-ketosteroids" is descriptive, designating compounds with a ketone group at the 17 position (C-17). The 17-KS are composed of the major urinary androgenic metabolites, but testosterone itself is not a 17-KS, and significant levles of testosterone may be associated with normal levels of 17-KS.

17-keto group

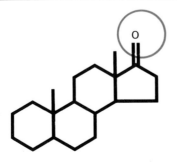

The commonly measured 17-ketosteroids are also known as the neutral 17-KS. Other compounds have a ketone group in the 17 position, but are not "neutral," for example, estrone. Estrone, due to its phenolic structure in ring A, is acidic, and therefore is removed from the urinary extract when washed with alkali in the procedure.

The 17-KS are divided into two groups: the major part being 11-deoxy-17-KS produced by the gonads and adrenal cortex, and the 11-oxy-17-KS, produced *only* by the adrenal cortex.

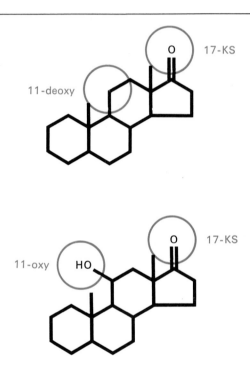

The three major urinary 11-deoxy-17-KS, and therefore, the three major urinary metabolites of androgens are: dehydroepiandrosterne (DHA), etiocholanolone, and androsterone. Note that the only difference between etiocholanolone and androsterone is the stereochemistry at the 5 position: alpha in androsterone and beta in etiocholanolone.

Dehydroepiandrosterone (DHA)

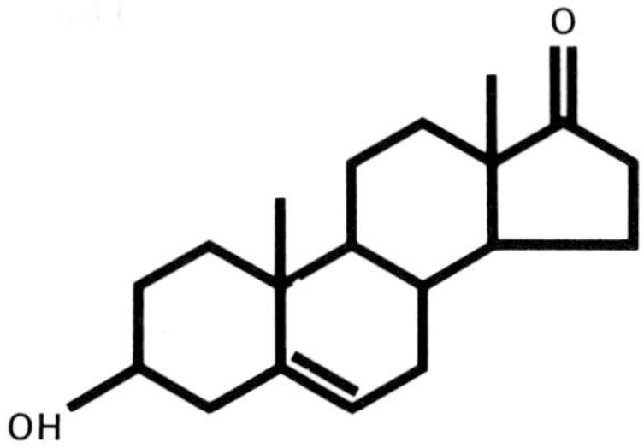

Etiocholanolone

Androsterone

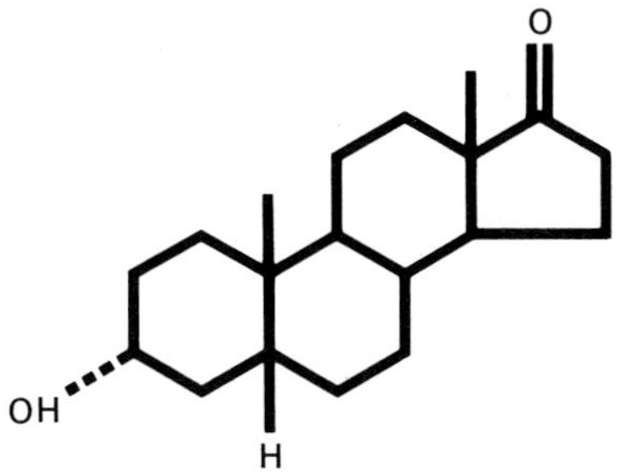

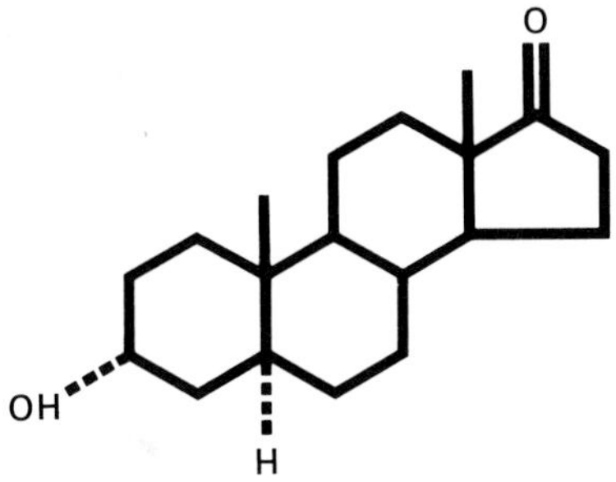

The major 11-oxy-17KS are of adrenal origin: 11-hydroxyetiocholanolone and 11-ketoetiocholanolone (metabolites of corticosteroids), and 11β-hydroxyandrosterone (metabolite of 11β-hydroxyandrostenedione).

11β-Hydroxyandrosterone

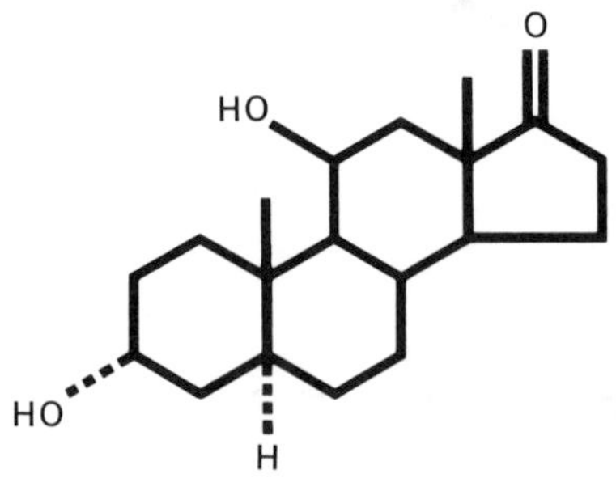

11-Hydroxyetiocholanolone

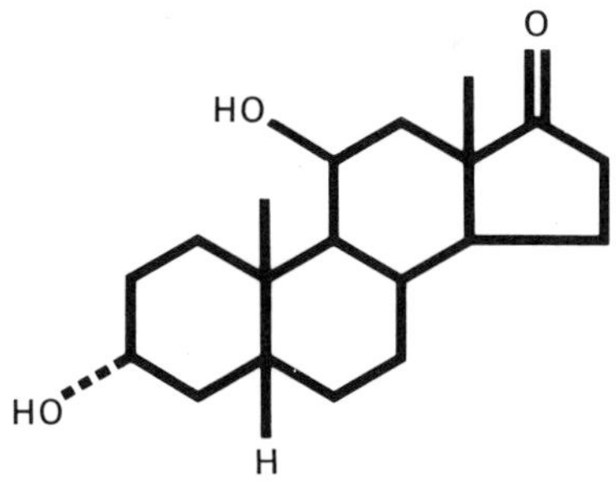

11-Ketoetiocholanolone

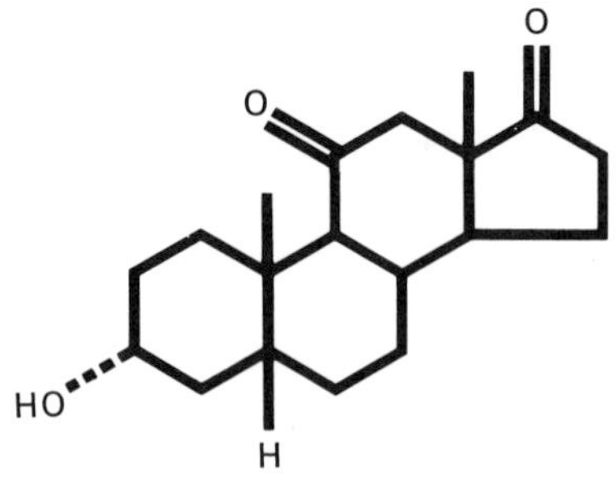

The majority of methods in clinical use for the assay of 17-KS include five major steps:

1. Hydrolysis of the 17-KS conjugates by acid in order to liberate the free steroids for extraction.

2. Extraction with organic solvents.

3. Removal of acidic material by washing with alkali.

4. Development of color, usually by the Zimmermann reaction (17-KS will give a purple color when treated with dinitrobenezene in the presence of alkali).

5. Measurement by colorimetric methods.

ormal 17-KS

The normal level of 17-ketosteroid excretion in a female is 10 ± 3 mg/24 hours. It should be kept in mind that excretion of 17-KS in the urine changes with age. This can be especially important in the evaluation of an elderly woman.

-KS
g/24 hrs

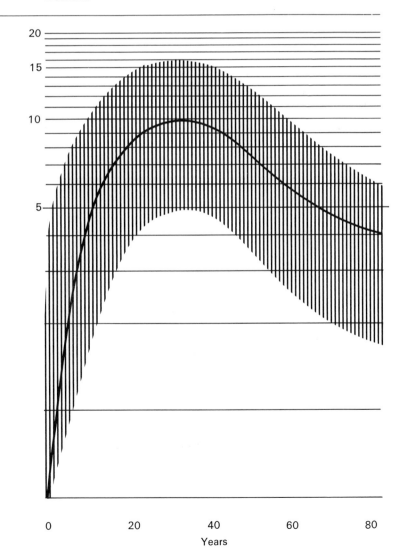

As stated above, the urinary 17-KS arise from precursors secreted by the adrenal cortex and the ovaries. In addition, a certain minimum of nonspecific pigments is present in every urine sample. The composition of normal 17-KS excretion is illustrated.

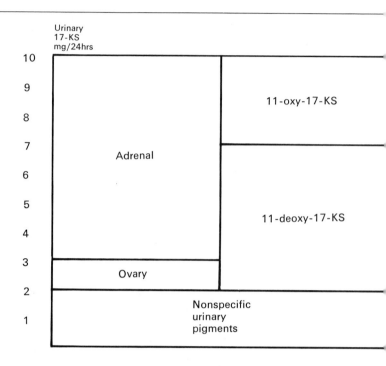

17-Ketogenic
Steroids and
17-Hydroxycortico-
steroids

17-Ketogenic steroid and 17-hydroxycorticosteroid (17-KG and 17-OHC) determinations measure urinary metabolites of glucocorticoids. There are significant differences in the two tests because more metabolites are measured by the 17-KG test.

The 17-KG and 17-OHC assays require the presence of a 17α-hydroxyl group. The mineralocorticoids [deoxycorticosterone (DOC), corticosterone (B), and aldosterone] do not have a 17-hydroxyl group, and therefore are not measured in 17-KG and 17-OHC assays.

17-hydroxyl group

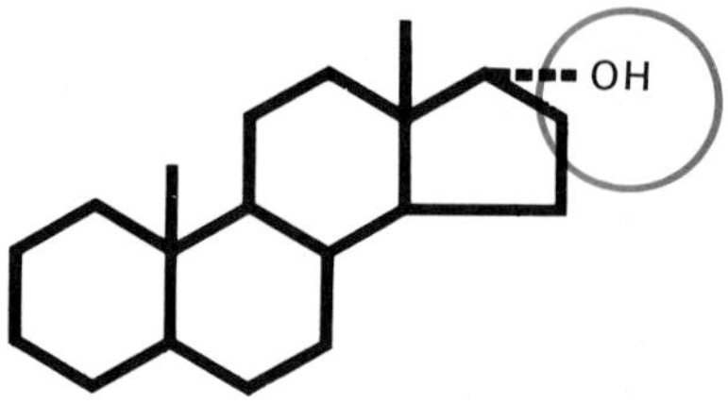

408

esoxycorticosterone
(DOC)

HCOH
|
C $=$ O

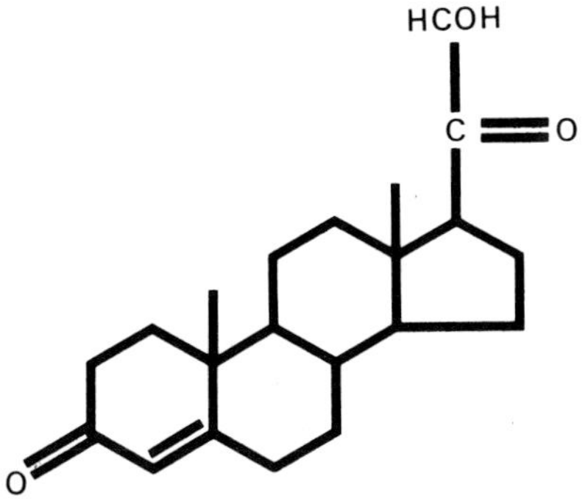

orticosterone
(B)

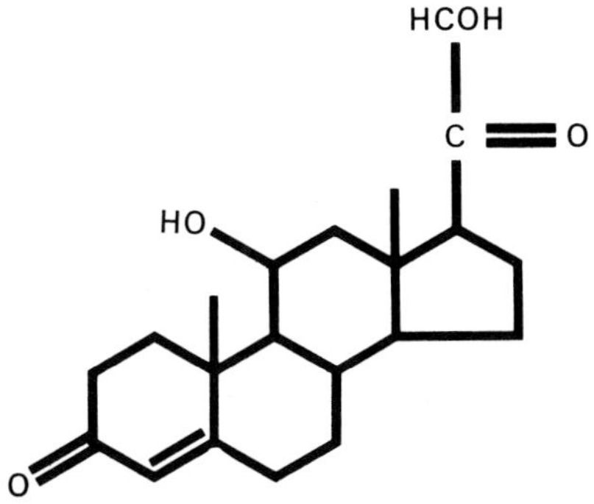

HCOH
|
C $=$ O

HO

Idosterone

HCOH
|
O   C $=$ O
‖   ‖
CH

HO

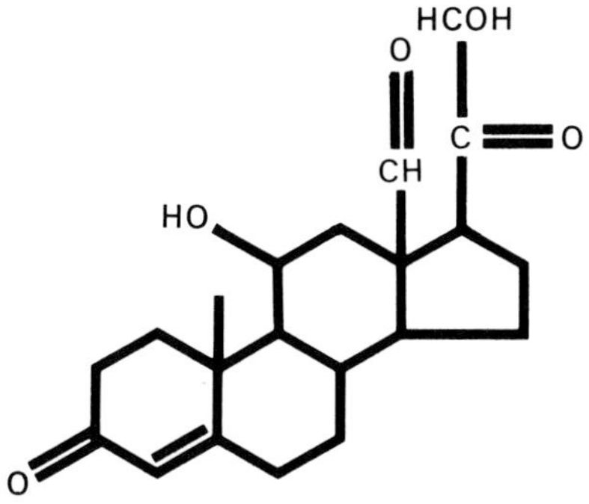

The principal glucocorticoid in the human is cortisol (hydrocortisone, Compound F). Cortisone (Compound E) is a metabolite of cortisol in the human.

Cortisol

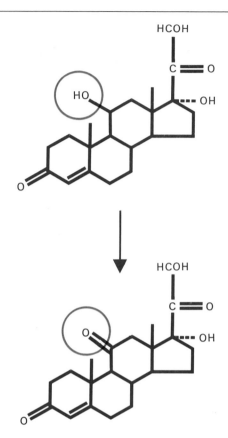

Cortisone

Enzymatic reductions produce the principal urinary metabolite of cortisol: tetrahydrocortisol.

Cortisol

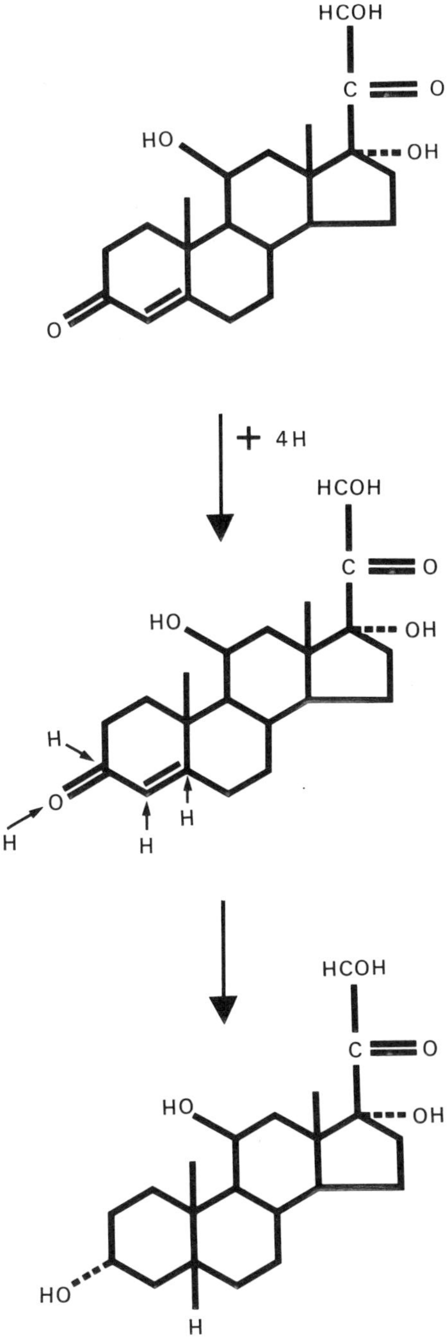

HCOH

C $\equiv$ O

HO

OH

O

$+$ 4H

HCOH

C $\equiv$ O

HO

OH

H

O

H

H

H

H

Tetrahydrocortisol

HCOH

C $\equiv$ O

HO

OH

HO

H

A similar reduction sequence applies to cortisone, yielding tetrahydrocortisone. Further reduction of tetrahydrocortisol and tetrahydrocortisone involves the ketone at the carbon-20 position, yielding cortol and cortolone.

Tetrahydrocortisol

Cortol

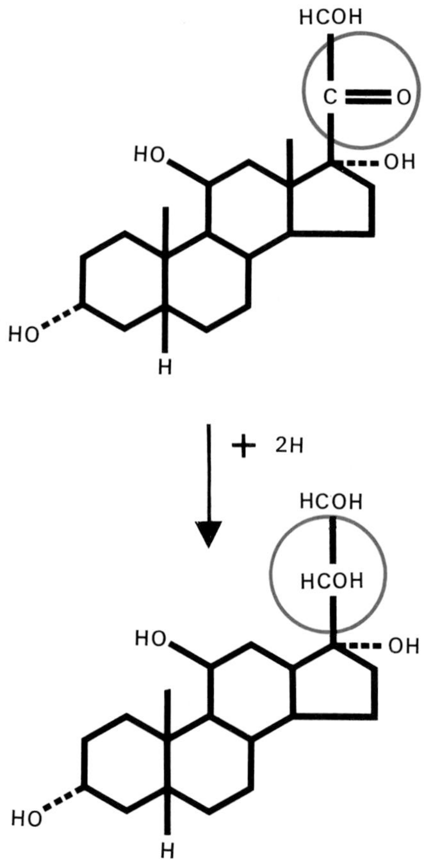

The Porter-Silber reaction produces a color with phenyl-hydrazine and sulfuric acid. The reaction requires an alpha ketolic group plus the 17-hydroxyl group. Therefore, a hydroxyl group must be at C-21 and C-17, and a ketone must be present at C-20. This reaction measures the 17-hydroxycorticosteroids, abbreviated as 17-OHC.

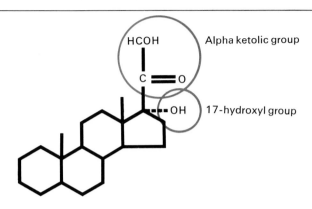

The 17-OHC assay, therefore, cannot measure cortol and cortolone, the further reduction products of tetrahydrocortisol and tetrahydrocortisone, because the C-20 group is reduced and is not a ketone. Nor can the 17-OHC assay measure pregnanetriol since the alpha ketolic group is not present.

Pregnanetriol

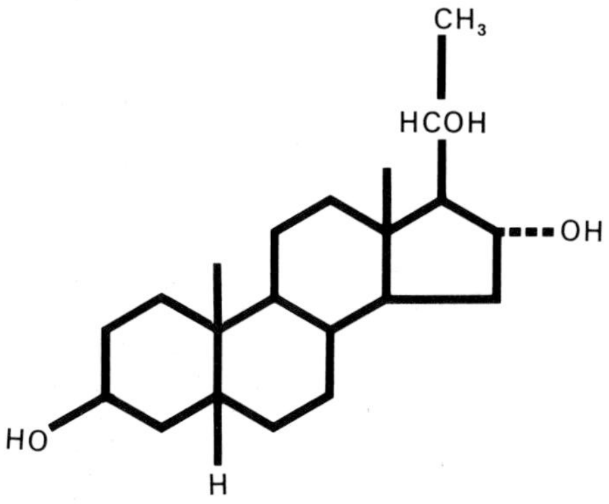

Normal 17-OHC

The normal urinary content of 17-hydroxycorticosteroids is 7 ± 3 mg/24 hours.

The 17-ketogenic steroids (17-KG) are compounds which, when oxidized with sodium bismuthate ($NaBiO_3$), give rise to 17-ketosteroids, which can then be measured by the Zimmermann reaction. The initial measurement of 17-KS is subtracted and the difference represents the 17-KG steroids. The requirement is a 17-hydroxyl group and a second hydroxyl group on either the C-20 or the C-21 position.

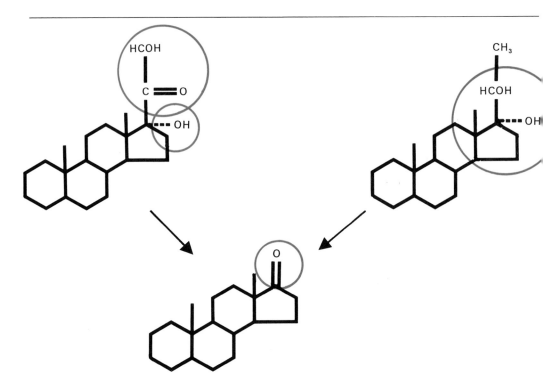

Therefore, the following compounds are measured: tetrahydrocortisol, tetrahydrocortisone, cortol, cortolone, and pregnanetriol (the latter three compounds are not measured in the 17-OHC assay). The compounds missing a 17-hydroxyl group, mainly mineralocorticoids (DOC, corticosterone, and aldosterone) will not be measured by either 17-OHC or 17-KG procedures.

Normal 17-KG

The normal urinary content of 17-ketogenic steroids is 10 ± 3 mg/24 hours. The measurement of additional steroids, when compared to the 17-OHC assay, may be troublesome in the adrenogenital syndrome where pregnanetriol excretion is elevated. Therefore, the 17-KG in the adrenogenital syndrome may be high, while the 17-OHC will be normal.

One should also keep in mind that values change with age.

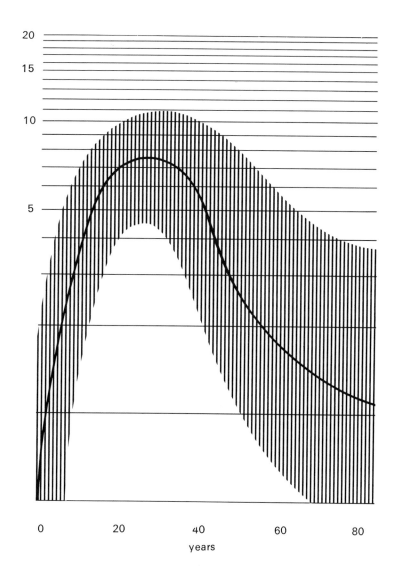

Thyroid Gland

Thyroid hormone synthesis depends in large part upon an adequate supply of iodine in the diet. In the small intestine iodine is absorbed as iodide, and is transported to the thyroid gland. Plasma iodide enters the thyroid under the influence of thyroid-stimulating hormone (TSH), the anterior pituitary thyrotropin hormone. Within the thyroid gland, iodide is oxidized and bound to tyrosine. Monoiodotyrosine and diiodotyrosine combine to form thyroxine (T_4) and triiodothyronine (T_3). These iodinated compounds are part of the thyroglobulin molecule, the colloid which serves as a storage depot for thyroid hormone. TSH induces a proteolytic process which results in the release of iodothyronines into the bloodstream as thyroid hormone. In the blood, thyroid hormone is tightly associated with a group of proteins chiefly thyroxine-binding globulin (TBG). Estrogen produces a rise in thyroxine-binding globulin capacity, and therefore thyroid function tests are affected by pregnancy and estrogen-containing medication. With the increase in TBG capacity, the maintenance of an euthyroid state depends upon the concept that free thryoxine concentration (unbound and metabolically active thyroid hormone) is within the normal range. Because of peripheral conversion of T_4 to T_3, the major activity at the cellular level is due to T_3.

Measurement of Protein-Bound Iodine (PBI)

The determination of the PBI involves precipitation of the serum proteins and measurement of the iodide present by a colorimetric reaction. Therefore, any iodide present will be measured, not only thyroid hormone iodide. The PBI can also be measured by applying the serum to a column ("thyroxine by column") and eliminating inorganic iodide. However, organic iodide contamination, as in x-ray contrast media, will be measured as protein-bound iodine. Water soluble contrast media are excreted by several weeks, while oil-soluble media may take months or years. Normal levels for the serum PBI are 4 to 8 μg/100 ml.

Thyroxine by Competitive Protein Binding

The protein used in this method of saturation analysis is thyroxine-binding globulin. The test measures thyroxine and not iodine, therefore iodine contamination will not interfere with the assay. The thyroxine level in pregnancy is elevated due to the rise in TBG, therefore the absolute amount of thyroxine by this assay will be elevated in pregnancy. Normal values are 3 to 6 μg/100 ml.

T_3 Red Cell or Resin Uptake

The patient's serum is incubated with radioactive T_3, and a weak T_3 binding agent (red blood cells or a resin). The amount of radioactive T_3 binding to the binding agent will be in proportion to the number of binding sites available on the TBG in the patient's serum. In hyperthyroidism, there is more thyroxine and less binding sites: therefore, more radioactive T_3 will be taken up by the binding agent—the T_3 uptake is increased in hyperthyroidism. Conversely in hypothyroidism there are more binding sites and the T_3 uptake is decreased. In pregnancy, with an increase in TBG, there are more binding sites and the T_3 uptake is decreased. Iodide contamination does not interfere with the assay, but compounds which increase TBG (estrogen, perphenazine) and compounds which decrease TBG-binding capacity (androgens, Dilantin) affect the T_3 uptake. The combination of an elevated PBI or free thyroxine and a decreased T_3 uptake is characteristic of pregnancy or estrogen therapy. Normal values vary according to the laboratory, but range from 25 to 36%.

The Free Thyroxine Index

This determination is now available in most laboratories, and represents the most useful measure of thyroid function in that it is not affected by organic or inorganic iodine, and it is corrected for changes in TBG. The free thyroxine is calculated by utilizing data from the measurement of thyroxine by saturation analysis and the T_3 uptake. The free thyroxine index gives the calculated measure of the amount of circulating thyroxine hormone.

Measurement of TSH

The radioimmunoassay of TSH is utilized to differentiate between primary and secondary hypothyroidism. It is a very sensitive measure of primary hypothyroidism, and therefore is a useful screening test (especially for infertility patients). The range of serum TSH is approximately nondetectable to 10 μU/ml.

Radioimmunoassay of T_3

This assay is important in diagnosing hyperthyroidism due to excessive production of T_3, with normal T_4 levels (T_3 toxicosis). The normal range for serum T_3 is 100–170 ng/100 ml.

ndex

bdominal pain, with clomiphene therapy, 382
bortion
  definition, 331
  due to inadequate luteal function, 14
  HCG levels following, 403
  habitual
    cure rate, 332
    definition, 332
    hormonal treatment, 332–333
    psychological aspects, 333
  rate with clomiphene therapy, 382
  septic and infertility, 322
bstinence, effect on sperm motility, 366
cetate, in cholesterol synthesis, 7, 8
cne
  and clomiphene citrate, 380
  and steroid contraceptives, 298
cromegaly
  and abnormal lactation, 177
  and hirsutism, 137
  symptoms in pituitary tumor, 112
CTH
  effect on excessive androstenedione production, 144
  excessive secretion in pituitary tumors, 112
  fetal, role in parturition, 210–211
  role in fetal adrenal gland, 191
  role in placenta, 203
ctinomycin D, inhibition of transcription, 22
ddison's disease, premature ovarian failure in, 112
denomatous hyperplasia, and anovulation, 378
denosine triphosphate (see ATP)
denylate cyclase in estradiol synthesis, 2
dipose tissue
  conversion of androstenedione to estrogen, 126
  fatty acid release, 274
  function, 272
doption, 334
drenal cortex, steroid hormone production, 15
drenal gland
  as source of androgens, 12
  fetal, 191–192
    activity, 187
    role in parturition, 210–211
  in anovulation, 132
  tumors
    and hirsutism, 138, 140, 141
    in hirsutism diagnosis, 147
drenal hyperplasia (see also Congenital adreno-genital syndrome)
  and pregnancy, 240
  congenital
    progestrone blood levels in, 14
  diagnosis, 247–249, 401
  in ambiguous genitalia, 236
  in Cushing's syndrome, 147
  pregnanetriol levels in, 14, 247
  with 17-hydroxylase deficiency, 246

Adrenogenital syndrome (see Adrenal hyperplasia)
Aging
  and steroid contraceptives, 302
  psychological aspects, 78
Albright's syndrome, 258
Aldosterone secretion in luteal phase, 60
Alcohol
  and abnormal semen, 366
  and impotence, 366
Allergic reactions as cause of male infertility, 365
Ambiguous genitalia
  diagnosis, 246–249
  fertility, 249–250
  sex assignment, 249–250
Amenorrhea
  and anorexia nervosa, 113
  and anovulation, 123, 128, 132
  and galactorrhea, 113, 174, 176
  and HMG therapy, 386
  and pituitary tumors, 113–115
  and stress, 116
  causes, 95–96
  definition, 94
  diagnosis, 97–106
  disorders of gonadal competence, 111–112
    gonadal agenesis, 112
    resistant ovary syndrome, 112
    mosaicism, 111
    Turner's syndrome, 111
  disorders of outflow tract or uterine target organ, 107–110
    Asherman's syndrome, 107
    Mullerian agenesis, 108–109
    Mullerian anomalies, 108
    testicular feminization, 109–110
  disorders of the hypothalamus, 116–118
    anorexia nervosa, 116–117
    anosmia, 118
  disorders of the pituitary, 112–116
    empty sella syndrome, 115–116
  in adrenal hyperplasia, 246
  in gonadal dysgenesis, 245
  on steroid contraceptives, 301
  postpill, 298–299
  prolactin levels in, 113, 174
  secondary, 113
    in gonadal dysgenesis, 245
  therapy
    effect on breast size, 169
    with ergot alkaloids, 178
Aminoglutethimide inhibition of steroidogenesis, 22
Amniotic fluid
  estetrol levels, 196
  estriol levels, 196
  prolactin levels, 170
Amphetamines in obesity management, 279
Ampicillin, effect on urine estrogen levels, 194–195
Anastomosis (see Tubal surgery, end to end anas-tomosis)

Androgen insensitivity (see Testicular feminization)
Androgens
  adrenal, role in puberty, 253
  as secretory product, 7
  cellular action, 22
  daily production levels in chronic anovulation, 129–131
  effect
    of abnormal levels, 55
    of fetal exposure, 234
    on hair growth, 137
  excessive, in anovulation, 127
  fetal, in estrogen synthesis, 189
  hypersensitivity in idiopathic hirsutism, 146
  inappropriate fetal exposure, 235–236
  increase and anovulation, 124
  metabolism, 15–17
  structure, 4
  synthesis, 7, 9
    abnormal, 243
    by corpus luteum, 57
    in follicular phase, 54
Androstanediol, 16
Androstane derivatives, 4
Androstenedione
  aromatization, 8
  blood levels
    in hirsutism, 144
    in hirsutism diagnosis, 141
  conversion to testosterone, 11
  daily production levels
    in chronic anovulation, 129
    in nonpregnant female, 13
  in females age 8 to 10, 44
  peripheral conversion to estrogens, 12
  postmenopause secretion, 10, 74
  secretion by stromal tissue, 10, 15, 54
Anemia and steroid contraceptives, 298
Anorchia, 244
Anorexia nervosa, 116–117
Anosmia and amenorrhea, 118
Anovulation (see also Infertility)
  adrenal gland involvement, 132
  and amenorrhea, 123, 128, 132
  and anorexia nervosa, 124
  and bleeding. 132, 160
  and breast disease, 128
  and cancer, 128
  and cancer risk, 123, 132
  and dysfunctional uterine bleeding, 128, 165, 166
  and endometrial abnormalities, 133
  and endometrial hyperplasia, 128
  and excessive androgen production, 127
  and follicular atresia, 127, 130
  and hirsutism, 123, 128, 132
  and hypoestrogen, 379
  and infertility, 128
  and obesity, 126, 132
  and polycystic ovaries, 128–132
  and stress, 124, 126
  at menarche, 254
  central defects, 124
    pituitary tumor, 124
  chronic, 123
    daily hormone levels, 129–131
  clinical presentations, 128
  endometrial biopsy prior to clomiphene therapy, 378
  etiology, 127–128
    due to anovulatory dysfunction, 128
    due to central failure, 128
    due to ovarian failure, 128
    impairment of estradiol clearance and metabolism, 125–126
  in amenorrhea diagnosis, 98
  in climacteric, 77
  inadequate estradiol levels, 126–127
  late and bleeding, 160
  loss of LH stimulation, 126–127
  ovarian biopsy, 379
  therapy, 133
    ergot alkaloids, 390
    GnRH, 389
    ovarian wedge resection, 383
Antibodies, agglutinizing in infertility, 329–331
Antibiotics in postoperative hydrotubation, 348
Anxiety, effect on fertility, 311
Appendix, ruptured and infertility, 322
Aromatization in estrogens conversion, 9
Artificial insemination
  donor, 370–372
  husband, 369
  split ejaculate, 370
  technique, 371
Ascheim and Zondek test for pregnancy, 401
Ascites in ovarian hyperstimulation, 387
Asherman's syndrome, diagnosis and treatment 107
Aspirin, effect in pregnancy, 221
Astrocytoma as cause of precocious puberty, 256
Atherosclerosis and estrogen therapy, 85
ATP, in steroidogenesis, 23–24
Atresia, follicular, 53–54
  effect of androgens, 54
  in anovulation, 127, 130
  in fetal life, 233
Atrophy, vaginal in climacteric, 78–80
Azospermia, 367

Basal body temperature
  for artificial insemination, 371
  in HMG therapy, 386
  in clomiphene therapy, 380, 381
  in ovulation determination, 326
Behavior, effect of menstrual cycle, 75
Bioassay for pituitary gonadotropins, 398
Binding globulin level, female androgen production, 15
Birth control pills (see Contraceptives, steroid)
Bleeding
  abnormal
    and steroid contraceptives, 299
    in climacteric, 79–80
  and obesity, 160
  and polycystic ovaries, 160
  anovulatory, 160
    treatment, 161–163
  breakthrough
    control in steroid contraceptives, 288
    in progestin therapy, 164, 165
    on steroid contraceptives, 301
  dysfunctional uterine, 151–166
    and anovulation, 165, 166
    control by oral contraceptives, 161–163
    in anovulation, 128
    treatment, 165–166
    treatment with D & C, 165, 166
  estrogen breakthrough, 158, 161
  estrogen withdrawal, 158, 159, 161
  heavy
    and steroid contraceptives, 298

in anovulation, 132
in estrogen therapy, 85
in postmenopausal women, 12
progesterone breakthrough, 158, 161
progesterone withdrawal, 158, 159, 161
prolonged, 160
uterine in salipingostomy, 346
Blindness in pituitary tumors, 113
Blood pressure, maternal role of prostaglandins, 220
Bone age
determination, 260
in precocious puberty, 256
Brain lesions as cause of precocious puberty, 256
Breast(s)
abnormal size and shape, 169
asymmetry, 169
cancer
and etiocholanolone excretion, 180
and steroid contraceptives, 289, 299
familial tendency, 180
hormonal treatment, 290
incidence, 179
increase with estrogen therapy, 83–84
relation of endogenous estrogen, 180–181
relation to cystic mastitis, 180
relation to estriol excretion, 180
relation to ovarian activity, 180
relation to prolactin levels, 181
relation to reproductive experience, 179–180
relation of thyroid hormone, 181
risk factors, 179–181
steroid therapy, 182
treatment, 181–182
development
by estrogen therapy, 118
at puberty, 253
disease in anovulation, 128
effect of steroids on development, 168
growth and development, 167–168
hormone therapy, effect on size, 169
in pregnancy, 170–174
tenderness in estrogen therapy, 85

Caffeine, effect on sperm motility, 369
Calcium, role in parturition, 222
Call-Exner body
formation, 68
in follicular maturation, 69
Cancer (see also Tumors and specific organs)
increase with estrogen therapy, 83–85
Carbohydrate metabolism and oral contraceptives, 293
Cardiac malformations
in Noonan's syndrome, 246
in Turner's syndrome, 246
Castration
effect
on gonadotropin levels, 102
on gonadotropin molecule size, 104
on hair growth, 137
Central nervous system
abnormalities and precocious puberty, 258
differentiation, 236
effect of fetal androgen exposure, 236
Cerebral abnormalities as cause of precocious puberty, 256
Cerebrovascular disease and oral contraceptives, 291
Cervix

inflammation from steroid contraceptive, 298
mucus
in post coital test, 317–322
treatment of poor, 319
Chloasma and steroid contraceptives, 297
Cholesterol
conversion to pregnenolone, 2, 7, 8
in progesterone synthesis by placenta, 186
in steroidogenesis, 7
levels effect of steroid contraceptives, 294
Chromosome(s)
abnormalities in male infertility, 367
Y, presence in amenorrhea, 103
Chymotrypsin, in postoperative hydrotubation, 345
Circadian cycle
effect on pineal gland, 42
female, sex steroids, 15
in pregnancy prolactin levels, 170
Cirrhosis and steroid contraceptives, 294
Climacteric (see also Menopause)
estrogen withdrawal, clinical implications, 76–80
frequent symptoms, 77–80
psychological aspects, 78
relationship of estrogen withdrawal, 72
symptoms treated by estrogen, 81–83
Clitorectomy
erotic response following, 240
in congenital adrenogenital syndrome, 240
Clitoris differentiation in ambiguous genitalia, 247
Clomid (see Clomiphene citrate)
Clomiphene citrate
administered with HMG, 389
and acne, 380
anti-estrogen effect, 22
complications, 382
for anosmia, 118
for hirsutism, 142
for hypoestrogenism, 379
for inadequate luteal phase, 329
for infertility treatment, 325
for low sperm counts, 367
inappropriate use, 380
ovulation induction in amenorrhea, 116
pharmacological effects, 376–378
psychological aspects of treatment, 381
selection of patients, 378–380
therapy results, 381–382
to delay ovulation, 379
treatment cycle 380–381
Coitus
frequency during clomiphene therapy, 380, 381
infrequent, 369
optimum frequency for fertility, 369
Colostrum in pregnancy, 171
Competitive protein binding (see Protein binding, competitive)
Condoms, therapy for sperm allergy, 329–330
Congenital adrenogenital syndrome (see also Adrenal hyperplasia)
and pregnancy, 240
description, 236–237
diagnosis, 239, 247–249
genetic aspects, 237
treatment, 240
Contraceptive, effect of lactation, 174
Contraceptives, steroid
age factors, 302
alternatives, 302–306
and amenorrhea, 301
and breakthrough bleeding, 301–302
and carbohydrate metabolism, 293

Contraceptives, steroids—*continued*
  and cerebrovascular disease, 291–292, 299
  and endometrial cancer, 84
  and epilepsy, 299
  and galactorrhea, 175
  and gallbladder disease, 295
  and gastrointestinal disturbances, 297
  and hypertension, 295–297, 299
  and lactation, 300
  and lipid metabolism, 294
  and myocardial infarction, 292
  and smoking, effect on stroke risk, 292
  and thromboembolic disease, 290–291, 299
  and varicose veins, 299
  carcinogenic effects, 288–290
  combination pill, pharmacology, 288
  common adverse effects, 297–298
  contraindications, 299–300
  discontinuance and amenorrhea, 298–299
  effect
    adrenal-pituitary gland, 292
    on depression, 76
    on dysmenorrhea, 76
    on libido, 54
    on lipoproteins, 294
    on liver, 294, 299
    on thyroid, 293
  estrogen dosage, 300
  steroids
  in amenorrhea diagnosis, 97
  in anovulation, 133
  in high 17-ketosteroid excretion, 144
  in hirsutism treatment, 142
  in hypothalamic amenorrhea therapy, 118
  in idiopathic hirsutism, 146
  metabolic effects, 288–298
  pharmacology, 284–288
  postcoital, 305
  preoperative treatment for endometriosis, 357
  progesterone and estrogen action, 39
  therapeutic use
    for anovulatory bleeding, 161, 163
    for depression, 76
    for dysfunctional uterine bleeding, 164, 165, 166
    for endometrioma, 360
    for endometriosis, 76, 356, 358–359
    in premenstrual tension, 76
    in prevention of endometriosis, 360
    in tubal implantation, 349, 351
Coronary heart disease
  and estrogen therapy, 82
  incidence in castrated women, 83
Corpus luteum
  formation following ovulation, 71
  role of HCG, 202
  secretions, 71
  synthesis of progesterone, 187
  synthesis of sex steroids, 57
Corticoid(s) structure, 4
Corticosteroids
  effect on urine estrogen levels, 194
  treatment in respiratory distress syndrome, 216
Corticosterone binding globulin (CBG) (see Transcortin)
Cortisol
  effect on breast development, 168
  effect on lactation, 171
  excess and short stature, 261
  in hirsutism treatment, 145
  in labor induction, 212
  levels
    activated by steroid contraceptives, 292
    in amniotic fluid at term, 212
    in placenta, 203
    in pregnancy, 170
    in umbilical cord blood, 211
  receptor-complex, 21
  structure, 410
  therapeutic use
  transcortin binding, 10
    in congenital adrenogenital syndrome, 240
    in 17-hydroxylase deficiency, 246
Cortisone, structure, 410
Cortol, 412
Cortolone, 412
Counseling, sexual, 369
Cranial trauma as cause of precocious puberty, 256
Craniopharyngioma as cause of precocious puberty, 256
Creatinine
  and estriol ratio in pregnancy, 195
  levels in diabetic pregnancy, 198
  urine levels in pregnancy, 193
Cryptorchidism, 366
Culdoscopy, for infertility diagnosis, 331
Curettage
  for anovulatory bleeding, 161
  for dysfunctional uterine bleeding, 165, 166
  in infertility investigation, 312
Cushing's disease
  and short stature, 261
  in hirsutism diagnosis, 140, 146, 147
  symptoms in pituitary tumor, 112
Cyclic AMP
  activation by tropic hormone, 23–25
  activation of prostaglandin synthesis, 24
  in estradiol synthesis, 2
  in steroidogenesis, 2
Cyclic guanosine 3'5' monophosphate, effect on cellular function, 24
Cyproterone acetate, in hirsutism therapy, 143
Cytomel for male infertility, 367

Danazol
  for endometriosis symptoms, 359
  for infertility, 359
Darkness, effect on pineal gland, 42
Dehydroepiandrosterone (DHA)
  in females age 6 to 8, 44
  in Δ^5-3β-hydroxy steroid pathway, 9
  levels in placental sulfatase deficiency, 201
  secretion by stromal tissue, 10
  synthesis, 8
  synthesis by ovary, 15
Dehydroepiandrosterone sulfate (DS)
  levels
    in assessing high risk pregnancy, 197
    in congenital adrenogenital syndrome, 239
    in hirsutism, 141
    in placental sulfatase deficiency, 201
  synthesis by fetal adrenal glands, 190
Depo Provera (see Medroxyprogesterone acetate)
Depression
  and steroid contraceptive use, 76, 298
  estrogen therapy, 81
  in climacteric, 77
Dexamethasone
  in hirsutism diagnosis, 140, 147
  in tubal surgery, 348

Diabetes mellitus
  and estrogen therapy, 85
  and fetal lung maturation, 216
  and pregnancy, 197–199
    and HPL levels in, 207
    child development prognosis, 200
    estriol assay, 198
    fetal loss risk, 197
  and retrograde ejaculation, 366
  and steroid contraceptives, 293
  mortality and obesity, 271
Diet in obesity management, 279
Diethylstilbestrol
  as postcoital contraceptive, 305
  for infertility, 321
  in treatment of tall stature, 262
Dihydrotestosterone (DHT)
  cellular action, 22
  in masculine differentiation, 16
  metabolism, 16, 17
Dilantin, effect on thyroxine-binding globulin, 417
Dilation and curettage (see Curettage)
Diuretics
  use in ovarian hyperstimulation, 388
  therapeutic use in premenstrual tension, 76
L-DOPA in treatment of galactorrhea, 178
Dopamine
  in hypothalamic regulation of gonadotropins, 37
  effect
    on GnRH, 37
    on LH and FSH release, 37
    in pituitary function, 37
    prolactin inhibition, 38
Doxycycline for mycoplasma, 329
Drug addiction, heroin and fetal lung maturation, 216
Drug effects on steroid hormone action, 22
Duct system, congenital absence, 366
Dysfunctional uterine bleeding (see Bleeding, dysfunctional uterine)
Dysmenorrhea
  and endometriosis, 356
  and steroid contraceptives, 298
  causes, 76
  surgery, 357
  therapy, 76
Dyspareunia in climacteric, 78–80

Edema in estrogen therapy, 85
Egg transport and fertilization, 314–316
Ejaculation
  premature, treatment by AIH, 369
  retrograde, 366
    treatment by AIH, 369
  split, 370
Electrolysis for hirsutism, 143, 144, 146
Embryology (see Sexual differentiation)
Emotional disturbances, cyclic, 75
Empty sella syndrome (see Sella turcica, empty)
Encephalitis as cause of precocious puberty, 256
Endocrine disorders in male infertility, 367–368
Endometrioma, treatment, 360
Endometriosis
  diagnosis, 356
  etiology, 355–356
  in anovulation, 127
  pregnancy rate following treatment, 358
  prevention, 360
  surgery, 357–358
  treatment, 356–360
Endometrium

adenocarcinoma, 163
and egg relationship, 156–158
biopsy
  for infertility, 327
  prior to clomiphene therapy, 378
breakdown phase, 155
changes in ovulatory cycle, 152–156
effect
  of estrogen therapy, 84–85
  of insufficient estrogen, 164
  of progesterone, 85
  of steroid contraceptives, 288
hyperplasia, 160
  and anovulation, 128
  following estrogen therapy, 84–85
  in estrogen therapy, 87
implantation phase, 155
menstrual, 152
neoplasia and steroid contraceptives, 289
proliferative phase, 153
secretory phase, 154
tuberculosis infection in, 107
Ephedrine, for retrograde ejaculation, 366
Epididymal obstruction, as cause for male infertility, 365
Epilepsy and steroid contraceptives, 299
Epinephrine, adipose tissue lipase stimulation, 274
17-epitestosterone and testosterone, 5
Ergot derivatives, clinical treatment of high prolactin levels, 38
Ergot alkaloids
  teratogenic effects, 178
  therapeutic use
    in amenorrhea, 178
    in anovulation, 390
    in galactorrhea, 178
    in pituitary tumors, 114, 115
    in prevention of postpartum milk secretion, 171
    side effects, 178
Erythroblastosis fetalis, diagnosis by estriol assay, 200
Estes procedure, 353
Estetrol
  levels in amniotic fluid, 196
  levels in placental sulfatase deficiency, 201
Estradiol
  administration and increase prostaglandins, 220
  and protein binding, 2
  biologic activity compared to estriol, 21
  conversion
    by aromatization, 9
    from androstenedione, 11
    from testosterone, 11
    to estriol, 3
    to estrone, 3
  daily production rate
    from testosterone, 13
    nonpregnant female, 13
  effect
    on FSH, 51–52
    on FSH and LH release, 55
    on human menstrual cycle, 60
    on production of RNA, 3
  follicular production in anovulation, 127
  inhibition of FSH stimulation, 125
  levels
    following ovulation, 57
    in positive feedback system, 53
    in pregnancy, 190
    lack of critical in anovulation, 126

Estradiol—*continued*
  levels—*continued*
    perimenopausal, 73
    postmenopause, 74
    prior to parturition, 212
  metabolism, 2, 3, 11
  role in normal menses, 124
  secretion in bloodstream, 2
  structure, 11
  synthesis, 1–3
    by follicular theca cells, 2, 9, 10
    by granulosa cells of corpus luteum, 2
    during follicular phase, 54
Estriol
  and creatine ratio in pregnancy, 195
  biologic activity compared to estradiol, 21
  excretion
    and breast cancer incidence, 180
    in diabetic pregnancy, 198
    in prolonged gestation, 200
  levels
    in amniotic fluid, 196
    in erythroblastosis fetalis, 200
    in intrauterine growth retardation, 200
    in placental sulfatase deficiency, 20
    in pregnancy, 195–196
    in toxemia diagnosis, 199
  low levels in pregnancy, child development prognosis, 200
  structure, 11
  synthesis by fetal adrenal gland, 189
  urine levels
    drug effects in pregnancy, 194–195
    in high risk pregnancy, 197
    in oxytocin-induced labor, 195
    in pregnancy, 192–194
    relation to fetal weight, 194
Estrogen
  administration
    in amenorrhea diagnosis, 98–99
    to prevent lactation, 171
  blood levels in pregnancy, 195–196
  breakthrough bleeding, 158
  conjugated
    excretion, 18
    for poor cervical mucus, 319
    in treatment of breakthrough bleeding in precocious puberty, 259
    in treatment of dysfunctional uterine bleeding, 164, 165, 166
    in treatment of short stature, 261
    in treatment of tall stature, 262
  daily production levels in chronic anovulation, 129–131
  in dependent neoplasms and steroid contraceptives, 299
  of lack during menopause, 77
  of steroid contraceptives, 288
  on breast cancer incidence, 180
  on breast growth, 168
  on egg release, 315
  on endometrial proliferative phase, 153
  on endometrial secretory phase, 154
  on endometrium shrinkage, 164, 165
  on fetal adrenal gland, 192
  on follicle maturation, 71
  on follicle selection for ovulation, 70
  on FSH, 52
  on gonadotropin release, 55
  on hair growth, 137
  on prolactin in pregnancy, 171
  on prostaglandin production, 208
  excessive in galactorrhea, 175
  excretion in pregnancy, 190
  in females age 10 to 12, 44
  in males, peripheral conversion from androgens, 12
  increase
    and progesterone withdrawl, 212–214
    and prostaglandin levels, 220
    in parturition, 208
  levels
    assessment in amenorrhea, 97–98
    in HMG therapy, 384, 385
    in ovarian hyperstimulation, 388
    in polycystic ovaries, 145
    in pregnancy, 170
    in pregnancy, 190
    laboratory measurement, 400
    postmenopause, 74–75
  mechanism of tissue reaction, 20
  menopausal production, 77
  metabolism, 11–13
  secretion by corpus luteum, 71
  structure, 4
  synthesis, 7
    by corpus luteum, 57
    by granulosa cells, 70
    in fetal-placenta unit, 188–190
    in thecal cells, 10, 70
  therapy
    administration and dosage, 86
    adverse effects, 80, 83–85
    after castration, 79
    and breast cancer risk, 181
    and gallbladder disease, 295
    and thromboembolic disease, 290
    contraindications, 80
    effect on breast size, 169
    effect on hair growth, 145
    in amenorrhea, 118
    in Asherman's syndrome, 107
    in breast development, 118
    in climacteric symptoms, 80–83
    in hirsutism, 142
    in osteoporosis, 80, 81–82
    postgonadectomy, 118
    supplemented with progesterone, 85
    metabolic effects, 85
  withdrawal
    bleeding, 158, 159
    effect on climacteric symptoms, 79–80
    rate factors, 80
  urine levels
    drug effects in pregnancy, 194–195
    in pregnancy, 192–194
Estrone
  and cancer, 86
  conversion by aromatization, 9
  conversion rate from androstenedione, 13
  in estradiol metabolism, 11
  levels in pregnancy, 190
  postmenopause levels, 74
  structure, 6, 11
Escherichia coli in sperm agglutination, 365
Ethinyl estradiol
  and pill related breakthrough bleeding, 301
  in breakthrough bleeding in precocious puberty, 259
  in oral contraceptives, 284
  in treatment of dysfunctional uterine bleeding, 164

Etiocholanolone excretion in breast cancer incidence, 180
Ethisterone, 285
Eunuchoidism in gonadal dysgenesis, 245

Fallopian tubes
　distal occlusion, 345
　infection from intrauterine insemination, 320
　pathology of, infertility, 343
　tests of patency, 322–325
Fat cells, 277
Fertilization
　in vitro, 316–317
　mechanisms, 313–317
Fetal distress, assessment with HPL levels, 207
Fetus
　anencephalic, 210
　effect of clomiphene therapy, 378
　lung development, 215–216
　macrosomia in diabetic pregnancy, 198
Fibrinogen, effect of oral contraceptives on, 298
Fimbrioplasty (see also Salpingostomy)
Follicle(s)
　atresia
　　during maturation phase, 69
　　in fetal life, 67–68
　attrition leading to menopause, 77
　development in adult, 69
　effect on estrogen withdrawal, 80
　estradiol production in anovulation, 127
　maturation, 68–69
　　gonadotropin effects, 69
　　role of estrogen, 71
　primordial, 67
　residual, 73
　selection for ovulation, 70
　steroid synthesis, 9
　stimulation in chronic anovulation, 130
Follicle-stimulating hormone (FSH)
　abnormalities in male infertility, 367
　daily production levels in chronic anovulation,
　　129–131
　effect
　　of clomiphene citrate, 377
　　of melatonin, 42
　　of steroid contraceptives, 288
　　on LH receptors, 55
　　on number of follicles maturing, 69
　inhibition by sustained estradiol levels, 125
　levels
　　in anorexia nervosa, 117
　　in fetus, 44
　　perimenopausal, 73
　releasing factors, 30
　role in menstrual cycle, 50–60
　secretion in fetus, 43
　serum levels in amenorrhea diagnosis, 101–105
Fructose production by seminal vesicles, 366
Furadantin and abnormal semen, 365

Galactorrhea, 174–179
　and amenorrhea, 174
　and amenorrhea, 176
　and elevated prolactin levels, 174
　and high prolactin levels, 113
　and hypothyroidism, 176
　and polytomography of sella turcica, 178
　and prolactin assay, 177
　and stress, 176

definition, 174
differential diagnosis, 175–176
drug-induced, 175
due to excessive estrogen, 175
due to hypothalamic lesions, 176
due to induced prolactin release, 175
due to PIH inhibition, 175, 176
due to pituitary tumors, 176, 177
in amenorrhea diagnosis, 98
treatment, 178–179
　with ergot alkaloids, 178
　with L-DOPA, 178
　with pyridoxine, 178
Gallbladder disease and steroid contraceptives,
　295
Genitalia
　ambiguous, 246–250
　external differentiation, 234–236
Gestation, prolonged, 200
　and anencephalic fetus, 210
　experimentally induced, 210
Glucocorticoids
　in progesterone withdrawal, 212–213
　synthesis, 7, 15
Glucosiduronate conjugates, structure, 18
Glucose
　as fetal fuel, 205, 206
　function, 273
　inadequate fetal supply, 206
Glucuro-conjugates in estradiol clearing, 3
Gonadal dysgenesis, 245
Gonad(s)
　agenesis, 112
　differentiation, normal, 232–233
　embryology and differentiation, 66
　tumor in Y chromosome presence, 103
Gonadotropin(s) (see also Follicle-stimulating hormone and Luteinizing hormone)
　effect
　　on follicle maturation, 69
　　of hypothalamus, 31
　　of progesterone, 56
　　on follicular growth, 51
　levels in amenorrhea diagnosis, 101–105
　molecule size, effect by castration, 104
　pituitary in fetus, 44
　radioimmunoassay for anovulation, 379
　radioimmunoassay techniques, 395, 398–399
　releasing factors for male infertility, 368
　secretion
　　in human life cycle, 43
　　in luteal phase, 56
Gonadotropin-releasing hormone (GnRH)
　as neurochemotransmitter, 29
　competition with oxytoxin, 35
　effect
　　of estradiol levels, 53
　　on FSH levels, 55
　　on pituitary gonadotropins, 38
　　on reproductive cycle, 35
　for anovulation therapy, 389
　in pineal gland, 42
　in pituitary disorder diagnosis, 105
　response to estrogen, 31
　role in anorexia nervosa, 117
　secretion
　　effect by dopamine, 37
　　effect by norepinephrine, 38
Gonorrhea as cause of male infertility, 366
Granulosa cells
　effect of FSH, 50

Granulosa cells—continued
  following ovulation, 57
  hypertrophy following ovulation, 71
  in corpus luteum, estradiol synthesis, 2
  luteinization, 54
  proliferation in follicular stage, 52
  proliferation during oocyte development, 67
  proliferation in oocyte development, 69
  steroid synthesis, 10
  tumors, 258
Growth
  adolescent spurt, 254
  Bayley-Pinneau tables, 260, 264–269
  short stature, 260–261
  tall stature, 261–262
Growth hormone
  effect on breast development, 168
  in treatment of short stature, 261
Gruelich-Pyle atlas, for bone age determination, 260

Hair
  axillary development, 253
  effect of castration, 137
  effect of nonhormonal factors, 138
  excessive, removal, 144
  growth, effect of estrogen therapy, 145
  hormonal influences, 137
  hypersensitivity in idiopathic hirsutism, 146
  loss with clomiphene therapy, 382
  pubic, development, 253
  structure and growth, 136–138
Hashimoto's thyroiditis, 245
Headaches
  and estrogens therapy, 81
  in climacteric, 78
  in pituitary tumors, 113
  migraine, and steroid contraceptives, 292, 299
  with clomiphene therapy, 382
Heat and abnormal semen, 365
Hepatitis and steroid contraceptives, 294
Hermaphrodism (see also Pseudohermaphrodite) 244
Hernia uteria inguinale (see Uterine hernia syndrome)
Hirsutism
  and abnormal lactation, 177
  and acromegaly, 137
  and adrenal involvement, 144–145
  and adrenal tumors, 138, 140, 141, 147
  and androgen-producing tumors, 145–146
  and anovulation, 123, 128
  and binding globulin level, 15–16
  and electrolysis, 143, 144, 146
  and steroid contraceptives, 298
  criteria for inpatient evaluation, 146
  diagnosis, 138–141
  effect
    of androgen therapy, 87
    of clomiphene citrate, 380
  hospital procedure for diagnosis, 147
  idiopathic, 15–16, 146
  suppression of testosterone in treatment, 143
  testosterone levels, 138–141
  therapy, 142–145
  X-linked transmission, 132
Hormone(s) (see also under specific names)
  bioassay, 389
  biosynthesis, 1–3
  cellular action, 18–25
  definition, 1
  effects
    biologic, 3
    metabolic, 3
  glycoprotein, 40
  polypeptide, 40
  steroid
    biosynthetic pathways, 7
    drug effect of action, 22
    excretion, 18
    laboratory measurement, 399
    mechanism of tissue reaction, 19–20
    nomenclature, 6
    nucleus, 4
    structure, 4–6
    synthesis, 9
  tropic, mechanism of cellular action, 23–25
Hot flashes, 77–80
Human chorionic gonadotropin (HCG)
  addition to clomiphene therapy, 380, 381
  and ovarian hyperstimulation, 388
  for inadequate luteal phase, 328–329
  effect on corpus luteum survival, 59
  effect on sexual differentiation, 44
  given with HMG therapy, 385
  in diagnosis of androgen-producing tumors, 146
  in hirsutism diagnosis, 147
  in obesity management, 279
  injections for sperm motility, 367
  laboratory measurement, 401–403
  role in fetal adrenal gland, 192, 211
  role in pregnancy, 202
  subunits, biological activity, 40
Human chorionic thyrotropin (HCT) in placenta, 202
Human menopausal gonadotropin (HMG)
  administered with clomiphene, 389
  administration and dosage, 384–386
  for anovulation therapy, 382–387
  for inadequate luteal phase, 329
  ovulation induction in amenorrhea, 116
  selection of patients for therapy, 383–384
Human placental lactogen (HPL)
  in breast development, 168
  in fetal fuel intake, 206
  levels in assessing fetal complications, 207
  levels in pregnancy, 170
  levels in prolonged gestation, 200
  role in placenta, 203
H-Y antigen, 232
Hydrocortisone in tubal surgery, 328
Hydrocephalus as cause of precocious puberty, 258
17-hydroxylase deficiency in adrenal hyperplasia, 246
20-hydroxylase enzymes in cholesterol conversion, 7–8
22-hydroxylase enzyme in cholesterol conversion, 7–8
16α-Hydroxyestrone, structure, 11
Δ5-3β-hydroxyl steroids in biosynthetic pathway, 9
17-hydroxypregnenolone, synthesis, 8
17α-hydroxy-progesterone
  blood levels, 14
  in Δ4-3-ketone pathway, 9
  rise in ovulatory phase, 56
  structure, 14
  synthesis, 8
Hypergonadotropic hypogonadism, ruling out in anovulation, 379
Hyperglycemia
  HPL levels in, 203
  in pregnancy, screening method, 197
Hyperinsulinemia in pregnancy, 170

Hyperkalemia in adrenal hyperplasia, 249
Hypermenorrhea in climacteric, 77
Hyperstimulation syndrome (see Ovary, hyperstimulation)
Hypertension
    and estrogen therapy, 85
    and steroid contraceptives, 292, 295–297, 299
    in adrenal hyperplasia, 237, 246
    in pregnancy
        estriol levels in, 199
        HPL levels in, 207
        prostaglandin levels in, 220
Hyperthecosis in chronic anovulation, 131
Hyperthyroidism
    and elevated HCG levels, 202
    diagnosis, 417
    impairment of estradiol metabolism, 126
Hypogonadism, treatment, 179
Hypogonadotropism, HMG therapy, 384
Hypoglycemia
    HPL levels in, 203
    in adrenal hyperplasia, 237
    in pregnancy, screening method, 197
Hypokalemic alkalosis in adrenal hyperplasia, 246
Hypomenorrhea (see Amenorrhea)
Hyponatremia in adrenal hyperplasia, 249
Hypophysectomy, effect on corpus luteum function, 58
Hypopituitarism and hair growth, 137
    and short stature, 261
Hypospadias and infertility, 366
Hypothalamus
    effect
        of clomiphene citrate, 376
        of progesterone, 39
        on gonadotropin function, 31
        on gonadotropin regulation, 37
        of pineal gland, 41–42
        on pituitary, 30–35
        of puberty, 44
        through cerebrospinal fluid, 33
    in sexual differentiation, 32
    lesions leading to galactorrhea, 176
    mechanisms of pituitary control, 29
    neurotransmitters, 29–30
    secretions in control of pituitary, 29
Hypothalamic-pituitary axis
    disorders in amenorrhea, 112–116
    disorders in anovulation, 124
    effect of steroid concentration, 53
    in normal ovulation, 123
Hypothyroidism
    and galactorrhea, 176
    and short stature, 261
    screening test, 417
    treatment and breast cancer incidence, 181
Hysterosalpingogram (HSG)
    and endometriosis, 357
    following tubal surgery, 352
    for infertility, 322–325
    in artificial insemination failure, 371
    therapeutic action, 324

Impotence and alcoholism, 366
Indomethacin, effect in pregnancy, 221
Infertility
    and adoption, 334
    and anovulation, 102, 123
    definition, 317
    due to endometriosis, 355, 356, 357
    due to inadequate luteal phase, 59–60
    due to mycoplasma, 329

due to ovulatory disorders, 325
due to sperm allergy, 329–331
effect of anxiety, 311
endometrial biopsy in, 327
endoscopy diagnosis, 331
following use of steroid contraceptives, 299
intrauterine insemination, 319–320
male
    due to abnormal semen, 364–366
    due to agglutination of sperm, 365
    due to coital timing, 366
    due to diabetes, 366
    due to ductal absence, 366
    due to ductal obstruction, 366
    due to endocrine disorders, 367–368
    due to failure of semen to liquify, 365
    due to hypospadias, 366
    due to Klinefelter's syndrome, 366
    due to retrograde ejaculation, 366
    due to testicular damage, 366
    due to tubal damage, 322–325
    due to varicocele, 368
    hormonal therapy, 367
    semen analysis, 363–366
    treated by artificial insemination, 369
    treatment with artificial insemination donor, 370
    treatment with clomiphene, 367
    treatment with Cytomel, 367
    treatment with prostaglandins, 372
    treatment with split ejaculate, 370
    post coital test, 318–322
    surgical treatment, 357
    testicular biopsy, 366
    treatment with Danazol, 359
    treatment by hysterosalpingography, 322–325
    tests of tubal patency
        hysterosalpingography, 322–325
        Rubin's test, 322
    tubal adhesions, surgery, 344
Insemination, artificial (see Artificial insemination)
Insomnia
    in climacteric, 78
    in estrogen therapy, 81
Insulin
    effect on breast development, 168
    effect of steroid contraceptives, 293
    in obesity, 278
    in pregnancy, effect of placental hormones, 205
    inhibition of lipase enzyme, 274
Intrauterine device (IUD)
    mechanism of action, 305–306
    use in Asherman's syndrome, 107
Intrauterine growth retardation, HPL levels in, 207
Iodine, protein-bound measurement, 416

Kallman's syndrome, 118
Karyotype
    in ambiguous genitalia, 249
    in amenorrhea diagnosis, 103
    in mosaicism diagnosis, 111
    in testicular feminization diagnosis, 109
    in Turner's syndrome diagnosis, 111
Δ^4-3-ketone in biosynthetic pathway, 9
17-ketosteroids
    blood levels in hirsutism, 138–141
    excretion in hirsutism diagnosis, 147
    high excretion, treatment, 144
    laboratory measurement, 403–415
    levels in congenital adrenogenital syndrome, 239
    normal urine levels, 407–408, 415
Klinefelter's syndrome, 366

Labor
induced by cortisol, 212
premature, preventive treatment, 214
prostaglandin levels in, 220
Lactation, 171–174
abnormal and acromegaly, 177
abnormal and hirsutism, 177
cessation, 174
contraceptive effect, 174
effect of steroid contraceptives, 300
inappropriate in pituitary tumors, 112
prevention
by ergot alkaloids, 171
by estrogen administration, 171
Laparoscopy for infertility diagnosis, 331
Laparotomy in ambiguous genitalia, 249
Lecithin, role in fetal lung development, 215–216
Libido
effect of androgens, 54
in climacteric, 78
increased with methyltestosterone, 87
Lipid metabolism and oral contraceptives, 294
Lipoproteins effect of steroid contraceptives, 294
Liver
adenomas and steroid contraceptives, 295
disease
and clomiphene therapy, 378
diseases
and steroid contraceptives, 294, 299
impairment of estradiol metabolism, 126
effect of steroid contraceptives, 294
Lubs syndrome, 242
Luteal phase
clinical measures of, 14
in perimenopausal period, 73
inadequate, 59–60
clomiphene therapy for, 380, 381
diagnosis, 328
in infertility, 327–329
treatment, 328–329
occurrence without ovum present, 381
Luteinizing hormone (LH)
abnormalities in male infertility, 367
activation of adenylate cyclase, 2, 23
and estradiol, 2
daily production levels in chronic anovulation, 129–131
effect
of melatonin, 42
of steroid contraceptives, 288
on corpus luteum function, 58
on number of follicles maturing, 69
on ovulation, 55
levels in anorexia nervosa, 117
levels in fetus, 44
loss of stimulation in anovulation, 126–127
releasing factors, 30
role in menstrual cycle, 50–60
secretion in fetus, 43
secretion in puberty, 44
serum levels in amenorrhea diagnosis, 101–105
steroidogenesis of estradiol, 54
stimulation, effect on steroid pathway, 7
subunits, biological activity, 40
suppression in hirsutism treatment, 142
synthesis, 40
Lysis of adhesions, 344

Macrosomia, HPL levels in assessing, 207
Malnutrition and delayed puberty, 259
Marijuana, effect on spermatogenesis, 365

Masculinized females
etiology, 241
fertility, 249
Mastitis, cystic, relation to breast cancer risk, 180
Mayer-Rokitansky-Kuster-Hauser Syndrome (see Mullerian tube, agenesis)
Medroxyprogesterone acetate
contraceptive use, 302–304
for emotional disturbances, 76
in amenorrhea diagnosis, 97
in dysfunctional uterine bleeding, 163
in treatment of amenorrhea, 118, 378–379
in treatment of anovulation, 133
in treatment of Asherman's syndrome, 107
in treatment of dysfunctional uterine bleeding, 166
in treatment of endometriosis, 359
in treatment of hirsutism, 143
in treatment of inadequate luteal phase, 329
in treatment of precocious puberty, 259
in treatment of short stature, 261
in treatment of tall stature, 262
in treatment of vasomotor symptoms, 87
Melatonin, effect on LH, 42
Menarche (see also Puberty)
age of onset, 45, 253–254, 255
anovulatory, 254
onset by estrogen production, 72
relation to growth spurt, 254
Meningitis as cause of precocious puberty, 258
Menopause (see also Climacteric)
age at occurrence, 76
bleeding, effect of stress, 80
effect of precocious puberty, 256
premature in mosaicism, 111
role of estrogen withdrawal, 72
Menstrual cycle
effect on behavior, 75
effect of pineal gland, 42
follicular phase, 49–53
length, 58
luteal phase, 55, 57–60
ovulation, 55–57
pituitary gonadotropin serum levels, 398
Menstruation
anovulation in, 45
basic principles, 95
duration of flow, 159
during lactation, 174
in climacteric, 77
Mental retardation in gonadal dysgenesis, 245
Messenger RNA in steroid hormone cellular action, 19–20
Mestranol
in oral contraceptives, 284
Methanimine mandelate, effect on urine estrogen levels, 194
Methyltestosterone treatment for endometriosis pain, 359
Mineralocorticoids, synthesis, 7, 15
Mitochondria
cholesterol conversion in, 7
Pregnenolone conversion in, 2
Mosaicism, 111
Mucus, cervical (see Cervix, mucus)
Müllerian duct
abnormal inhibiting factor, 244
development in bilateral dysgenetic testes, 244
embryonic development, 234
Müllerian tube
agenesis, 108–109

anomalies in amenorrhea, 108
Mumps and abnormal semen, 365
Myalgia in climacteric, 78
Mycoplasma and infertility, 329
Myocardial infarction and steroid contraceptives, 292

Noonan's syndrome, 246
Norepinephrine
  adipose tissue lipase stimulation, 274
  effect on GnRH, 38
  in melatonin synthesis, 41
Nortestosterone (see Testosterone, progestational derivatives)
Neurophysin
  estrogen, 35
  nicotine, 35
  secretion, 34
Nicotine and abnormal semen, 366
Nutrition, maternal and fetal lung maturation, 216

Obesity
  and anovulation, 126,132
  and bleeding, 160
  and brain center, 275
  and empty sella syndrome, 116
  correlation with endometrial cancer, 74
  endocrine changes in, 277–278
  experimental, 278–279
  management, 279–280
  mortality, 271
  presenting with short stature, 261
  psychological factors, 276
Oligomenorrhea (see also Amenorrhea)
  X-linked transmission, 132
Oligo-ovulation (see Anovulation)
Oocyte(s)
  during follicle maturation, 67
  expulsion mechanism, 70
Oogenesis in fetus, 44
Oogonia during follicle formation, 67
Optic glioma as cause of precocious puberty, 256
Oral contraceptives (see Contraceptives, steroids)
Orchiditis as cause of male infertility, 366
Ornade, for retrograde ejaculation, 366
Osteoporosis
  causes, 80
  effect on lower back pain, 78
  estrogen therapy, 81–82
Ova
  embryology, 66
  post-fertilization, 156
Ovarian failure (see Hypogonadotropic hypogonadism)
Ovariectomy (see Castration)
Ovary(ies)
  at birth, 68
  at puberty, 68
  atrophy, 77
  biopsy for anovulation, 379
  development, 66–75
  embryology and differentiation, 66–68, 232–233
  enlargement with clomiphene therapy, 382
  excessive androgens, 145
  hyperstimulation, 387–389
  in duct system differentiation, 234
  in peripheral conversion of estrogens, 12
  polycystic, 128–132
    and bleeding, 160
    elevated estrogen levels in, 145
    in chronic anovulation, 131–132

relation to breast cancer, 180
size in anovulation, 131–132
steroidogenesis, 70
surgical removal, estrogen therapy following, 79
synthesis
  androgens, 7
  biosynthetic pathways, 9
  estrogens, 7
  progestin, 7
tumor, 15
  in precocious puberty, 258
  nonendocrine, 55
  wedge resection, 383
Ovral, 359
Ovulation (see also Anovulation), 57
  basal body temperature in, 326
  clinical measures of, 14
  correlation with dysmenorrhea, 76
  experiments, hypothalamic stimulation, 29
  induction
    in hypothalamic amenorrhea, 116
    in ovarian failure, 378
    in pituitary tumors, 115
Oxytocin
  challenge test in prolonged gestation, 200
  competition with GnRH, 35
  effect of suckling, 171, 173
  effect on parturition, 208–209
  in milk ejection, 173
  induced labor, urine estriol levels in, 195
  secretion, 34
  secretion in parturition, 222

Palpitations in climacteric, 78
Parturition, endocrinology, 208–222
Pelvic inflammatory disease and infertility, 322
Penis differentiation in ambiguous genitalia, 247
Pergonal (see Human menopausal gonadotropins)
Perhydrocyclopentanephenanthrene in steroid hormone structure, 4
Phenolphthalein, effect on urine estrogen levels, 194
Phenothiazines and elevated prolactin levels, 175
Phospholipid levels effect of steroid contraceptives, 294
Pineal gland
  effect
    of light, 42
    on gonadal function, 41
    on hypothalamus, 41
    on menstrual cycle, 42
    on reproductive function, 42
  tumor
    as cause of precocious puberty, 256
    effect on gonadal function, 41
Pituitary
  anterior
    blood flow, 28
    mechanisms of hypothalamic control, 29
    prolactin secretion, 29
  effect of progesterone, 40
  effect on milk production, 171
  fetal secretions, 208
  gonadotropins
    laboratory measurement, 398–399
    response to GnRH, 38
  implantation of pineal products, 42
  non-neoplastic masses, 113
  posterior in hypothalamic pathway, 34
  transplantation, 29

Pituitary—*continued*
    tumors
        and amenorrhea, 113–115
        and in anovulation, 124
        and galactorrhea, 176–177
        and increased prolactin secretion, 176, 177
        diagnosis, 104–107
        diagnosis in amenorrhea, 98
        in male infertility, 367
        in pregnancy, 113, 115, 179
        prolactin levels in, 113–115
        surgical management, 114
        treatment, 178–179
Placenta
    hormones effect on maternal insulin, 205
    progesterone synthesis in, 186–187
    secretion of glycoprotein hormones, 40
    steroidogenesis in, 59
    synthesis of estrogen, 188–190
Placental sulfatase deficiency, 201
Polyostotic fibrous dysplasia, 258
Polytomography
    in pituitary tumor diagnosis, 104–105, 114–115
    of sella turcica in galactorrhea, 178
Pomeroy ligation (see Sterilization, tubal)
Porphyria and steroid contraceptives, 298
Portal vessels, hypothalamic-pituitary linkage, 28
Porter-Silber reaction, 413
Postmenopause
    estrogen suppression, 56
    hormone levels, 74
Postoperative hydrotubation, 345, 346
Pre-eclampsia, child development prognosis, 200
Prednisone in hirsutism diagnosis, 140
Pregnancy
    and adrenal hyperplasia
    and clomiphene therapy, 378
    and congenital adrenogenital syndrome, 240
    and contraceptives, steroid, 299
    and diabetes mellitus, 197
        child development prognosis, 200
        HPL levels in, 207
    and galactorrhea, 178
    and hyperglycemia, 197
    and hypertension, 199
    and hypoglycemia, 197
    and ovarian hyperstimulation, 388
    and pituitary tumors, 113, 115, 179
    and pre-eclampsia, child development prognosis, 200
    and toxemia, estriol levels, 199
    drug effects, 221
    ectopic
        and infertility, 322
        following tubal surgery, 352
    effect
        diabetogenic, 205
        of fasting state, 206
        on breast cancer risk, 180
        on breasts, 170–174
        on hair growth, 137
    estrogen levels in, 190
    following HSG, 324–325
    following tubal surgery, 344–345, 348, 351, 352, 353
    high risk
        DS levels in, 197
        estriol levels in, 197
    low estriol levels in, child development prognosis, 200
    multiple

        with clomiphene therapy, 381–382
        with HMG therapy, 383, 386
    progesterone levels in, 187
    optimum exposure for achieving, 369
    rate
        after varicocele surgery, 368–369
        by artificial insemination, 369, 370, 371
        for clomiphene therapy, 380
        in endometriosis, 358
        with clomiphene therapy, 381–382
        with HMG therapy, 383, 385–387
    synthesis of estrogen, 188–190
    thyroxine levels in, 416
    urine levels of estriol/creatine ratio, 193–195
Pregnane derivatives, 4
Pregnanediol
    excretion in habitual abortion, 332
    levels to document pregnancy, 400
    structure, 14
Pregnanediol glucuronide, urine excretion rates, 13
Pregnanetriol
    excretion
        in adrenal hyperplasia, 247
    in congenital adrenogenital syndrome, 237, 239
    in adrenogenital syndrome, 14
    structure, 14
Pregnenolone
    conversion from cholesterol, 2, 8
    conversion to progesterone, 9
    in progesterone synthesis by placenta, 186
Premarin (see Estrogen, conjugated)
Premenstrual tension, treatment, 76
Progestational agents
    anti-estrogen effect, 22
    in premature labor, 214
Progesterone
    blood levels, 14
        following ovulation, 57
    breakthrough bleeding, 158, 161
    daily production rates, nonpregnant female, 13
    decrease
        and estrogen increase, 212–214
        and fetal growth, 212
        in parturition, 208
    effect
        on breast development, 168
        on endometrial secretory phase, 154
        on endometrium growth, 85
        on FSH and LH release, 55–56
        on hypothalamus, 39
        on pituitary, 40
    in amenorrhea diagnosis, 97
    in Δ^4-3-ketone pathway, 9
    in tissue response to estrogen, 21
    interference with aldosterone secretion, 60
    levels
        during ovulation, 57
        in pregnancy, 170, 187
        to document pregnancy, 400
    mechanism of tissue reaction, 21
    metabolism, 13–14
    receptor complex, 21
    role in pregnancy, 187
    secretion
        by corpus luteum, 71
        in inadequate luteal phase, 59
    structure, 5, 6, 14
    synthesis, 8
        by corpus luteum, 187
        in fetal-placenta unit, 186–187

in granulosa cells, 10
vaginal suppositories for inadequate luteal phase, 328
withdrawal bleeding, 158, 159, 161
Progestins
compounds
in pregnancy, 241
effect on hair growth, 137
in oral contraceptives, 285–287
in prevention of endometriosis, 360
levels in pregnancy, 170
treatment
and breakthrough bleeding, 164, 165
for dysfunctional uterine bleeding, 164, 165, 166
for habitual abortion, 332–333
for precocious puberty, 259
structure, 4
synthesis, 7
by corpus luteum, 57
Prolactin
assay in galactorrhea, 177
effect
in menstrual cycle, 58
of dopamine, 38
of estrogen in pregnancy, 171
of suckling, 171
on breast development, 168
elevated in male infertility, 367
fetal role in parturition, 211
increased secretion in pituitary tumors, 176, 177
induced release in galactorrhea, 175
levels
in amenorrhea, 113, 115
in inadequate luteal phase, 60
postpartum, 171
relation to breast cancer, 181
secretion
from anterior pituitary, 29
in premature breast development, 253
serum levels
in amenorrhea, 98
in pituitary tumor diagnosis, 105
synthesis in chorionic tissue, 170
Prolactin-inhibiting factor, 29
inhibition and galactorrhea, 175, 176
Prolactin releasing hormone (PRH), 173–174
Promethazine in tubal surgery, 348
Prostatectomy and retrograde ejaculation, 366
Prostaglandin E relationship to infertile males, 372
Prostaglandin F, regulation of corpus luteum in non-primates, 58
Prostaglandins
as cause of dysmenorrhea, 76
effect in parturition, 208
in cyclic AMP mechanism, 24
levels in labor, 220
nomenclature, 216–217
role in labor, 221
role in utero-placental blood flow, 219–220
synthesis, 217–219
in follicle, 70
in parturition, 210, 221–222
treatment for male infertility, 372
vasodilator effects, 219
Protein(s)
intracellular synthesis, steroid hormone regulation of, 20
synthesis
production by messenger RNA, 3
in steroidogenesis, 2

Protein binding
competitive, 397
radioimmunoassay, 394–397
iodine, 416
Provera (see Medroxyprogesterone acetate)
Pruritus
in climacteric, 78–80
from steroid contraceptives, 294
Pseudohermaphrodite in testicular feminization, 109
Pseudovaginal perineoscrotal hypospadias, 242
Puberty
and breast development, 168
delayed, 259
environmental factors, 255
normal, 253–255
onset role of adrenal steroids, 44
precocious, 45, 255–259
and virilization, 256
diagnosis, 256
due to gonadotropin secretion, 256–258
due to ovarian tumor, 258
etiology, 256–258
in CNS abnormalities, 258
treatment, 259
sequence, 45
Pyridoxine (Vitamin B$_6$), treatment in galactorrhea, 178

Radiation and abnormal semen, 365
Radioimmunoassay
basic principles, 394
for human chorionic gonadotropin, 401
for pituitary gonadotropins, 398–399
techniques, 395–397
Reifenstein syndrome, 242
Renin-angiotensin system, and hypertension, 295–297
Religious requirements, interference for fertilization, 379
Resistant ovary syndrome, 112
Respiratory distress syndrome
cortisol levels in, 212
description, 215
lecithin/sphingomyelin ratio in, 215–216
preventive treatment, 216
Rhinorrhea in empty sella syndrome, 116
RNA (see Messenger RNA)
Rubin's test for tubal patency, 322

Salpingitis isthmica nodosum diagnosis, 324
Salpingolysis, 344
Salpingostomy, 344–348
Salt-wasting, in adrenal hyperplasia, 237
Saturation analysis
basic principles, 394
methodology, 395–397
Schistosomiasis as cause of amenorrhea, 107
Sella turcica
abnormal and galactorrhea, 113
empty, in amenorrhea, 115–116
in pituitary tumor diagnosis, 104–107
polytomography in galactorrhea, 178
Semen
abnormal, 364–366
agglutination of sperm, 365
analysis, 363–366
effect of varicocele, 368
ejaculate volume, 363–364
examination in infertility, 317
failure to liquify, 365
split for insemination, 370

Sertoli cells embryology, 232
Sex
  assignment for rearing, 249–250
  changes, 250
Sex characteristics
  effect of estrogen, 71
  secondary
    atrophy in climacteric, 72
    development, 253
Sexual differentiation
  abnormal, 236–250
  central nervous system, 236
  duct system, 234
  external genitalia, 233–234
  gonads, 232–233
  normal, 232–236
Sexual precocity (see Puberty, precocious)
Sex hormone binding globulin (SHBG), in blood
    transport of steroids, 10
Sheehan's syndrome
  and amenorrhea, 113
  postpartum symptoms, 173
Silastic hood in salpingostomy, 344–345
Smoking
  and abnormal semen, 365
  and steroid contraceptive risk, 302
Sperm
  agglutination, 365
  antibodies
    and infertility, 329–331
    in agglutination, 365
  autoimmunity, 365
  count, 364
    and testosterone rebound therapy, 368
    raised with clomiphene, 367
  embryology, 66
  in post coital test, 320, 321
  intrauterine insemination, 319–320
  motility
    after varicocele surgery, 368
    effect of caffeine, 369
    effect of freezing, 369
    increase with HCG injections, 367
  transport and capacitation, 313–314
Spermatic vein varicocele, 368
Spermatogenesis, effect
  of heat, 365
  of marijuana, 365
Spironolactone, prevention of translocation of hor-
    mone-receptor complex, 22
Spotting (see Bleeding, breakthrough)
Stein-Leventhal syndrome (see Ovary, polycystic)
Sterility (see Infertility)
Sterilization, tubal, reversal, 351–351
Steroid hormone(s) (see Hormone(s) steroid and
    specific names)
Steroid therapy for breast cancer, 182
Steroids (see Hormones, steroid)
Steroidogenesis, 2, 7–10
  cholesterol in, 7
  effect of HCG, 59
  in fetal-placenta unit, 185–194
  in menstrual cycle, 50
  increased by phosphorylation, 24
  inhibition by drugs, 22
Stress
  and amenorrhea, 116
  and anovulation, 126
  and galactorrhea, 176
  and increase estrogen production, 126
  effect on late menopausal bleeding, 80

Stroke and oral contraceptives, 291–292
Stromal tissue
  androgen secretion, 15
  androgen synthesis in follicular phase, 54
  androstenedione secretion, 10
  DHA secretion, 10
  hyperplasia, 55
    in chronic anovulation, 131
  in endometrial implantation phase, 155
  in endometrial proliferative phase, 153
  in endometrial secretory phase, 154
  secretions, 9
    effect on estrogen withdrawal, 80
    in chronic anovulation, 131
  testosterone secretion, 10
Suicide, correlation with menstrual cycle, 75
Sulfate conjugates, structure, 18
Sulfo-conjugate(s) in estradiol clearing, 3
Suprasellar teratoma as cause of precocious pu
    berty, 256
Swyer syndrome, 244

Tanycytes, 33
Testes
  bilateral dysgenic (see Swyer syndrome)
  differentiation in ambiguous genitalia, 247
  embryonic differentiation, 66, 232
  functional, in ambiguous genitalia, 246
  in mixed gonadal dysgenesis, 245
  injury as cause of male infertility, 365
Testicular feminization, 109–110, 241–243
  congenital androgen insensitivity, 22
  diagnosis, 247–249
Testosterone
  abnormalities in male infertility, 367
  and 17-epitestosterone comparison, 5
  aromatization, 8
  binding capacity, 15
    in hirsutism, 141
  blood levels
    in androgen-producing tumors, 145–146
    in hirsutism, 138–141
    sampling, 15
  cellular action, 22
  conversion from androstenedione, 11
  daily production rate
    female, 16
    in chronic anovulation, 129–131
    premenopausal peripheral conversion, 13
  effect on breast size and shape, 169
  fetal levels, 44
  in duct system differentiation, 234
  in masculine differentiation, 16
  in sexual differentiation, 32
  levels in anovulation and polycystic ovaries, 141
  metabolism, 3
    structure, 17
  postmenopausal level, 74
  progestational derivatives, 285–286
  rebound therapy, 368
  secretion by stromal cells, 10
  structure, 6
  synthesis, 9
    abnormal, 243
    by adrenal, 16
    by ovary, 16
    by stromal tissue, 54
  therapeutic use
    for endometriosis pain, 359
    of short stature, 261

Tetrahydrocortisol
  measurement by Zimmermann reaction, 414
  reduction, 411
  structure, 411
Tetrahydrocortisone (see Tetrahydrocortisol)
Theca cells
  differentiation in follicular phase, 52
  effect of ovulation, 71
  follicular, estradiol synthesis, 2
  formation, 69
  steroid synthesis, 10
  tumors, 258
Theca interna at ovulation, 70
Thelache (see Breast(s), development and Puberty)
Thromboembolic disease
  contraindication
    of estrogen replacement therapy, 80
    for steroid contraceptives, 299
  relationship to steroid contraceptives, 290–291
Thyroid gland
  autoimmunity, 245
  effect of steroid contraceptives, 293
  function tests, 416–417
    effects of estrogen, 416
  hormone
    and reversal of galactorrhea, 176
    and hair growth, 137
    effect on breast development, 168
    effect on lactation, 171
    laboratory measurement, 416–417
    levels in hyperthyroidism, 416
    levels in hypothyroidism, 417
    levels in pregnancy, 416
  hormone synthesis, 416
Thyroid stimulating hormone (TSH)
  relation to breast cancer, 181
  subunits, biological activity, 40
Thyrotropin-releasing hormone, 29
Thyroxine (see Thyroid gland, hormone)
Thyroxin-binding globulin (TGB), effect
  of androgens, 417
  of Dilantin, 417
  of estrogen, 293, 416, 417
  of perphenazine, 417
Toxemia in pregnancy
  estriol levels in, 199
  role of prostaglandins, 220
Transcortin
  estrogen effect, 293
  in blood transport of steroids, 10
Triglyceride levels, effect of steroid contraceptives, 294
Triiodothyronine, 416, 417
Tubal surgery, 343–353
  ectopic pregnancy, 352
  end to end anastomosis, 351–352
  Estes procedure, 353
  fimbrioplasty, 344–348
  lysis of adhesions, 344
  salpingostomy, 344–348
  selection of cases, 343, 352–353
  tubal implantation, 348–351
    causes of failure, 348–349
Tuberculosis
  as cause of amenorrhea, 107
  as cause of ductal obstruction, 366
Tumors (see also specific sites)
  estrogen dependent,
    contraindication for estrogen replacement therapy, 80

  contraindication for steroid contraception, 299
  estrogen producing in precocious puberty, 258
Turner's syndrome
  amenorrhea in, 94
  description, 111
  genotype, 245
  karyotype, 111
  male, (see Noonan's syndrome)
  thyroid autoimmunity, 245
Twins (see Pregnancy, multiple)

Urethra, caruncles in climeractic, 78
Urinary chorionic gonadotropin test, 401
Urinary difficulties, in climacteric, 78–80
Urinary tract
  atrophy, estrogen therapy, 83
  infections and steroid contraceptives, 298
Uterine hernia syndrome, 244
Uterus
  bleeding (see Bleeding)
  cancer and steroid contraceptives, 288–289, 299
  contractions
    role of calcium, 222
    endocrinology, 208
    role of oxytocin, 222
    role of prostaglandins, 222
  leiomyomata and steroid contraceptives, 299
  suspension in infertility, 312
  synthesis of prostaglandins, 210

Vagina
  absence of, 94, 108–109
  atrophy, estrogen therapy, 83
  discharge in estrogen therapy, 85
  hypoplasia of, 108–109
  tissue atrophy in climacteric, 78–80
Valsalva maneuver, 369
Vanishing testis syndrome (see Anorchia)
Varicocele as cause of male infertility, 368
Varicose veins and steroid contraceptives, 299
Vas ligation reanastomosis, 365
Vasomotor reactions
  control by estrogen therapy, 81
  control by medroxyprogesterone, 87
  secretion, 34
Virilism (see also Hirsutism), 135
  and binding globulin levels, 15–16
Virilizing adrenal hyperplasia (see Congenital adrenogenital syndrome)
Visual disturbances
  in pituitary tumors, 113–114
  with clomiphene therapy, 382
von Recklinghausen's disease as cause of precocious puberty, 258

Weight
  ideal, 272
  gain and steroid contraceptives, 297
  loss
    and anorexia, 116–117
    and anovulation, 124
Wolffian duct system
  embryonic development, 234
  development in testicular feminization, 243
  dependence on testosterone, 16

Zimmermann reaction, 414
Zona pellucida, formation, 69